Register Now for Online Access to Your Book!

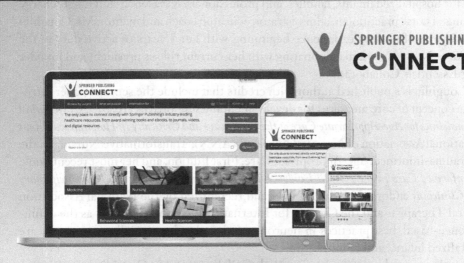

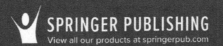

Mary E. Coughlin, MS, NNP, RNC-E, is a global leader in neonatal nursing and has pioneered the concept of trauma-informed, age-appropriate care as a biologically relevant paradigm for hospitalized infants, families, and professionals. A seasoned staff nurse, charge nurse, neonatal nurse practitioner, administrator, educator, coach and mentor, Ms. Coughlin has over 35 years of nursing experience beginning with her 7 years of active duty in the U.S. Air Force Nurse Corp and culminating with her current role as president and founder of Caring Essentials Collaborative.

Ms. Coughlin is a published author with credits that include the seminal paper introducing the concept of core measures for developmentally supportive care, the 2011 *Clinical Practice Guidelines for Age-Appropriate Care of the Premature and Critically Ill Hospitalized Infant* for the National Association of Neonatal Nurses (NANN); Transformative Nursing in the NICU: Trauma-Informed, Age-Appropriate Care, First Edition, and her most recent book: *Trauma-Informed Care in the NICU: Evidence-Based Practice Guidelines for Transdisciplinary Neonatal Clinicians* endorsed by the NANN and recognized by the National Association of Neonatal Therapists and the Council for International Neonatal Nurses as the definitive, evidence-based, best practices in neuroprotective, developmentally supportive care for hospitalized infants and families.

In her role as president of Caring Essentials Collaborative, Ms. Coughlin has educated, inspired, and empowered close to 10,000 interdisciplinary NICU clinicians from over 14 countries to transform the experience of care for the hospitalized infant and family in crisis. She works with individuals, teams, and organizations committed to improving the experience of care for hospitalized newborns, infants, and families.

From speaking engagements and keynote presentations to individual coaching, master classes, and unit-based/organizational quality-improvement initiatives, Mary presents the biologic and existential relevance of trauma-informed, age-appropriate care engaging the hearts and minds of her clients and learners for measurable and sustainable results.

Transformative Nursing in the NICU

Trauma-Informed, Age-Appropriate Care

SECOND EDITION

Mary E. Coughlin, MS, NNP, RNC-E

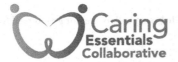
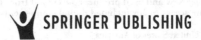

Springer Publishing Company, LLC
11 West 42nd Street, New York, NY 10036
www.springerpub.com
connect.springerpub.com/

Acquisitions Editor: Rachel X. Landes
Compositor: Transforma

ISBN: 978-0-8261-5419-4
ebook ISBN: 978-0-8261-5432-3
DOI: 10.1891/9780826154323

20 21 22 23 24/ 5 4 3 2 1

The author and the publisher of this Work have made every effort to use sources believed to be reliable to provide information that is accurate and compatible with the standards generally accepted at the time of publication. Because medical science is continually advancing, our knowledge base continues to expand. Therefore, as new information becomes available, changes in procedures become necessary. We recommend that the reader always consult current research and specific institutional policies before performing any clinical procedure or delivering any medication. The author and publisher shall not be liable for any special, consequential, or exemplary damages resulting, in whole or in part, from the readers' use of, or reliance on, the information contained in this book. The publisher has no responsibility for the persistence or accuracy of URLs for external or third-party Internet websites referred to in this publication and does not guarantee that any content on such websites is, or will remain, accurate or appropriate.

Medicine is an ever-changing science. Research and clinical experience are continually expanding our knowledge, in particular our understanding of proper treatment and drug therapy. The authors, editors, and publisher have made every effort to ensure that all information in this book is in accordance with the state of knowledge at the time of production of the book. Nevertheless, the authors, editors, and publisher are not responsible for any errors or omissions or for any consequence from application of the information in this book and make no warranty, expressed or implied, with respect to the content of this publication. Every reader should examine carefully the package inserts accompanying each drug and should carefully check whether the dosage schedules therein or the contraindications stated by the manufacturer differ from the statements made in this book. Such examination is particularly important with drugs that are either rarely used or have been newly released on the market.

Library of Congress Cataloging-in-Publication Data
Names: Coughlin, Mary, author.
Title: Transformative nursing in the NICU : trauma-informed, age-appropriate care / Mary E. Coughlin.
Description: Second edition. | New York, NY : Springer Publishing Company, LLC, 2020. | Includes
    bibliographical references and index. | Summary: "Each core measure chapters begins with an overview of
    the subject but then dives into the relevance of the core measure first for the clinician, then the family and
    finally the infant. Unless the nurse is whole and healthy, physically, emotionally and spiritually s/he is unable to
    meet the needs of the infant and family in crisis. This work isn't about doing more, and in truth, in many ways
    it's an invitation to do less and 'be' more"–Provided by publisher.
Identifiers: LCCN 2020039374 (print) | LCCN 2020039375 (ebook) | ISBN 9780826154194 (paperback) |
    ISBN 9780826154323 (ebook)
Subjects: MESH: Neonatal Nursing–methods | Neonatal Nursing–standards | Intensive Care,
    Neonatal–psychology | Stress, Psychological–nursing | Infant, Newborn–psychology | Family Health
Classification: LCC RJ253 (print) | LCC RJ253 (ebook) | NLM WY 157.3 | DDC 618.92/01–dc23
LC record available at https://lccn.loc.gov/2020039374
LC ebook record available at https://lccn.loc.gov/2020039375

Publisher's Note: New and used products purchased from third-party sellers are not guaranteed for quality, authenticity, or access to any included digital components.

Printed in the United States of America.

Contents

Foreword

I have been a neonatal nurse and educator for almost 40 years. I have written over 100 articles and approximately 30 textbooks, many on neonatal care, including developmental care, and I am honored to write the foreword for this new edition of *Transformative Nursing in the NICU: Trauma-Informed, Age-Appropriate Care*.

I met Mary Coughlin through my work with the National Association of Neonatal Nurses and saw her passion for supporting positive infant growth and development and parental emotional support. She has made substantial contributions to my textbooks and journal writings. Always adding a fresh, new dimension to neonatal and family-centered care, Mary's high energy and innovative thinking have led health professionals and families to voice the need for a trauma-informed approach to care in the NICU. This approach acknowledges the traumatic stress associated with the NICU experience.

A trauma-informed approach recognizes that trauma comes in many forms—physical, psychological, and emotional. Yet until recently, trauma-informed care was limited to populations outside the NICU. This text is the culmination of Mary's most important work and reflects her years of experience championing the needs of hospitalized infants and their families. This second edition highlights the relevance of trauma-informed care for infants, their families, and the clinicians.

I have seen firsthand the impact our NICUs have on infants and their families. Families are traumatized first by the birth of a small or sick newborn and then by entry into a strange environment called a *NICU*. Acknowledging that this "trauma" experience is unique to each infant and family is part of the approach labeled "trauma-informed" care. Although not a new concept, it still lacks universal support for its implementation in neonatal care. Yet, a trauma-informed approach is exactly what infants and families need. This book addresses the most important issues impacting neonatal care practices.

It also recognizes that the NICU environment impacts health professionals. Compassion fatigue, burnout, and staff turnover are all facets of work in healthcare today, especially in a fast-paced, emotionally charged environment. Frontline workers are faced daily with making difficult decisions and having difficult conversations with families. This work takes a toll on the clinician and is traumatic. This text stresses care for the health professional and the need for self-care. During these challenging times of the pandemic, self-care is critical for health professionals.

Since publication of the first edition, this book has changed the course of neonatal care globally. It gave nurses hope that they could return to the type of care they always desired to render: high-quality, culturally sensitive, individualized, family-centered, developmentally appropriate care. Mary demonstrates to the reader why trauma-informed care is as critical as any other aspect of the treatment plan. She makes the case for how promotion of a healing environment will positively impact neonatal and family outcomes.

Using evidence, which is increasingly robust, to support interventions and competencies to measure care and health professionals' performance outcomes, may increase the implementation of trauma-informed care. Trauma-informed care supports infant and family integrative developmental care in which health professionals across disciplines and families work together to provide safe, effective, high-quality care. Use of an individualized approach that focuses on attaining the best possible outcome for infants and their families is essential in providing neonatal care today. A trauma-informed approach makes that possible. This book needs to be in the toolkit of every clinician and neonatal educator.

Carole Kenner, PhD, RN, FAAN, FNAP, ANEF
Carol Kuser Loser Dean and Professor
The School of Nursing, Health, and Exercise Science
The College of New Jersey
Chief Executive Officer
Council of International Neonatal Nurses, Inc.

Preface

Research without advocacy is just a dusty journal on someone's shelf. Advocacy without research is just a temper tantrum.
—Rebecca Shlafer

When Springer Publishing reached out to me about writing a second edition to *Transformative Nursing in the NICU*, I was very flattered. But, if I am honest with you, as grateful as I was for the invitation, I was not excited about the prospect of writing another book. It's a *lot of work*.

It was January of 2019 (feels like a lifetime ago now). I was so busy: gearing up for our second Annual Science and Soul Congress on Trauma-informed Care in Bruges, Belgium; working with the team from Baptist Memorial in Tennessee on a SURGE workshop; and had myriad speaking engagements booked throughout the year. In addition, Aberdeen Maternity Hospital, yes, in Aberdeen, Scotland, had contracted a 6-month Quantum Caring program with me, focusing on the Pain and Stress core measure.

How would I ever write a book? I just couldn't imagine having enough bandwidth, between me, myself, and I, to write *and* run the business of changing the world (insert smiley face).

My lovely and incredibly patient and supportive publisher suggested maybe she could find someone else to write the book and, initially I thought, sure, that sounds great. However, after a series of phone calls and lots of internal discussions with my team (me, myself, and I), we agreed that a second edition made sense and I should write it. After all, since the first book came out in 2014 the concept of trauma-informed care in the NICU has evolved significantly. My vision of what it meant to be trauma informed has undergone dramatic evolution. The concept has transitioned from a focus on the infant exclusively with a peripheral nod to the family, to an all-out awareness that the experience of the NICU is traumatic to everyone: the infant, family, AND clinician—this message needs to be disseminated globally!

As I drafted the outline for this second edition I could feel myself getting very excited. There was so much to share. The research has been growing exponentially and, as I became increasingly aware, I also have been growing and evolving exponentially. I began this journey with the idea that I had to convince everyone about the science behind trauma-informed care. I believed if I just curated enough evidence, then everyone would be onboard; we would eradicate trauma in the NICU forever!

What I discovered is the secret to the transformation I was so desperately searching for did not lie in the science, but in the balance of science and soul. Within our beating hearts, our deep knowledge of our shared humanity, lies the essence of transformation. We must balance the scales. Science does not have all the answers. We must reconnect with our inner wisdom and employ all ways of knowing if we are to help the infant and family in crisis transcend their suffering, their trauma.

It is this essence of knowing that I have woven throughout this second edition. It is knowing that we cannot give what we do not have; we cannot give compassion to others if we are not compassionate with ourselves. We cannot give love, if we do not love ourselves. Trauma-informed care begins with *you*.

Each core measure chapter begins with an overview of the subject and then dives into the relevance of the core measure, first for the clinician, then the family, and finally the infant. Unless the nurse is whole and healthy, physically, emotionally, and spiritually, the nurse is unable to meet the needs of the infant and family in crisis. This work isn't about doing more, and in truth, in many ways it's an invitation to do less and "be" more.

Be more mindful, more present, more compassionate, and more patient. To begin the journey to a trauma-informed paradigm, knowledge is the foundation, but it must be complemented by a healing intention and personal wholeness. Courage is key; the courage to break free of the status quo, to ask the difficult questions, and to become a leader for change!

My hope is that as you read this book something inside you will be awakened, the words and the message will resonate with you and you will answer the call to join this movement to becoming trauma informed. Thank you.

Mary E. Coughlin

Section I

Quality Healthcare: A Global Initiative

1

What Is Quality Healthcare?

Unless someone like you cares a whole awful lot, nothing is going to get better. It's not.
—Dr. Seuss, *The Lorax*

The history of healthcare quality improvement began over a century ago, beginning in the 19th century with champions, such as Dr. Ignaz Semmelweis, an obstetrician who championed handwashing in medical care, and Florence Nightingale, who identified the association between poor living conditions and high death rates among soldiers treated in Army hospitals. Dr. Ernest Codman pioneered the creation of hospital standards to assess healthcare outcomes. And so began the pursuit of quality health care.

The Institute of Medicine (2001) defines *quality* as the degree to which health services for individuals and populations increase the likelihood of desired health outcomes and are consistent with current professional knowledge. Despite the existence of global healthcare standards, evidence-based best practices, accreditation requirements, countless reports and government regulations, quality healthcare continues to elude the majority of patients and healthcare consumers. This reality begs the question: "Why has quality healthcare been so difficult to achieve?" The answer may be as simple as refocusing healthcare from the conventional question, "What is wrong with you?" to the question "What happened to you?" McCannon et al. (2019) delineate a list of 10 lessons from healthcare on quality improvement that may give us some insight as to where we can begin to do better (Table 1.1).

VALUE-BASED HEALTHCARE

Value focuses on improving patient health outcomes; it is the measured improvement relative to the cost required to achieve the desired outcomes (Teisberg et al., 2020). Health outcomes are described in terms of capability, comfort, and calm (Table 1.2). These dimensions of health outcomes describe the results from an efficacious and empathetic point of view, rather than by focusing on the hospitality aspects of the healthcare experience (Teisberg et al., 2020).

Table 1.1 10 Lessons From Healthcare on Quality Improvement

1. Avoid systems myopia.	*Myopia* refers to ocusing on improvement in hospitals and specialty areas, while failing to understand the larger societal factors responsible for unequal outcomes and skyrocketing costs (including the undue power of health insurers and hospitals, underinvestment in communities and public health, lack of access to healthy food and transportation, and deep racial bias)
2. Start with the customer.	Deeply understand what patients, families, and community members value and dislike; ensure processes serve beneficiaries; eliminate activities that do not add value for the end user and orient the system away from self-serving, idiosyncratic concerns of those who hold the purse strings
3. Track rate of learning.	Study the rate at which new innovations are trialed to learn what works; become trailblazers and generators of new knowledge
4. Emphasize adaptation, not fidelity.	Encourage and celebrate context-appropriate adjustments to evidence-based ideas and innovations
5. Design measurement systems for the front line.	The first design principle of any effective measurement system is this: Put timely, easy-to-interpret data in the hands of those who can make day-to-day change, including doctors, nurses, patients, and families
6. Embrace nuance in evaluation.	Thoughtful researchers have come to understand that there are many approaches to learning and evaluation, and each is appropriate at different times; when spreading an innovation that already has sound evidence, it is not necessary to reassess its impact; instead, we should be studying local implementations and adaptations that will facilitate broader adoption
7. Live in the field.	A good measurement system doesn't provide conclusions; it provides clues; use data as a prompt to go out to visit communities, hospital units, and other care settings; understand what is really happening in all of its texture, harvesting the wisdom of those giving and receiving care and then actively removing impediments to their progress

(continued)

Table 1.1 10 Lessons From Healthcare on Quality Improvement *(continued)*

8. Understand the psychology of change.	Technical work that fails to connect with the reasons people are called to their professions soon becomes drudgery; tapping into the huge stores of peoples' passion and creativity and applying that to improvement leads to success
9. Approach payment incentives with caution.	Doctors and nurses are endlessly ranked and rated, and compensated accordingly, but there is very little evidence to suggest that this leads to better outcomes for patients; possible reasons for the failure of pay-for-performance programs include the fact that they make faulty comparisons between dissimilar organizations, induce groups to misreport their performance, and belittle and discourage care providers, resting on the problematic assumption that financial incentives are what drive behavior
10. Address inequity proactively	Major racial disparities in health and discrimination in the provision of health care services persists; organizations must pursue interventions that target injustice, and any quality project must solve for the needs of oppressed groups first, studying stratified data on progress in addition to overall changes in outcomes

Source: Adapted from McCannon, J., Delgado, P., & Bisognano, M. (2019, August 23). *10 lessons from health care on quality improvement.* https://ssir.org/articles/entry/10_lessons_from_health_care_on_quality_improvement

Table 1.2 Dimensions of Health Outcomes and Examples From the NICU

Health-Outcome Dimensions	Clinical Example
Capability—*The ability of patients to do the things that define them as individuals and enable them to be themselves*	• Age-appropriate care, based on the infant's developmental competence • Unrestricted, nurturing time with parents • Age-appropriate playful encounters with loving adults and siblings • Experiencing consistently reliable relief of physical pain and pain-related stress • Unrestricted access to family • Social encounters that respect the dignity and personhood of the infant

Source: Adapted from Teisberg, E., Wallace, S., & O'Hara, S. (2020). Defining and implementing value-based health care: A strategic framework. *Academic Medicine, 95*(5), 682–685. https://doi.org/10.1097/ACM.0000000000003122

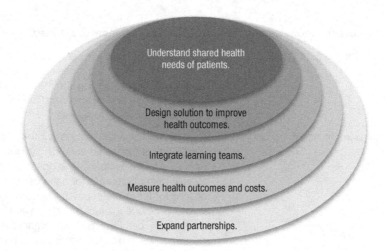

Figure 1.1 Strategic framework for value-based healthcare implementation to achieve better patient outcomes.

Source: Teisberg, E., Wallace, S., & O'Hara, S. (2020). Defining and implementing value-based health care: A strategic framework. *Academic Medicine, 95*(5), 682–685. https://doi.org/10.1097/ACM.0000000000003122 Reprinted with permission from Wolters Kluwer Health, Inc.

Better outcomes reduce spending and decrease the need for ongoing care as a consequence of healthcare-acquired morbidity. Value-based healthcare aligns with the aspirational goals of the Institute for Healthcare Improvement's "Triple Aim." These goals aim to improve the patient experience of care and reduce per capita costs while improving population health (refer to Chapter 3). Population health is the focus of value-based healthcare and is achievable through the adoption of a clear framework to create the desired and necessary transformation (Figure 1.1; Teisberg et al., 2020).

Transformation begins when an organization recognizes and understands the unique shared needs of its patient population and develops a comprehensive evidence-based solution to meet those needs. Speaking in terms of the NICU, the populations served are newborns and infants. The unique shared needs of these patient populations include being showered with love and attention; enjoying age-appropriate play such as being read to, sung to, talked to; being held, cuddled, and kissed; enjoying pleasurable eating experiences; having one's basic needs met; and living a pain- and stress-free existence.

This is the value proposition of trauma-informed care. When an infant's disease-independent, developmental needs are met consistently and reliably, the infant is at a significantly reduced risk for short-term and long-term morbidity associated with NICU hospitalization (Montirosso et al., 2017). Reducing morbidity and modulating the epigenetic, hormonal, and biologic adaptations that influence the developmental trajectory of the infant's physical and mental health decreases healthcare costs while enhancing quality of life for the infant and family (Kommers et al., 2016; Montirosso et al., 2016; Provenzi et al., 2018).

Table 1.3 Categories of Hospital-Acquired Conditions

1. Foreign object retained after surgery 2. Air embolism 3. Blood incompatibility 4. Stage III and IV pressure ulcers 5. Falls and trauma 6. Manifestations of poor glycemic control 7. Catheter-associated UTI	8. Vascular catheter-associated infection 9. Surgical site infection, mediastinitis following CABG 10. Surgical site infection following bariatric surgery for obesity 11. Surgical site infection following certain orthopedic procedures	12. Surgical site infection following CIED 13. DVT/PE following certain orthopedic procedures 14. Iatrogenic pneumothorax with venous catheterization

CABG, coronary artery bypass graft; CIED, cardiovascular implantable electronic device; DVT, deep vein thrombosis; PE, pulmonary embolism; UTI, urinary tract infection.

Source: Centers for Medicare & Medicaid Services. (n.d.). *Centers for Medicare and Medicaid Services.* www.cms.gov/Medicare/Medicare-Fee-for-Service-Payment/HospitalAcqCond/Hospital-Acquired_Conditions

Table 1.4 Examples of "Other Injuries" Associated With NICU Hospitalization

Developmental	Mental Health	Neurological
• Motor delay • Language delays	• Behavioral problems • Executive dysfunction • Attention deficit disorder • Autism spectrum • Anxiety/depression	• Minor cognitive deficits • Learning disabilities • Visual motor perceptual difficulties • Cortical vision impairment • Auditory dys-synchrony

HOSPITAL-ACQUIRED CONDITIONS

Hospital-acquired conditions (HAC) are (a) high cost, high volume, or both; (b) result in the assignment of a diagnosis-related group that has a higher payment when present as a secondary diagnosis; and (c) could reasonably have been prevented through the application of evidence-based guidelines. Common HACs are listed in Table 1.3. Several of these categories have subcategories within them to provide more accurate clarification. For example, under category number 5, there is a subcategory described as "other injuries."

Examining this subcategory through a trauma-informed lens, "other injuries" takes on a whole new meaning within the context of the NICU. The critically ill infant may incur "other injuries" as a consequence of the NICU experience related to unmanaged or undermanaged pain, fragmented and/or inadequate sleep, clinician-directed "feeding" practices, maternal separation and deprivation, postural malalignment, and more. In the wake of mounting evidence and evidence-based guidelines for trauma-informed care, these "other injuries" (Table 1.4) could reasonably have been prevented, or at the very least mitigated, through the application of evidence-based guidelines in trauma-informed, age-appropriate care (Coughlin, 2016).

EVIDENCE-BASED PRACTICE AND CLOSING THE GLOBAL QUALITY CHASM

Evidence-based practice involves the conscientious, explicit, and judicious use of current best evidence to make decisions about the care of patients (Belita et al., 2020). Evidence-informed decision-making is a process whereby high-quality research, local data, and patient and professional experiences are synthesized and applied to decision-making for clinical practice (Belita et al., 2018). Nurses play a key role globally in building evidence and working with interdisciplinary teams to accelerate the implementation of evidence-based nursing practice (Correa-de-Araujo, 2016).

Despite the key role nurses play in healthcare, three immediate and international challenges impede nursing's ability to provide evidence-based care (Box 1.1; Correa-de-Araujo, 2016). Demands for accountability in safety and quality healthcare are raising awareness of these barriers, and policy makers and leaders are beginning to take notice. This, however, does not suggest that the work of nurses championing best practices is done. Much more work is needed to address the global gaps in quality and patient safety.

BOX 1.1 LIMITATIONS TO NURSES' ABILITY TO PROVIDE EVIDENCE-BASED PRACTICE

1. Limitations within healthcare systems, leading to decreased support for their education and development
2. Prejudice against their intent to advance their practice
3. Issues associated with workforce reduction

Source: Adapted from Correa-de-Araujo, R. (2016). Evidence-based practice in the United States: Challenges, progress, and future directions. *Health Care for Women International,* 37(1), 2–22. https://doi.org/10.1080/07399332.2015.1102269

Redesigning healthcare systems to meet the needs of underserved and vulnerable populations and families is critical. This redesign requires creativity and mastery in teamwork. Educating the future workforce and upskilling the existing workforce is imperative to raise awareness, increase skills, and empower clinicians to improve systems of care in the NICU and beyond.

SUMMARY

The very nature of this challenge is what calls us to our higher purpose. It can feel vulnerable, bearing witness to tragedy, but when you lean in to suffering, even for a moment, you transform the darkness into love. To engage the hearts and minds of our clinician colleagues around the globe, we must be grounded in science and guided by our moral compass to lead and become agents of change today and leaders for tomorrow. It takes time, reflection, revisions, challenges, and sometimes opposition to create something that is transformational and sustainable.

Empowerment, at the end of the day, comes from refocusing health care from the conventional question of "What is the matter with you?" to the modern question of "What matters to you?"
—DiGloia, Clayton, and Giarrusso

REFERENCES

Belita, E., Squires, J. E., Yost, J., Ganann, R., Burnett, T., & Dobbins, M. (2020). Measures of evidence-informed decision-making competence attributes: A psychometric systematic review. *BMC Nursing, 19,* 44. https://doi.org/10.1186/s12912-020-00436-8

Belita, E., Yost, J., Squires, J. E., Ganann, R., Burnett, T., & Dobbins, M. (2018). Measures assessing attributes of evidence-informed decision-making (EIDM) competence among nurses: A systematic review protocol. *Systematic Reviews, 7*(1), 181. https://doi.org/10.1186/s13643-018-0849-8

Correa-de-Araujo, R. (2016). Evidence-based practice in the United States: Challenges, progress, and future directions. *Health Care for Women International, 37*(1), 2–22. https://doi.org/10.1080/07399332.2015.1102269

Coughlin, M. (2016). *Trauma-informed care in the NICU: Evidence-based practice guidelines for neonatal clinicians.* Springer Publishing Company.

DiGloia, A. M., Clayton, S. B., & Giarrusso, M. B. (2016) "What matters to you?": A pilot project for implementing patient-centered care. *Patient Experience Journal, 3*(2), 7. https://doi.org/10.35680/2372-0247.1121

Institute of Medicine. (2001). *Crossing the quality chasm: A new health system for the 21st century* (Committee on Quality of Health Care in America, ed.). National Academies Press.

Kommers, D., Oei, G., Chen, W., Feijs, L., & Oetomo, S. B. (2016). Suboptimal bonding impairs hormonal, epigenetic and neuronal development in preterm infants, but these impairments can be reversed. *Acta Paediatrica, 105*(7), 738–751. https://doi.org/10.1111/apa.13254

McCannon, J., Delgado, P., & Bisognano, M. (2019, August 23). *10 lessons from health care on quality improvement.* https://ssir.org/articles/entry/10_lessons_from_health_care_on_quality_improvement

Montirosso, R., Giusti, L., Del Prete, A., Zanini, R., Bellu, R., Borgatti, R.; NEO-ACQUA Study Group. (2016). Does developmental care in NICUs affect health-related quality of life in 5-years-old children born preterm? *Pediatric Research, 80,* 824–828. https://doi.org/10.1038/pr.2016.158

Montirosso, R., Tronick, E., & Borgatti, R. (2017). Promoting neuroprotective care in neonatal intensive care units and preterm infant development: Insights from the Neonatal Adequate Care for Quality of Life Study. *Child Development Perspectives, 11*(1), 9–15. https://doi.org/10.1111/cdep.12208

Provenzi, L., Guida, E., & Montirosso, R. (2018). Preterm behavioral epigenetics: A systematic review. *Neuroscience and Biobehavioral Reviews, 84,* 262–271. https://doi.org/10.1016/j.neubiorev.2017.08.020

Teisberg, E., Wallace, S., & O'Hara, S. (2020). Defining and implementing value-based health care: A strategic framework. *Academic Medicine, 95*(5), 682–685. https://doi.org/10.1097/ACM.0000000000003122

2

Neuroscientific Consequences of NICU Trauma

I swore never to be silent whenever and wherever human beings endure suffering and humiliation. We must take sides. Neutrality helps the oppressor, never the victim. Silence encourages the tormentor, never the tormented.
    —Elie Wiesel

WHAT IS *NEUROSCIENCE*?

Neuroscience is the study of the nervous system. It encompasses anatomy, physiology, biochemistry, molecular and developmental biology, cytology and psychology. Over the past century, researchers have discovered that *neuroplasticity* is a fundamental property of the nervous system and consequently, neuroscience (Mateos-Aparicio & Rodriguez-Moreno, 2019). The concept that "neurons that fire together, wire together" represents neuroplasticity. Neuroplasticity has unique relevance during critical and time-sensitive periods of brain development (Ismail et al., 2017; Nist et al., 2019).

Ismail et al. (2017) describe five patterns of neuroplasticity (Figure 2.1). Neuroplasticity does not always result in beneficial adaptations (Ismail et al., 2017). Biological adversity, such as exposure to toxic stress, malnutrition, infection, pain, and maternal deprivation, disrupt brain development by limiting experience-expectant plasticity. The results are structural changes to brain architecture (Figure 2.2; DeMaster et al., 2019). Abnormal neuroplasticity is linked with several pediatric disorders of the central nervous system mediated by adverse early-life experiences (Box 2.1).

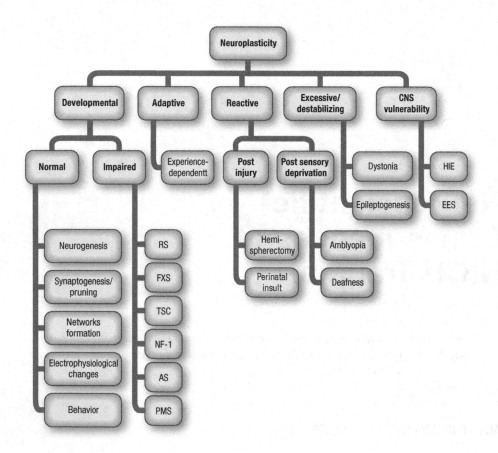

Figure 2.1 Patterns of neuroplasticity.

AS, Angelman syndrome; CNS, central nervous system; EES, epileptic encephalopathy syndromes; FXS, Fragile X syndrome; HIE, hypoxic ischemic encephalopathy; NF-1, neurofibromatosis syndrome; PMS, Phelan–McDermid syndrome; RS, Rett syndrome; TSC, tuberous sclerosis syndrome.
Source: Ismail, F. Y., Fatemi, A., & Johnston, M. V. (2017). Cerebral plasticity: Windows of opportunity in the developing brain. *European Journal of Paediatric Neurology, 21*(1), 23–48. doi: 10.1016/j.ejpn.2016.07.007 Reprinted with permission from Elsevier.

Early-life adversity becomes biologically embedded at a cellular level, derailing healthy development and long-term health and wellness (refer to Chapter 5; Nist, 2017). Nist et al. (2019) put forth a conceptual model describing the biological embedding of neonatal stress exposure in the NICU that impacts brain architecture. Figure 2.3 represents the confluence of multiple biologic systems affected by neonatal stress modulated by the prenatal environment and maternal–infant interactions (refer to Chapter 9 for more information; Nist et al., 2019). Brain plasticity, or the way experiences shape the development of the brain, can be leveraged to improve outcomes (DeMaster et al., 2019).

Critical and sensitive periods of development create windows of opportunity for neuromodulatory interventions that may augment neuroplasticity and improve clinical

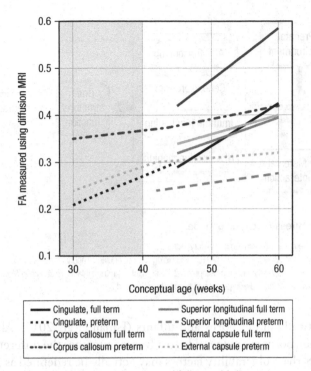

Figure 2.2 White matter changes following preterm and full-term births.

FA, fractional anisotropy.
Source: DeMaster, D., Bick, J., Johnson, U., Montroy, J. J., Landry, S., & Duncan, A. F. (2019). Nurturing the preterm infant brain: Leveraging neuroplasticity to improve neurobehavioral outcomes. *Pediatric Research, 85*, 166–175. doi: 10.1038/s41390-018-0203-9 Reprinted with permission from Springer Nature.

BOX 2.1 PEDIATRIC DISORDERS OF THE CENTRAL NERVOUS SYSTEM RELATED TO NEUROPLASTICITY

- Hypoxic–ischemic encephalopathy
- Cerebral palsy
- Epilepsy and epileptic encephalopathies
- Dystonia
- Intellectual disabilities
- Autism spectrum disorders
- Attention deficit disorder
- Schizophrenia

Source: Adapted from Ismail, F. Y., Fatemi, A., & Johnston, M. V. (2017). Cerebral plasticity: Windows of opportunity in the developing brain. *European Journal of Paediatric Neurology, 21*(1), 23–48.

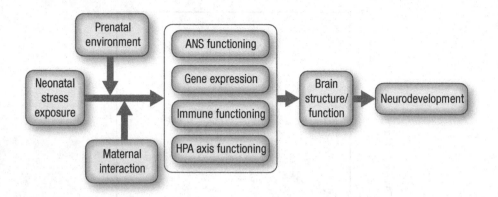

Figure 2.3 Neonatal Stress-Embedding model.

ANS, autonomic nervous system; HPA, hypothalamic–pituitary–adrenal.
Source: Nist, M. D., Harrison, T. M., & Steward, D. K. (2019). The biological embedding of neonatal stress exposure: A conceptual model describing the mechanisms of stress-induced neurodevelopmental impairment in preterm infants. *Research in Nursing & Health, 42*(1), 61–71. doi: 10.1002/nur.21923 Reprinted with permission from John Wiley and Sons.

outcomes for critically ill newborns and infants (Ismail et al., 2017). Although preterm and critically ill newborns are vulnerable to adverse outcomes the differential susceptibility model suggests that vulnerability factors may actually be redefined as plasticity factors (DeMaster et al., 2019). Differential susceptibility suggests that individuals are susceptible to both the negative and positive aspects of an environment. Leveraging plasticity factors by mitigating toxic stress and enriching the environment (refer to Chapter 10) improves long-term outcomes in this fragile population across sensory motor, cognitive, and behavioral domains (DeMaster et al., 2019).

WHAT IS *TRAUMA*?

Trauma results from an event or a series of events experienced by an individual as physically and/or emotionally harmful or life-threatening. These experiences overwhelm the individual's ability to cope and have lasting adverse implications for the person's physical, psychosocial–emotional, spiritual, and even existential health and well-being. Trauma can result from experiences that induce powerlessness, fear, and recurrent hopelessness and create a constant state of vigilance. Traumatic experiences can be dehumanizing, shocking, or terrifying, representing a singular event or multiple compounding events over time. Trauma often includes the betrayal of a trusted person or institution and the loss of a felt sense of safety.

   Implications of trauma for critically ill preterm and term infants are pervasive and exemplified in the image of the trauma tree (Figure 2.4). Similar to a tree, injuries and traumatic experiences that occur early in development, like the roots of a tree, compromise the lifelong developmental potential of the individual (or the tree). Childhood trauma,

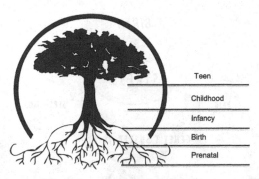

Teen

Childhood

Infancy

Birth

Prenatal

Figure 2.4 Trauma tree. This image has been adapted to exemplify the metaphor of the trauma tree and human development.

mediated by toxic stress, deranges the individual's developmental trajectory with lifelong consequences to physical and mental health (Dowd, 2017; Franke, 2014; Shonkoff et al., 2012; Weber & Harrison, 2019).

Pediatric medical traumatic stress includes the physiological and psychological responses of children to painful procedures; serious illness; frightening environments; separation from parent; and feelings of fear, terror, helplessness, and isolation (Kassam-Adams & Butler, 2017). D'Agata et al. (2016) proposed a conceptual model of infant medical trauma in the NICU (IMTN; Figure 2.5). In the IMTN model the brain is the dynamic locus of susceptibility influenced by the infant's genetic predisposition as well as environmental and experiential factors (D'Agata et al., 2016).

NICU-related factors, best characterized as stressors, are complex, multisensory, and painful, resulting in physiologic and psychological perturbations (D'Agata et al., 2016; Montirosso & Provenzi, 2015; Weber & Harrison, 2019). Montirosso and Provenzi (2015) define preterm birth as an early adverse experience due to the infant's exposure to high levels of toxic stress and limited experiences with maternal care. Figure 2.6 represents a proposed model for preterm behavioral epigenetic studies. The model highlights the impact of prenatal adversities, NICU-related stressors, and the quality of NICU-related care (modifiable factors), mediated by epigenetic mechanisms, on the phenotype of the hospitalized infant (Montirosso & Provenzi, 2015).

In addition to the intrinsic vulnerability and susceptibility of hospitalized infants to medical trauma during their inpatient experience, these infants also are at high risk for nonaccidental trauma and abuse hospitalization in the postdischarge period (Doud et al., 2015; Puls et al., 2019). Prematurity and neonatal comorbidities have been identified as risk factors for abuse hospitalization within the first year postdischarge (Doud et al., 2015). Puls et al. (2019) created a nationally representative U.S. birth cohort of 3.7 million newborns to examine the prevalence of risk factors for abuse and newborn risk for physical abuse hospitalization. Prematurity, low birth weight (LBW), and intrauterine drug exposure were independently associated with abuse hospitalization in the first 6 months following discharge (Puls et al., 2019). Poverty and living in rural settings, combined

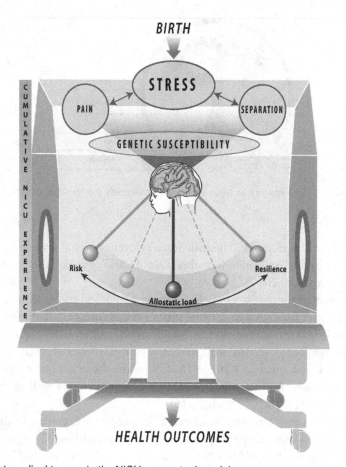

Figure 2.5 Infant medical trauma in the NICU conceptual model.

Source: D'Agata, A. L., Young, E. E., Cong, X., Grasso, D. J., & McGrath, J. M. (2016). Infant medical trauma in the neonatal intensive care unit (IMTN): A proposed concept for science and practice. *Advances in Neonatal Care, 16*(4), 289–297. doi: 10.1097/ANC.0000000000000309 Reprinted with permission from Wolters Kluwer.

with prematurity and LBW, increased the infant's risk for abuse hospitalization 10-fold (Puls et al., 2019).

NICU TRAUMA AND BRAIN ARCHITECTURE

The primary source of infant trauma in the NICU is maternal separation. Maternal separation and socio-emotional neglect alter brain structures responsible for processing stress and threat (Debiec, 2018). This remodeling leads to a loss of flexibility in regulating emotion and responding to danger. Consequently, the ability to "unlearn" threats or extinguish fear is compromised (Debiec, 2018). Maternal separation has been linked to neuropsychiatric disorders in adulthood, particularly depression and anxiety-like behaviors (Boulanger-Bertolus et al., 2017; Roque et al., 2014).

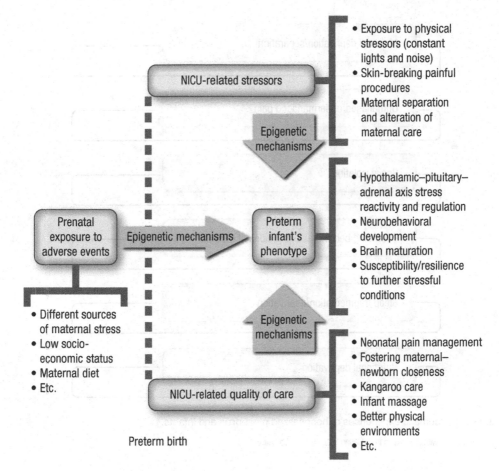

Figure 2.6 A prospective model to inform preterm birth behavioral epigenetic studies.

Source: Montirosso, R., & Provenzi, L. (2015). Implications of epigenetics and stress regulation on research and developmental care of preterm infants. *Journal of Obstetric, Gynecologic & Neonatal Nursing, 44*(2), 174–182. doi: 10.1111/1552-6909.12559 Reprinted with permission from Elsevier.

Csaszar-Nagy and Bokken (2018) report the negative effect of a 2-hour mother–infant separation immediately after birth in healthy term infants. The separated mother–infant dyads were compared to dyads that experienced continuous skin-to-skin contact. The mother–infant couplets that were separated for 2 hours postbirth demonstrated a higher risk for poor maternal bonding at 1-year of age despite having roomed-in for the remainder of their hospital stay. Newborns separated from their mother spent more time crying with a higher frequency of cries and had a significant elevation in their salivary cortisol levels than the skin-to-skin newborns (Csaszar-Nagy & Bokken, 2018). Neurological sequelae associated with reduced maternal contact and care includes decreased total gray and white matter volumes with increased volumes in the amygdala (Mooney-Leber & Brummelte, 2017).

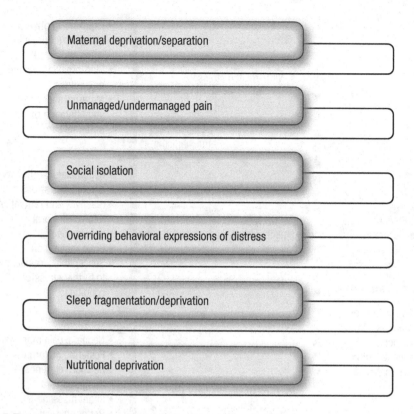

Figure 2.7 Traumatic experiences of hospitalized newborns and infants.

Source: Reprinted with permission from Caring Essentials Collaborative, LLC.

In addition to maternal separation and maternal deprivation there are several other facets to the NICU experience that are traumatic to the developing human and that alter brain architecture (Figure 2.7). Unmanaged and/or undermanaged pain during the newborn period is associated with reduced cortical thickness at 7 years of age (Ranger et al., 2013). Experience-induced plasticity associated with early procedural pain markedly decreases thalamic growth, which has been linked to impaired cognitive and motor outcomes at 3 years' corrected age (Duerden et al., 2018). Figure 2.8 highlights discrete regions of the brain that are specifically impacted by invasive procedures and surgeries and areas influenced by infant clinical factors and genotypes (Chau et al., 2019). Refer to Chapter 9 for more information about pain and stress for the infant, the family and the clinician.

The detriments of social isolation are similar to maternal separation and deprivation (Box 2.2). Social isolation trauma increases the infant's risk for neurodevelopmental disorders by reducing exposure to the neuroprotection that is offered through social caregiver–infant contact (Colonnello et al., 2017). Humans have an inherent need to belong (Baumeister & Leary, 1995; Colonnello et al., 2017; Comparetti, 1986; Over, 2016). A sense of belonging

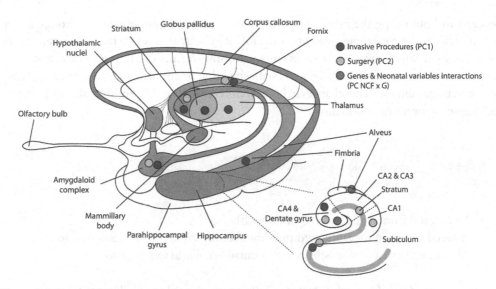

Figure 2.8 Reduced regional volumes in the limbic system, basal ganglia, and thalamus.

CA, cornus ammonis; NCF, neonatal clinical factors; PC, principle component.
Source: Chau, C. M. Y., Ranger, M., Bichin, M., Park, M. T. M., Amaral, R. S. C., Poskitt, K., Synnes, A. R., Miller, S. P., & Grunau, R. E. (2019). Hippocampus, amygdala, and thalamus volumes in very preterm children at 8 years: Neonatal pain and genetic variation. *Frontiers in Behavioral Neuroscience, 13*, 51. https://doi.org/10.3389/fnbeh.2019.00051

begins before birth through the psychophysiological connection between mother and her developing fetus (Allen, 2019; Comparetti, 1986). Consequences of social isolation include activation of the stress response system as well as changes to the frontotemporal–thalamic– cerebellar network, with decreased cerebellum volume and cerebellar neurotransmitter dysfunctions (Adamaszek et al., 2017; Sanders & Hall, 2018).

BOX 2.2 EXAMPLES TO MITIGATE SOCIAL ISOLATION TRAUMA IN THE CLINICAL SETTING

- Facilitate parents' access to their baby, regardless of scheduled care times.
- Greet the infant with soft, reassuring vocalization prior to a caring encounter.
- Establish a synchronous rapport with the infant during the caring encounter, responding to the infant's behavioral communication throughout.
- Engage with the infant in a respectful and meaningful way.
- Speak with the infant during caring encounters.

Specific neuroarchitectural aberrations related to overriding an infant's behavioral expressions of distress have not been described in the literature. Overriding infant cues in relation to feeding has been shown to have a negative impact on feeding success. Many care practices proceed without taking the infant's response to the encounter into account. Although it is a best practice to pace care engagement on the infant's ability to tolerate the encounter, this is inconsistent in clinical practice. All stress is not pain, however, pain and stress share very similar biobehavioral responses. It has been well established that infant pain and stress are associated with functional and anatomic changes in brain architecture (Box 2.3; Smith et al., 2011). Refer to Chapter 9 for more information.

BOX 2.3 STRUCTURAL AND FUNCTIONAL CHANGES IN BRAIN ARCHITECTURE ASSOCIATED WITH STRESS

- Decreased frontal and parietal brain width
- Altered diffusion measures and functional connectivity in the temporal lobes
- Abnormalities in motor behavior on neurobehavioral examination

Source: Smith, G. C., Gutovich, J., Smyser, C., Pineda, R., Newnham, C., Tjoeng, T. H., Vavasseur, C., Wallendorf, M., Neil, J., & Inder, T. (2011). NICU stress is associated with brain development in preterm infants. *Annals of Neurology, 70*(4), 541–549. doi: 10.1002/ana.22545

Sleep fragmentation and sleep deprivation undermine brain growth, maturation, and development. Sleep is the predominate behavioral state of newborns. The amount of time an infant spends in sleep increases with decreasing gestational age (refer to Chapter 8 for more information about sleep). Impaired sleep is associated with disturbances in myelination and changes in micro- and macro sleep architecture, both of which contribute to altered neurodevelopmental outcomes (Bennet et al., 2018; Kurth et al., 2016).

Nutritional deprivation trauma is not just about intake, but energy expenditure. Nutrients needed for normal brain development are highlighted in Figure 2.9 and are juxtaposed with the causes of energy deficiency reported in the preterm infant (Figure 2.10). The developing brain is responsible for 60% of total body energy requirements (Tan et al., 2018; refer to Chapter 5 for additional information on energy expenditure). Energy imbalance increases adenosine triphosphate utilization, resulting in increased epochs of hypoxia and oxidative stress. These factors wreak havoc on somatic and brain growth and development leading to increased risk for neurodevelopmental compromise.

CONSEQUENCES OF NICU TRAUMA

Although the incidence of major morbidity associated with prematurity is stable to slightly decreasing with advancing gestational age, the frequency of minor morbidities is on the rise across all gestational ages (Table 2.1; Johnson & Marlow, 2017; Manuck et al., 2016). Infants born at less than 32 weeks of gestation have an increased risk for cognitive and

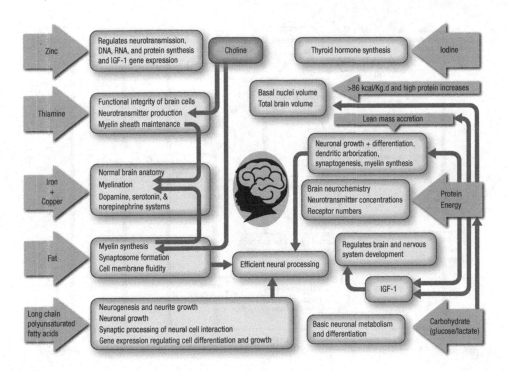

Figure 2.9 Nutrients needed for normal brain development.

IGF-1, insulin-like growth factor 1.
Source: Cormack, B. E., Harding, J. E., Miller, S. P., & Bloomfield, F. H. (2019). The influence of early nutrition on brain growth and neurodevelopment in extremely preterm babies: A narrative review. *Nutrients, 11*(9), 2029. https://doi.org/10.3390/nu11092029

socioemotional problems as well as an increased risk for psychiatric disorders that persist into adolescence and adulthood (Linsell et al., 2019; Montagna & Nosarti, 2016). These individuals are four times more likely to have behavioral problems that negatively impact home life, friendships, and school and leisure activities (Linsell et al., 2019). The majority of former preterm infants do not experience marriage or cohabitate in a committed relationship and are less likely to have children (Johnson & Marlow, 2017; Linsell et al., 2019).

The quality of parental caregiving has lifelong implications for the infant's mental health (Kundakovic & Champagne, 2015). The attachment relationship can either foster resilience to psychological distress or contribute to an increased risk for psychopathology. Low-quality maternal care reduces frontal electroencephalographic asymmetry, increases fear responses, and increases the infant's negative affect at 9 months of age persisting through 2 to 3 years of age (Figure 2.11; Kundakovic & Champagne, 2015).

A 20-year longitudinal study examining trajectories for psychopathology in extremely LBW infants revealed that both internalizing and externalizing problems persist into adolescence and adulthood (Table 2.2; Mathewson et al., 2017; Van Lieshout et al., 2018). Johnson and Marlow (2017) report outcomes of extremely preterm individuals

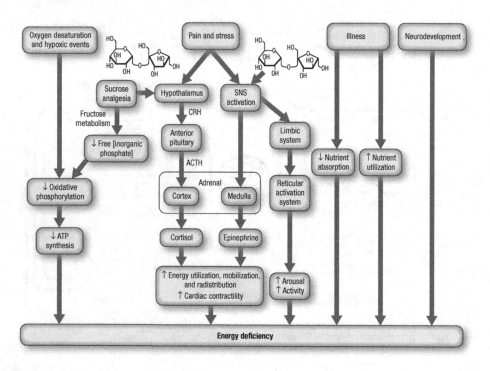

Figure 2.10 Causes of energy deficiency in the premature infant.

ATP, adenosine triphosphate; CRH, corticotropin-releasing factor; SNS, sympathetic nervous system.
Source: Tan, J. B. C., Boskovic, D. S., & Angeles, D. M. (2018). The energy costs of prematurity and the neonatal intensive care unit (NICU) experience. *Antioxidants, 7*(3), 37. https://doi.org/10.3390/antiox7030037

Table 2.1 Major and Minor Neonatal Morbidities

Major Neonatal Morbidities	Minor Neonatal Morbidities	
• Bronchopulmonary dysplasia • Periventricular brain injury • Retinopathy of prematurity • Sepsis • Necrotizing enterocolitis	• Minor cognitive deficits • Learning disabilities • Executive dysfunction • Motor delay • Visual motor perceptual difficulties • Attention deficit disorder	• Language delays • Behavioral problems • Cortical vision impairment • Auditory dys-synchrony • Autism spectrum • Anxiety/depression

into adulthood, demonstrating that adults do not outgrow their cognitive and behavioral challenges. Adolescents with a history of preterm birth experience have reduced social interactions, increased risk-taking behaviors, introversion, and neuroticism (Johnson & Marlow, 2017; Van Lieshout et al., 2018). In addition to intellectual disabilities in adults

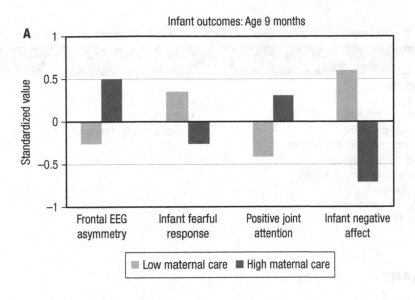

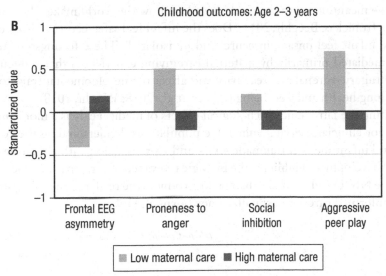

Figure 2.11 Impact of low- versus high-quality maternal care in humans on (A) infant and (B) childhood outcomes.

Source: Kundakovic, M., & Champagne, F. A. (2015). Early-life experience, epigenetics, and the developing brain. *Neuropsychopharmacology Reviews, 40,* 141–153. doi: 10.1038/npp.2014.140 Reprinted with permission from Springer Nature.

born extremely premature, these individuals are more likely to experience psychiatric disorders, such as acute stress disorder, attention deficit hyperactivity disorder, and mood disorders, that persist from childhood (Johnson & Marlow, 2017).

Table 2.2 **Examples of Internalizing and Externalizing Behaviors**

Internalizing Behaviors	Externalizing Behaviors
• Depression • Anxiety • Social withdrawal • Substance abuse • Feelings of loneliness or guilt • Feelings of sadness • Nervousness and irritability • Fearfulness • Difficulty concentrating • Negative self-talk	• Aggression • Disruption • Acting out • Destruction of property

SUMMARY

Infants make meaning out of the world based on how the world makes them feel (Korl et al., 2019; Tronick & Beeghly, 2011). Does the infant feel safe, secure, and/or connected; or does the infant feel unsafe, insecure, and/or isolated? These feelings create cellular memories mediated primarily by maternal caregiving experiences that influence hypo-thalamic–pituitary–adrenal axis reactivity and affect the developmental trajectory of the infant's lifelong health and well-being (Lester et al., 2018; Wright, 2018).

Mitigating the iatrogenic psychological effects of medical care is a moral and ethical imperative for clinicians serving vulnerable populations. Understanding the concepts of pediatric and infant medical traumatic stress and its association with alterations in brain growth and development highlights the biologic relevance of a trauma-informed approach to care in the NICU and beyond. Chapter 3 introduces the reader to the value proposition of trauma-informed care for hospitalized newborns and infants.

It's not about what it is, it's about what it can become.
—Dr. Seuss, *The Lorax*

READER RESOURCE

Adverse childhood experiences (ACEs): Impact on brain, body and behavior: www.youtube.com/watch?v=W-8jTTIsJ7Q

REFERENCES

Adamaszek, M., D'Agata, F., Ferrucci, R., Habas, C., Keulen, S., Kirkby, K. C., Leggio, M., Marien, P., Molinari, M., Moulton, E., Orsi, L., Van Overwalle, F., Papadelis, C., Priori, A., Sacchetti, B.,

Schutter, D. J., Styliadis, C., & Verhoeven, J. (2017). Consensus paper: Cerebellum and emotion. *Cerebellum, 16*(2), 552–576. https://doi.org/10.1007/s12311-016-0815-8

Allen, K.-A. (2019, June 20). The importance of belonging across life: A developmental perspective of our need to belong. *Psychology Today*. https://www.psychologytoday.com/us/blog/sense-belonging/201906/the-importance-belonging-across-life

Baumeister, R. F., & Leary, M. R. (1995). The need to belong: Desire for interpersonal attachments as a fundamental human motivation. *Psychological Bulletin, 117*(3), 497–529. https://doi.org/10.1037/0033-2909.117.3.497

Bennet, L., Walker, D. W., & Horne, R. S. C. (2018). Waking up too early—The consequences of preterm birth on sleep development. *Journal of Physiology, 596*(23), 5687–5708. https://doi.org/10.1113/JP274950

Boulanger-Bertolus, J., White, A. M., & Debiec, J. (2017). Enduring neural and behavioral effects of early life adversity in infancy: Consequences of maternal abuse and neglect, trauma and fear. *Current Behavioral Neuroscience Reports, 4*, 107–116. https://doi.org/10.1007/s40473-017-0112-y

Chau, C. M. Y., Ranger, M., Bichin, M., Park, M. T. M., Amaral, R. S. C., Poskitt, K., Synnes, A. R., Miller, S. P. & Grunau, R. E. (2019). Hippocampus, amygdala, and thalamus volumes in very preterm children at 8 years: Neonatal pain and genetic variation. *Frontiers in Behavioral Neuroscience, 13*, 51. https://doi.org/10.3389/fnbeh.2019.00051

Colonnello, V., Petrocchi, N., Farinelli, M., & Ottaviani, C. (2017). Positive social interactions in a lifespan perspective with a focus on opioidergic and oxytocinergic systems: Implications for neuroprotection. *Current Neuropharmacology, 15*(4), 543–561. https://doi.org/10.2174/1570159X14666160816120209

Comparetti, A. M. (1986). Fetal and neonatal origins of being a person and belonging to the world. *Italian Journal of Neurological Sciences, 5*, 95–100.

Csaszar-Nagy, N. & Bokken, I. (2018). Mother–newborn separation at birth in hospitals: A possible risk for neurodevelopmental disorders? *Neuroscience and Biobehavioral Reviews, 84*, 337–351. https://doi.org/10.1016/j.neubiorev.2017.08.013

D'Agata, A. L., Young, E. E., Cong, X., Grasso, D. J., & McGrath, J. M. (2016). Infant medical trauma in the neonatal intensive care unit (IMTN): A proposed concept for science and practice. *Advances in Neonatal Care, 16*(4), 289–297. https://doi.org/10.1097/ANC.0000000000000309

Debiec, J. (2018, June 21). A sudden and lasting separation from a parent can permanently alter brain development. *The Conversation*. https://theconversation.com/a-sudden-and-lasting-separation-from-a-parent-can-permanently-alter-brain-development-98542

DeMaster, D., Bick, J., Johnson, U., Montroy, J. J., Landry, S., & Duncan, A. F. (2019). Nurturing the preterm infant brain: Leveraging neuroplasticity to improve neurobehavioral outcomes. *Pediatric Research, 85*, 166–175. https://doi.org/10.1038/s41390-018-0203-9

Doud, A. N., Lawrence, K., Goodpasture, M., & Zeller, K. A. (2015). Prematurity and neonatal comorbidities as risk factors for nonaccidental trauma. *Journal of Pediatric Surgery, 50*(6), 1024–1027. https://doi.org/10.1016/j.jpedsurg.2015.03.029

Dowd, M. D. (2017). Early adversity, toxic stress, and resilience: Pediatrics for today. *Pediatric Annals, 46*(7), e246–e249. https://doi.org/10.3928/19382359-20170615-01

Duerden, E. G., Grunau, R. E., Guo, T., Foong, J., Pearson, A., Au-Young, S., Lavoie, R., Chakravarty, M. M., Chau, V., Synnes, A., & Miller, S. P. (2018). Early procedural pain is associated with regionally specific alterations in thalamic development in preterm infants. *Journal of Neuroscience, 38*(4), 878–886. https://doi.org/10.1523/JNEUROSCI.0867-17.2017

Franke, H. A. (2014). Toxic stress: Effects, prevention and treatment. *Children, 1*(3), 390–402. https://doi.org/10.3390/children1030390

Ismail, F. Y., Fatemi, A., & Johnston, M. V. (2017). Cerebral plasticity: Windows of opportunity in the developing brain. *European Journal of Paediatric Neurology, 21*(1), 23–48. https://doi.org/10.1016/j.ejpn.2016.07.007

Johnson, S., & Marlow, N. (2017). Early and long-term outcome of infants born extremely preterm. *Archives of Disease in Childhood, 102*, 97–102. https://doi.org/10.1136/archdischild-2015-309581

Kassam-Adams, N. & Butler, L. (2017). What do clinicians caring for children need to know about pediatric medical traumatic stress and the ethics of trauma-informed approaches? *AMA Journal of Ethics, 19*(8), 793–801. https://doi.org/10.1001/journalofethics.2017.19.8.pfor1-1708

Krol, K. M., Moulder, R. G., Lillard, T. S., Grossmann, T., & Connelly, J. J. (2019). Epigenetic dynamics in infancy and the impact of maternal engagement. *Science Advances, 5*(10), eaay0680. https://doi.org/10.1126/sciadv.aay0680

Kundakovic, M. & Champagne, F. A. (2015). Early-life experience, epigenetics, and the developing brain. *Neuropsychopharmacology Reviews, 40*, 141–153. https://doi.org/10.1038/npp.2014.140

Kurth, S., Dean III, D. C., Achermann, P., O'Muircheartaigh, J., Huber, R., Deoni, S. C. L., & LeBourgeois, M. K. (2016). Increased sleep depth in developing neural networks: New insights from sleep restriction in children. *Frontiers in Human Neuroscience, 10*, 456. https://doi.org/10.3389/fnhum.2016.00456

Lester, B. M., Conradt, E., LaGasse, L. L., Tronick, E. Z., Padbury, J. F., & Marsit, C. J. (2018). Epigenetic programming by maternal behavior in the human infant. *Pediatrics, 142*(4), e20171890. https://doi.org/10.1542/peds.2017-1890

Linsell, L., Johnson, S., Wolke, D., Morris, J., Kurinczuk, J. J., & Marlow, N. (2019). Trajectories of behavior, attention, social and emotional problems from childhood to early adulthood following extremely preterm birth: A prospective cohort study. *European Child & Adolescent Psychiatry, 28*(4), 531–542. https://doi.org/10.1007/s00787-018-1219-8

Manuck, T. A., Rice, M. M., Bailit, J. L., Grobman, W. A., Reddy, U. M., Wapner, R. J., Thorp, J. M., Caritis, S. N., Prasad, M., Tita, A. T. N., Saade, G. R., Sorokin, Y., Rouse, D. J., Blackwell, S. C., & Tolosa, J. E. (2016). Preterm neonatal morbidity and mortality by gestational age: A contemporary cohort. *American Journal of Obstetrics and Gynecology, 215*(1), 103.e1–103.e14. https://doi.org/10.1016/j.ajog.2016.01.004

Mateos-Aparicio, P., & Rodriguez-Moreno, A. (2019). The impact of studying brain plasticity. *Frontiers in Cellular Neuroscience, 13*, 66. https://doi.org/10.3389/fncel.2019.00066

Mathewson, K. J., Chow, C. H. T., Dobson, K. G., Pope, E. I., Schmidt, L. A., & Van Lieshout, R. J. (2017). Mental health of extremely low birth weight survivors: A systematic review and meta-analysis. *Psychological Bulletin, 143*(4), 347–383. https://doi.org/10.1037/bul0000091

Montagna, A. & Nosarti, C. (2016). Socio-emotional development following very preterm birth: Pathways to psychopathology. *Frontiers in Psychology, 7*, 80. https://doi.org/10.3389/fpsyg.2016.00080

Montirosso, R., & Provenzi, L. (2015). Implications of epigenetics and stress regulation on research and developmental care of preterm infants. *Journal of Obstetric, Gynecologic & Neonatal Nursing, 44*(2), 174–182. https://doi.org/10.1111/1552-6909.12559

Mooney-Leber, S. M., & Brummelte, S. (2017). Neonatal pain and reduced maternal care: Early-life stressors interacting to impact brain and behavioral development. *Neuroscience, 342*, 21–36. https://doi.org/10.1016/j.neuroscience.2016.05.001

Nist, M. D. (2017). Biological embedding: Evaluation and analysis of an emerging concept for nursing scholarship. *Journal of Advanced Nursing, 73*(2), 349–360. https://doi.org/10.1111/jan.13168

Nist, M. D., Harrison, T. M., & Steward, D. K. (2019). The biological embedding of neonatal stress exposure: A conceptual model describing the mechanisms of stress-induced neurodevelopmental impairment in preterm infants. *Research in Nursing & Health, 42*(1), 61–71. https://doi.org/10.1002/nur.21923

Over, H. (2016). The origins of belonging: Social motivation in infants and young children. *Philosophical Transactions Royal Society of London Biological Sciences, 371*(1686), 20150072. https://doi.org/10.1098/rstb.2015.0072

Puls, H. T., Anderst, J. D., Bettenhausen, J. L., Clark, N., Krager, M., Markham, J. L., & Hall, M. (2019). Newborn risk factors for subsequent physical abuse hospitalization. *Pediatrics, 143*(2), e20182108. https://doi.org/10.1542/peds.2018-2108

Ranger, M., Chau, C. M. Y., Garg, A., Woodward, T. S., Beg, M. F., Bjornson, B., Poskitt, K., Fitzpatrick, K., Synnes, A. R., Miller, S. P., & Grunau, R. E. (2013). Neonatal pain-related stress predicts cortical thickness at age 7 years in children born very preterm. *PLoS One, 8*(10), e76702. https://doi.org/10.1371/journal.pone.0076702

Roque, S., Mesquita, A. R., Palha, J. A., Sousa, N., & Correia-Neves, M. (2014). The behavioral and immunological impact of maternal separation: A matter of timing. *Frontiers in Behavioral Neuroscience, 8*, 192. https://doi.org/10.3389/fnbeh.2014.00192

Sanders, M. R., & Hall, S. L. (2018). Trauma-informed care in the newborn intensive care unit: Promoting safety, security and connectedness. *Journal of Perinatology, 38*(1), 3–10. https://doi.org/10.1038/jp.2017.124

Shonkoff, J. P., Garner, A. S.; The Committee on Psychosocial Aspects of Child and Family Health, Committee on Early Childhood Adoption, and Dependent Care and Section on Developmental and Behavioral Pediatrics, Siegel, B. S., Dobbins, M. I., Earls, M. F., McGuinn, L., Pascoe, J., & Wood, D. L. (2012). The lifelong effects of early childhood adversity and toxic stress. *Pediatrics, 129*(1), e232–e246. https://doi.org/10.1542/peds.2011-2663

Smith, G. C., Gutovich, J., Smyser, C., Pineda, R., Newnham, C., Tjoeng, T. H., Vavasseur, C., Wallendorf, M., Neil, J., & Inder, T. (2011). Neonatal intensive care unit stress is associated with brain development in preterm infants. *Annals of Neurology, 70*(4), 541–549. https://doi.org/10.1002/ana.22545

Tan, J. B. C., Boskovic, D. S., & Angeles, D. M. (2018). The energy costs of prematurity and the neonatal intensive care unit (NICU) experience. *Antioxidants, 7*(3), 37. https://doi.org/10.3390/antiox7030037

Tronick, E., & Beeghly, M. (2011). Infants' meaning-making and the development of mental health problems. *American Psychologist, 66*(2), 107–119. https://doi.org/10.1037/a0021631

Van Lieshout, R. J., Ferro, M. A., Schmidt, L. A., Boyle, M. H., Saigal, S., Morrison, K. M., & Mathewson, K. J. (2018). Trajectories of psychopathology in extremely low birth weight survivors from early adolescence to adulthood: A 20-year longitudinal study. *Journal of Child Psychology & Psychiatry, 59*(11), 1192–1200. https://doi.org/10.1111/jcpp.12909

Weber, A., & Harrison, T. M. (2019). Reducing toxic stress in the neonatal intensive care unit. *Nursing Outlook, 67*, 169–189. https://doi.org/10.1016/j.outlook.2018.11.002

Wright, R. O. (2018). "Motherless children have the hardest time": Epigenetic programming and early life environment. *Pediatrics, 142*(4), e20181528. https://doi.org/10.1542/peds.2018-1528

3

The Value Proposition of Trauma-Informed Care

We're all human, aren't we? Every human life is worth the same, and worth saving.
—J. K. Rowling, *Harry Potter and the Deathly Hallows*

WHAT IS THE VALUE EQUATION?

Total global healthcare expenditure is roughly 9% of the world's gross domestic product (GDP). GDP represents the total monetary, or market value, of all finished goods and services produced in a country and functions as a scorecard of a country's economic health. In 2018, the United States spent 16% of its GDP on healthcare; twice as much as any other high-income country in the world (Figure 3.1; Tikkanen & Abrams, 2020). Annually, $935 billion of U.S. healthcare expenditure is spent on ineffective care that provides minimal benefit to the patient (Tikkanen & Abrams, 2020). Moreover, Americans have the lowest life expectancy and the highest suicide rate across 36 high-income countries (Tikkanen & Abrams, 2020). Premature birth survivors contribute to both the shortened life expectancy and the high suicide rate (Crump, 2020; Risnes et al., 2016).

Gestational age is inversely correlated with all causes of death between the ages of 0 and 45 years in men and women to include cardiovascular, respiratory, endocrine, neurological, cancer, and external causes (Crump, 2020). External causes, defined as accidents or violence, suicide, and substance abuse/overdoses, are responsible for the majority of deaths among preterm birth survivors (Risnes et al., 2016). Addressing the psychosocio–emotional and spiritual needs of critically ill infants and their families requires an actionable prevention strategy that enriches the value of neonatal care by mitigating the long-term consequences associated with prematurity and NICU hospitalization (Lean, Rogers, Pail, & Gerstein, 2018).

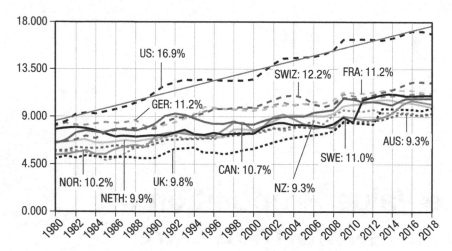

Figure 3.1 Healthcare spent as a percentage of gross domestic product adjusted for differences in cost of living 2018; Organization for Economic Co-operation and Development average = 8.8%.

Source: Tikkanen, R., & Abrams, M. K. (2020, January 30). *U.S. health care from a global perspective, 2019: Higher spending, worse outcomes?* https://www.commonwealthfund.org/publications/issue-briefs/2020/jan/us-health-care-global-perspective-2019

Value-based care shifts the paradigm from volume to value, with an emphasis on quality, safety, efficacy, and cost. The goal of a value-based healthcare system is to cocreate and measure outcomes meaningful for patients and their families with value expressed as the best health outcomes achieved per dollar spent (Marzorati & Pravettoni, 2017). Value is an important feature of quality healthcare. However, a consensus on the meaning of value and what constitutes value in healthcare remains elusive for many key stakeholders (Table 3.1; Marzorati & Pravettoni, 2017).

Dukhovny et al. (2016) introduced a value equation to examine the quality, efficacy, and safety of various interventions in neonatology juxtaposed to the costs, direct and indirect, associated with care delivery. The goal is to eradicate wasteful expenditure and ensure safe quality care:

$$Value = Outcomes \div Costs.$$

Waste refers to elements that incur costs but provide no benefit, such as duplicated services, poor care coordination, and so forth. Improving outcomes without increasing costs eradicates waste.

Improving outcomes almost always reduces costs in neonatology, both direct hospital costs and indirect costs such as lost productivity with regard to the infant's and/or family's present and future contributions to society (Dukhovny et al., 2016). Optimizing value doesn't need to be complicated, but does require a paradigm shift from "routine care" to value-based care and minimizing harm in the short term and long term (Profit et al., 2019).

Table 3.1 **Healthcare Stakeholders**

Stakeholder	Value Attributes
Clinicians	• Appropriateness of care • Effectiveness • Evidence-based
Payers/hospital administrators	• Clinical benefit achieved for the money spent • Patient satisfaction • Reduced length of stay
Policy makers	• Sustainability • Equanimity • Cost-effective
Patients	• Satisfies health goals • Improved health-related quality of life • Respectful, transparent, and consistent communication • Shared decision-making

Source: Adapted from Marzorati, C., & Pravettoni, G. (2017). Value is the key concept in the health care system: How it has influenced medical practice and clinical decision-making processes. *Journal of Multidisciplinary Healthcare, 10,* 101–106. doi: 10.2147/JMDH.S122383

Aligning evidence-based practice and evidence-based economics with quality- improvement processes creates the value road map that supports quality, safety, and efficacy for families in crisis (Dukhovny et al., 2016).

Value-conscious care begins with evidence-based practice. Despite the plethora of systematic reviews and meta-analyses highlighting the benefits and value of developmentally supportive, trauma-informed care for hospitalized infants and their families, translation into clinical practice remains troublesome. Bridging this gap requires an understanding of organizational culture and the knowledge, skills, and attitudes of clinicians toward evidence-based practice and cultural transformation.

Evidence-based economics suggest that economic phenomena, such as production, distribution, and consumption of goods and services, are not binary. Both direct and indirect costs contain many facets that must be understood to fully grasp their relationship to value. For example, the economic implications of pain management or two-person care may not be obvious, but that does not mean they do not bring value to the patient, family, and staff experience.

Quality improvement or the adoption of evidence-based best practices in the clinical setting brings the concept of value to life. Using the Plan–Do–Study–Act Model for Improvement, clinicians evaluate the effectiveness, quality, and safety of potentially better practices from a quantitative and qualitative perspective. Successful quality-improvement initiatives understand and address the social and behavioral components of change in order to establish accountability and sustainability, bringing value to the patient–family dyad, the clinician, and healthcare systems at large.

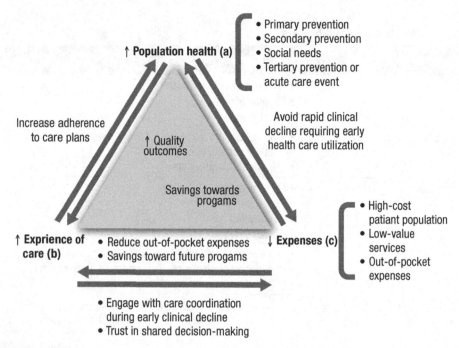

Figure 3.2 Triple Aim and its relationship among healthcare value components.

Source: Gupta, R. (2019). Health care value: Relationships between population health, patient experience and costs of care. *Primary Care: Clinics in Office Practice, 46*(4), 603–622. doi: 10.1016/j.pop.2019.07.005 Reprinted with permission from Elsevier.

THE INSTITUTE FOR HEALTHCARE IMPROVEMENT'S TRIPLE AIM

The Institute for Healthcare Improvement's (IHI) Triple Aim is a unique framework developed to optimize health system performance through (a) the pursuit of improved population health, and (b) experience of care (c) while reducing costs (Figure 3.2). *Population health* refers to the quality of health for a specific population that includes both healthcare and the social determinants of health (SDOH; Gupta, 2019). Quality of healthcare is defined by its safety, patient-centeredness, effectiveness, timeliness, and equity.

SDOH include health and healthcare, neighborhoods and the built environment, economic stability, education, and social and community context. These determinants take on new meaning within the context of the NICU and influence lifelong health and wellness for this fragile and vulnerable population (Table 3.2). Where you live affects your health and well-being. For the NICU population, living in the NICU environment for days, weeks, and months, influences the developmental trajectory of the infant—family dyad in meaningful and measurable ways across the life span.

Since the introduction of the IHI's Triple Aim in 2008, there has been some criticism that the framework fails to explicitly acknowledge the critical role of the clinical

Table 3.2 **Social Determinants of Health Within the NICU Context**

SDOH	NICU Context
Health and healthcare	• Medical practices and NICU-related quality of care to include (but not be limited to) pain-management practices, sleep protection, diet, postural support, skin care, etc.
Neighborhood and built environment	• Physical environment of the NICU to include (but not be limited to) sensory, spacial, and aesthetic dimensions; urban versus rural setting; academic versus private-practice models of care delivery; etc.
Economic stability	• Economics of the facility influencing staffing patterns and resources • Family economics, i.e., food and/or housing insecurity, transportation and parking, childcare resources, health insurance, etc.
Education	• Organizational investment in continuous professional development for staff • Individual clinician investment in ongoing professional education • Parent knowledge/education regarding parenting skills, breastfeeding benefits, skin-to-skin care, importance of parental presence and emotional closeness, etc.
Social and community context	• Organizational catchment area and commitment to meeting the unique needs of demographics served; organizational culture and leadership model • Clinicians' knowledge, skills and attitudes regarding caring encounters with infants and families; reading infant behavioral cues to provide responsive contingent care • Family culture; social support network and resources; trauma-history; knowledge, skills, and attitudes about parenting their hospitalized infant

SDOH, social determinants of health.

workforce in achieving healthcare transformation (Sikka et al., 2015). The IHI introduced a framework for "joy in work" in 2017 in response to escalating rates of clinician burnout. Finding purpose and joy in work are crucial for the physical, psychological, and emotional health and well-being of healthcare professionals (Galuska et al., 2018; Sikka et al., 2015). Experts recommend expanding the IHI's Triple Aim framework to include "joy in work"—a

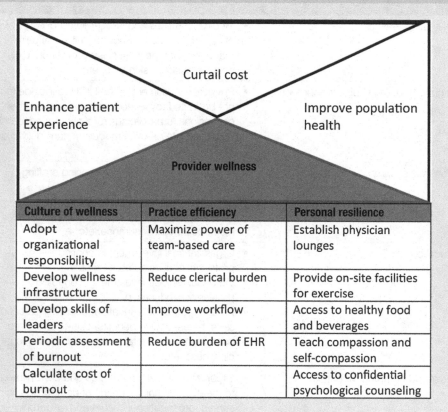

EXHIBIT 3.1 QUADRUPLE AIM WITH RECIPROCAL DOMAINS OF CLINICIAN WELL-BEING

EHR, electronic health record.

Source: Anandarajah, A. P., Quill, T. E., & Privitera, M. R. (2018). Adopting the Quadruple Aim: The University of Rochester Medical Center experience: Moving from physician burnout to physician resilience. *American Journal of Medicine*, *131*(8), 979–986. doi: 10.1016/j.amjmed.2018.04.034 Reprinted with permission from Elsevier.

Quadruple Aim (Anandarajah et al., 2018; Galuska et al., 2018; Sikka et al., 2015). Adding this fourth element enhances teamwork, improves efficiencies, results in high-quality patient care, and greatly improves job satisfaction (Exhibit 3.1).

The concept of population health and experience of care underpins the core measures for trauma-informed care in the NICU (Figure 3.3). The core measures are disease-independent domains that address the human needs of the patient and family (refer to chapters in Section II). These measures emphasize prevention and protection as turnkey for safe, quality healthcare and lifelong health and wellness. Preventive and protective

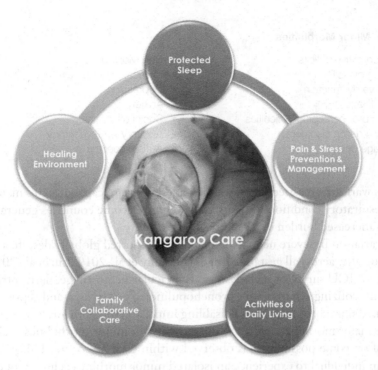

Figure 3.3 Core measures for trauma-informed care. Kangaroo care, or skin-to-skin care, is the quintessential care practice impacting each core measure.

Source: Reprinted with permission from Caring Essentials Collaborative, LLC.

healthcare practices that mitigate and minimize toxic stress reduce morbidity, increase value, and enrich the individual's quality of life.

Attending to an infant's basic needs as a developing human being is a primary prevention strategy in the hospital setting. Intensive care and primary preventive care do not need to be mutually exclusive in the NICU. Through experience-dependent and experience-expectant neural activity, newborns and infants learn about their world and their value in the world. All mammals, including humans, have a biological imperative for social connectedness (Sanders & Hall, 2018). This biologic realty must be prima facie for all hospitalized newborns and infants to ensure the highest standard for population health.

REDUCING THE GLOBAL BURDEN OF PRETERM BIRTH AND NEONATAL COMPLICATIONS

Approximately 15 million infants are born prematurely around the globe. Prematurity is the leading cause of death in children under the age of 5 years. In low-income countries, half of infants born at less than 32 weeks' gestation die due to a lack of appropriate cost-effective

Table 3.3 Minor Morbidities

• Minor cognitive deficits	• Behavioral problems
• Learning disabilities	• Cortical vision impairment
• Executive dysfunction	• Depression
• Motor delays	• Anxiety
• Visual motor perceptual difficulties	• Social difficulties
• Attention deficit disorders	• Auditory dys-synchrony
• Language delays	• Autism spectrum

care such as warmth, breastfeeding resources, and basic care capabilities to manage infections and respiratory conditions. Infants born in high-income countries generally survive but with an increased burden of disability and morbidity.

Wide variation in severe neonatal morbidity is reported globally despite a decline in neonatal mortality across all gestational ages (Bonamy et al., 2019; Liu et al., 2019). Major morbidity in NICU survivors includes intraventricular hemorrhage, periventricular leukomalacia, necrotizing enterocolitis, bronchopulmonary dysplasia, and sepsis (Anderson et al., 2016). Major morbidities have a disabling impact on the survivor; however, for those who escape major morbidity, many are diagnosed with minor morbidities (Table 3.3). A spectrum of outcome possibilities is observed within each minor morbidity category. It is rare for an individual to experience an isolated minor morbidity; clusters of conditions are more common. These clustered conditions impact the affected individual and family physically, socially, emotionally, cognitively, and psychologically.

Reducing the burden of these minor morbidities and possibly influencing the evolution of many of the major morbidities mediated by inflammation requires attention to managing the infants experience of toxic stress and pain (Kuhlman et al., 2020; Patra et al., 2017; Weber & Harrison, 2019). High circulating levels of inflammatory mediators are linked to increased risk of many adult diseases (David et al., 2017; Kuhlman et al., 2020). Epidemiological and epigenetic studies reveal early-life adversity, such as preterm birth and other perinatal conditions, interact with the epigenome and microbiome altering developmental programming (refer to Chapter 4; Fumagalli et al., 2018; Lu & Claud, 2019; Montirosso et al., 2016; Provenzi et al., 2017, 2018). Early prevention and optimal nutrition are effective interventions to preserve long-term health and wellness (Simeoni et al., 2018).

Buffering early-life toxic stress reduces the burden of disease associated with the NICU experience (Weber & Harrison, 2019). Parental presence must be actively pursued and supported by healthcare organizations. Creating welcoming, comfortable, and suitable accommodations for parents and families of hospitalized newborns is a first step in preserving the integrity of the family in crisis and buffer the toxic stress experience of the infant (refer to Chapter 7). Parental presence and parental holding are related to improved neurodevelopmental outcomes in preterm infants through ages 4 to 5 years (Pineda et al., 2018; Reynolds et al., 2013).

The buffering effect of maternal presence is operationalized through skin-to-skin care and breastfeeding experiences. In addition to improved neurodevelopmental outcomes, skin-to-skin care and breastfeeding results in significant cost savings (Lowson et al., 2015; Stuebe et al., 2017). Skin-to-skin care and breastfeeding are associated with a reduced length of hospital stay and a decrease in subsequent re-hospitalizations resulting in cost savings in excess of nearly $905,000 (Lowson et al., 2015). Stuebe et al. (2017) reported a 5% increase in breastfeeding rates statistically significantly reduced the incidence of infectious morbidity over the first year of life using a simulation model with staggering medical cost savings.

THE VALUE PROPOSITION OF TRAUMA-INFORMED CARE IN THE NICU

The degree to which every aspect of the NICU experience prompts a stress response is the degree to which the value of service can be improved by mitigating and managing traumatic stress. Chronic early-life stress is associated with lifelong increased risk for psychopathology and chronic health problems mediated by dysregulation of the hypothalamic–pituitary–adrenal (HPA) axis (refer to Chapter 4; Bunea et al., 2017). Dysregulation of the HPA axis is linked to asthma, chronic pain syndromes, impaired cognitive and emotional capacity, depression, anxiety, as well as social and behavioral difficulties (Agorastos et al., 2018; Burke et al., 2017; Chen & Baram, 2016; Rosa et al., 2018).

Nurses have the power to shape the care environment and care experience for hospitalized infants and their families (Weber et al., 2018). Supporting activation of the oxytocin (OT) system disarms the stress response, cultivates social connectedness, and is a necessary and critical component for optimal neurodevelopment of all infants (Figure 3.4; Weber et al., 2018). Facilitating caring encounters that activate the OT system, such as skin-to-skin care, breastfeeding, social vocalizations, holding, and positive touch, become therapeutic strategies creating a socially supportive milieu for the infant and family in crisis (Scatliffe et al., 2019; Weber et al., 2018). Weber et al. (2018) present examples of nursing diagnosis and potential nursing interventions that mediate OT activity (Table 3.4)

Toxic stress is a mediator between early-life adversity and suboptimal outcomes in learning, behavior, and health. Social supportive and nurturing interactions counteract the stress response and cultivate connectedness and resilience. Understanding the biology underlying early-life stress and social, nurturing interactions opens up new opportunities for primary prevention and earlier intervention for infants and families in the NICU and beyond.

Adhering to the admonishment "first, do no harm," the value proposition of trauma-informed care is clear. Changing the routine care paradigm to a trauma-informed approach requires a cultural shift that recognizes the importance and value of compassionate, person-centered, family-collaborative care. Many healthcare professionals are unfamiliar with the

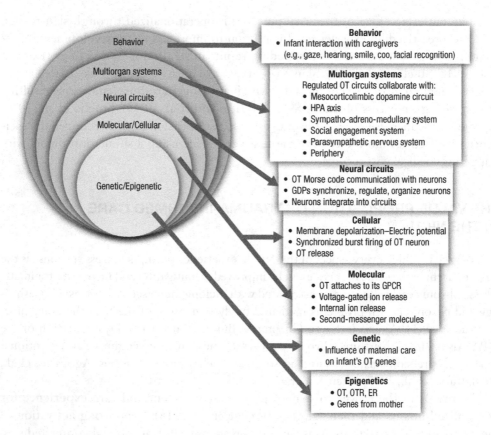

Figure 3.4 Nested hierarchies of effects of oxytocin.

ER, estrogen receptors; GDP, giant depolarizing potentials; GPCR, G-protein-coupled receptors; HPA, hypothalamic–pituitary–adrenal; OT, oxytocin; OTR, oxytocin receptors.
Source: Weber, A. M., Harrison, T. M., & Steward, D. K. (2018). Expanding regulation theory with oxytocin: A psychoneurobiological model for infant development. *Nursing Research, 67*(2), 133–145. doi: 10.1097/NNR.0000000000000261 Reprinted with permission from Wolters Kluwer Health, Inc.

concept of trauma-informed care. Engaging subject matter experts in trauma-informed cultural transformation (Caring Essentials Collaborative, LLC, is the definitive resource for trauma-informed education and cultural transformation for organizations serving newborns and infants) will support your organization's journey to deliver value-conscious care in the NICU.

SUMMARY

Given what is now known about the biological implications of early-life adversity and traumatic stress in the NICU (refer to Chapter 2and Chapter 4), there are clear opportunities to eliminate waste, improve outcomes, and reduce costs through the adoption of a trauma-informed

Table 3.4 Nursing Diagnoses and Interventions Related to Oxytocin Processes

Focus	Nursing Diagnosis/Nursing Interventions	Underlying OT-Based Process
Infant	Pain: Chronic/acute • Assess pain using developmentally appropriate tools. • Use nonpharmacologic interventions to reduce pain (e.g., nonnutritive sucking, breastfeeding, kangaroo care, facilitated tucking).	• OT nerves in spine andperipheral nervous system regulate pain. • OT reduces pain thresholds, pain perception.
Infant	Disorganized behavior • Use consistent nurturing response. • Assist parents; modify environment for appropriate stimulation (e.g., lighting, sound). • Model caregiving: Support infant behavioral organization (e.g., hand containment, facilitated tucking, nonnutritive sucking).	• Physical contact increases OT release. • Infant sleep, arousal, and hunger regulate the OT system. • Regulation of basic infant behaviors is the cornerstone for supportive social interaction.
Infant	Delayed development: Risk • Assess risk factors (e.g., prematurity, genetic disorders). • Identify/use educational resources to facilitate infant development. • Implement neuroprotective interventions (e.g., kangaroo care, breastfeeding, stress reduction, modification of environmental stimuli, minimize parent–infant separation).	• OT is necessary for neurodevelopmental processes. • We hypothesize that neuroprotective nursing interventions facilitate OT-based neurobiological processes in the infant.
Mother	Anxiety • Assess level of and physical reactions to anxiety (heart racing, sleeplessness). • Encourage positive self-talk (e.g., "I can do this one step at a time"). • Use empathy to validate feelings. • Minimize the number of professionals with whom the parents have contact. • Reduce parent–infant separation (which increases parental anxiety). • Provide anticipatory guidance on infant care plan.	• Divergent effects of OT in stress response systems produce engagement or avoidance/aggression with appropriate anxiety responses to stress. • OT decreases social anxiety to facilitate socially based behaviors during maternal–infant interaction.

(continued)

Table 3.4 Nursing Diagnoses and Interventions Related to Oxytocin Processes *(continued)*

Focus	Nursing Diagnosis/Nursing Interventions	Underlying OT-Based Process
Mother	Powerlessness: Risk • Assess parental satisfaction with the infant's care. • Encourage parents to participate in family-centered rounds. • Assist parents in making decisions regarding infant treatment schedule. • Encourage parents to fully participate in the infant's care. • Establish a routine for daily phone calls; initiate calls. • Provide a sense of control by having parents plan infant care/activities.	• Mothers are at risk for alteration in parental role, ineffective parental performance, impaired parent–infant interaction, and impaired maternal–infant attachment when they do not feel valuable and in control of infant care, which we theorize results in dysregulation of the maternal OT system.
Mother	Role strain: Parent/caregiver • Provide a consistent, encouraging, nonjudgmental environment. • Involve in activities with the infant they can successfully achieve. • Provide a "homelike" environment (e.g., family personalizes infant room/space). • Provide positive feedback for supportive parenting behaviors.	• Empowering mothers to own their parental role results in sensitive parenting behaviors, higher levels of OT in mother and infant, and greater brain activation and connectivity in OT-based networks.
Mother	Parental performance: Ineffective • Use active listening: Explore understanding of developmental needs, expectations. • Examine parenting style, behaviors (e.g., psychosocial environment at home, attribution of negative traits to infant, involvement with infant care). • Assess maternal depression, stress, and anxiety. • Plan education directed toward parental concerns. • Model developmentally appropriate caregiving skills (e.g., gentle touch, soft voice, containment, nonnutritive sucking, contingent responses to infant cues).	• Maternal OT is associated with supportive maternal behaviors and coordination of social interactions with the neonate's alert state. • Parenting behaviors that release infant OT include comforting touch, soft voice, gaze, contingent responses, high quality affect. • Parents who display more affectionate touch increase their OT levels after interaction with their infant.

(continued)

Table 3.4 Nursing Diagnoses and Interventions Related to Oxytocin Processes *(continued)*

Focus	Nursing Diagnosis/Nursing Interventions	Underlying OT-Based Process
	• Acknowledge, praise parenting strengths. • Initiate referrals to agencies (e.g., Help me Grow, March of Dimes), parent education programs, social support groups (e.g., NICU Peer Parent Support groups).	
Dyad	Breastfeeding: Ineffective • Provide lactation counseling and breastfeeding assistance. • Provide parent education. • Infant engaging in nonnutritive sucking at breast.	• OT levels are higher in breastfeeding mothers than in formula-feeding mothers. • Human milk OT levels are higher after breastfeeding.
Dyad	Family processes: Interrupted • Assist parents in identifying and prioritizing family strengths and needs. • Promote positive attitudes by communicating what skills parents already do well. • Help parents identify appropriate support systems (e.g., extended family, friends, social worker) and community resources (e.g., faith groups, volunteers, respite care). • Identify social services (e.g., transportation, finances).	• Ensuring that family's needs are met relieves parental anxiety, allows parents to maximize time in the NICU. • When family processes are restored, parents are less stressed, more likely to engage in supportive social interactions with their infants, which cause release of OT.
Dyad	Parent–infant interaction: Impaired • Assess parent–infant interactions, especially during feeding and care. • Model consistent, nurturing behaviors when caring for and interacting with infant. • Foster developmentally supportive parenting behaviors.	• Early, consistent, developmentally supportive interactions regulate infant OT brain biology, emotions, and social behaviors that emerge from that biology.

(continued)

Table 3.4 **Nursing Diagnoses and Interventions Related to Oxytocin Processes** *(continued)*

Focus	Nursing Diagnosis/Nursing Interventions	Underlying OT-Based Process
Dyad	Maternal–infant attachment impaired: Risk • Minimize parent–infant separation immediately after birth. • Identify infant's strengths and vulnerabilities. • Educate parents regarding infant growth and development, clarifying expectations. • Invite parents to spend the night (e.g., Ronald McDonald House, hospital room). • Provide infant photos, mementos (e.g., outgrown blood pressure cuff, hat), journal developmental milestone reports to celebrate progress, promote normalcy. • Suggest parents provide a photo and/or audiotape of themselves.	• Synchronized, supportive interactions foster attachment, which is facilitated by the OT system. • OT coordinates with the social engagement system, which produces the physiologic states, emotions, and engagement cues that encourage dyadic attachment.

OT, oxytocin.

Source: Weber, A. M., Harrison, T. M., & Steward, D. K. (2018). Expanding regulation theory with oxytocin: A psychoneurobiological model for infant development. *Nursing Research, 67*(2), 133–145. doi: 10.1097/NNR.0000000000000261 Reprinted with permission from Wolters Kluwer Health, Inc.

paradigm. A trauma-informed approach in the NICU promotes a sense of safety, security, and connectedness while cultivating resilience for infants and families in crisis with far-reaching implications for health and well-being (Coughlin, 2017; Crump, 2020; Sanders & Hall, 2018). The value trauma-informed care confers on infants, families, and clinicians is priceless.

> *It is an absolute human certainty that no one can know his own beauty or perceive a sense of his own worth until it has been reflected back to him in the mirror of another loving, caring human being.*
> —John Joseph Powell

READER RESOURCES

Brain hero: www.youtube.com/watch?v=s31HdBeBgg4

Triple Aim: www.youtube.com/watch?time_continue=89&v=a_QskzKFZnI&feature=emb_logo

REFERENCES

Agorastos, A., Pervanidou, P., Chrousos, G. P., & Kolaitis, G. (2018). Early life stress and trauma: Developmental neuroendocrine aspects of prolonged stress system dysregulation. *Hormones, 17,* 507–520. https://doi.org/10.1007/s42000-018-0065-x

Anandarajah, A. P., Quill, T. E., & Privitera, M. R. (2018). Adopting the quadruple aim: The University of Rochester Medical Center experience: Moving from physician burnout to physician resilience. *American Journal of Medicine, 131*(8), 979–986. https://doi.org/10.1016/j.amjmed.2018.04.034

Anderson, J. G., Baer, R. J., Partridge, J. C., Kuppermann, M., Franck, L. S., Rand, L., Jelliffe-Pawlowski, L. L., & Rogers, E. E. (2016). Survival and major morbidity of extremely preterm infants: A population-based study. *Pediatrics, 138*(1), e20154434. https://doi.org/10.1542/peds.2015-4434

Bonamy, A. K. E., Zeitlin, J., Piedvache, A., Maier, R. F., van Heijst, A., Varendi, H., Manktelow, B. N., Fenton, A., Mazela, J., Cuttini, M., Norman, M., Petrou, S., van Reempts, P., Barros, H., & Draper, E. S. (2019). Wide variation in severe neonatal morbidity among very preterm infants in European regions. *Archives of Disease in Childhood-Fetal and Neonatal Editions, 104*(1), F36–F45. https://doi.org/10.1136/archdischild-2017-313697

Bunea, I. M., Szentagotai-Tatar, A., & Miu, A. C. (2017). Early-life adversity and cortisol response to social stress: A meta-analysis. *Translational Psychiatry, 7,* 1274. https://doi.org/10.1038/s41398-017-0032-3

Burke, N. N., Finn, D. P., McGuire, B. E., & Roche, M. (2017). Psychological stress in early life as a predisposing factor for the development of chronic pain: Clinical and preclinical evidence and neurobiological mechanisms. *Journal of Neuroscience Research, 95*(6), 1257–1270. https://doi.org/10.1002/jnr.23802

Chen, Y., & Baram, T. Z. (2016). Toward understanding how early-life stress reprograms cognitive and emotional brain networks. *Neuropsychopharmacology, 41*(1), 197–206. https://doi.org/10.1038/npp.2015.181

Coughlin, M. (2017). Trauma-informed, neuroprotective care for hospitalized newborns and infants. *Infant, 13*(5), 176–179.

Crump, C. (2020). Preterm birth and mortality in adulthood: A systematic review. *Journal of Perinatology, 40*(6), 833–843. https://doi.org/10.1038/s41372-019-0563-y

David, J., Measelle, J., Ostlund, B., & Ablow, J. (2017). Association between early life adversity and inflammation during infancy. *Developmental Psychobiology, 59*(6), 696–702. https://doi.org/10.1002/dev.21538

Dukhovny, D., Pursley, D. M., Kirpalani, H. M., Horbar, J. H., & Zupancic, J. A. F. (2016). Evidence, quality, and waste: Solving the value equation in neonatology. *Pediatrics, 137*(3), e20150312. https://doi.org/10.1542/peds.2015-0312

Fumagalli, M., Provenzi, L., De Carli, P., Dessimone, F., Sirgiovanni, I., Giorda, R., Cinnante, C., Squarcina, L., Pozzoli, U., Triulzi, F., Brambilla, P., Borgatti, R., Mosca, F., & Montirosso, R. (2018). From early stress to 12-month development in very preterm infants: Preliminary findings on epigenetic mechanisms and brain growth. *PLoS One, 13*(1), e0190602. https://doi.org/10.1371/journal.pone.0190602

Galuska, L., Hahn, J., Polifroni, E. C., & Crow, G. (2018). A narrative analysis of nurses' experiences with meaning and joy in nursing practice. *Nursing Administration Quarterly, 42*(2), 154–163. https://doi.org/10.1097/NAQ.0000000000000280

Gupta, R. (2019). Health care value: Relationships between population health, patient experience and costs of care. *Primary Care: Clinics in Office Practice, 46*(4), 603–622. https://doi.org/10.1016/j.pop.2019.07.005

Kuhlman, K. R., Horn, S. R., Chiang, J. J., & Bower, J. E. (2020). Early life adversity exposure and circulating markers of inflammation in children and adolescents: A systematic review and meta-analysis. *Brain, Behavior, and Immunity, 86*, 30–42. https://doi.org/10.1016/j.bbi.2019.04.028

Lean, R. E., Rogers, C. E., Pail, R. A., & Gerstein, E. D. (2018). NICU hospitalization: Long-term implications on parenting and child behaviors. *Current Treatment Options in Pediatrics, 4*(1), 49–69.

Lowson, K., Offer, C., Watson, J., McGuire, B., & Renfrew, M. J. (2015). The economic benefits of increasing kangaroo skin-to-skin care and breastfeeding in neonatal units: Analysis of a pragmatic intervention in clinical practice. *International Breastfeeding Journal. 10*, 11. https://doi.org/10.1186/s13006-015-0035-8

Lu, J., & Claud, E. C. (2019). Connection between gut microbiome and brain development on preterm infants. *Developmental Psychobiology, 61*(5), 739–751. https://doi.org/10.1002/dev.21806

Lui, K., Lee, S. K., Kusuda, S., Adams, M., Vento, M., Reichman, B., Darlow, B. A., Lehtonen, L., Modi, N., Norman, M., Hakansson, S., Bassler, D., Rusconi, F., Lodha, A., Yang, J., Shah, P. S.; on behalf of the International Network for Evaluation of Outcomes (iNeo) of neonates investigators. (2019). Trends in outcomes for neonates born very preterm and very low birth weight in 11 high-income countries. *Journal of Pediatrics, 215*, 32–40. https://doi.org/10.1016/j.jpeds.2019.08.020

Marzorati, C., & Pravettoni, G. (2017). Value is the key concept in the health care system: How it has influenced medical practice and clinical decision-making processes. *Journal of Multidisciplinary Healthcare, 10*, 101–106. https://doi.org/10.2147/JMDH.S122383

Montirosso, R., Provenzi, L., Fumagalli, M., Sirgiovanni, Giorda, R., Pozzoli, U., Beri, S., Menozzi, G., Tronick, E., Morandi, F., Mosca, F., & Borgatti, R. (2016). Serotonin transporter gene (*SLC6A4*) methylation associates with neonatal intensive care unit stay and 3-month-old temperament in preterm infants. *Child Development, 87*(1), 38–48. https://doi.org/10.1111/cdev.12492

Patra, A., Huang, H., Bauer, J. A., & Giannone, P. J. (2017). Neurological consequences of systemic inflammation in the premature neonate. *Neural Regeneration Research, 12*(6), 890–896. https://doi.org/10.4103/1673-5374.208547

Pineda, R., Bender, J., Hall, B., Shabosky, L., Annecca, A., & Smith, J. (2018). Parent participation in the neonatal intensive care unit: Predictors and relationships to neurobehavior and developmental outcomes. *Early Human Development, 117*, 32–38. https://doi.org/10.1016/j.earlhumdev.2017.12.008

Profit, J., Scheid, A., & Ridout, E. (2019, October 30). *First, do no harm: Value-driven patient safety in the neonatal intensive care unit*. https://psnet.ahrq.gov/perspective/first-do-no-harm-value-driven-patient-safety-neonatal-intensive-care-unit

Provenzi, L., Fumagalli, M., Giorda, R., Morandi, F., Sirgiovanni, I., Pozzoli, U., Mosca, F., Borgatti, R., & Montirosso, R. (2017). Maternal sensitivity buffers the association between SLC6A4 methylation and socio-emotional stress response in 3-mont-old full term, but not very preterm infants. *Frontiers in Psychiatry, 8*, 171. https://doi.org/10.3389/fpsyt.2017.00171

Provenzi, L., Guida, E., & Montirosso, R. (2018). Preterm behavioral epigenetics: A systematic review. *Neuroscience & Biobehavioral Reviews, 84*, 262–271. https://doi.org/10.1016/j.neubiorev.2017.08.020

Reynolds, L. C., Duncan, M. M., Smith, G. C., Mathur, A., Neil, J., Inder, T., & Pineda, R. G. (2013). Parental presence and holding in the neonatal intensive care unit and associations with early neurobehavior. *Journal of Perinatology, 33*(8), 636–641. https://doi.org/10.1038/jp.2013.4

Risnes, K. R., Pape, K., Bjorngaard, J. H., Moster, D., Bracken, M. B., & Romundstad, P. R. (2016). Premature adult death in individuals born preterm: A sibling comparison in a prospective nation-wide follow-up study. *PLoS One*, *11*(11), e0165051. https://doi.org/10.1371/journal.pone.0165051

Rosa, M. J., Lee, A., & Wright, R. J. (2018). Evidence establishing a link between prenatal and early life stress and asthma development. *Current Opinions in Allergy and Clinical Immunology*, *18*(2), 148–158. https://doi.org/10.1097/ACI.0000000000000421

Sanders, M. R., & Hall, S. L. (2018). Trauma-informed care in the newborn intensive care unit: Promoting safety, security and connectedness. *Journal of Perinatology*, *38*, 3–10. https://doi.org/10.1038/jp.2017.124

Scatliffe, N., Casavant, S., Vittner, D., & Cong, X. (2019). Oxytocin and early parent–infant interactions: A systematic review. *International Journal of Nursing Studies*, *6*(4), 445–453. https://doi.org/10.1016/j.ijnss.2019.09.009

Sikka, R., Morath, J. M., & Leape, L. (2015). The Quadruple Aim: Care, health, cost and meaning in work. *BMJ Quality and Safety*, *24*(10), 608–610. https://doi.org/10.1136/bmjqs-2015-004160

Simeoni, U., Armengaud, J.-B., Sideek, B., & Tolsa, J.-F. (2018). Perinatal origins of adult disease. *Neonatology*, *113*, 393–399. https://doi.org/10.1159/000487618

Stuebe, A. M., Jegier, B. J., Schwarz, E. B., Green, B. D., Reinhold, A. G., Colaizy, T. T., Bogen, D. L., Schaafer, A. J., Jegier, J. T., Green, N. S., & Bartick, M. C. (2017). An online calculator to estimate the impact of changes in breastfeeding rates on population health and costs. *Breastfeeding Medicine*, *12*(10), 645–658. https://doi.org/10.1089/bfm.2017.0083

Tikkanen, R., & Abrams, M. K. (2020, January 30). *U.S. health care from a global perspective, 2019: Higher spending, worse outcomes?* https://www.commonwealthfund.org/publications/issue-briefs/2020/jan/us-health-care-global-perspective-2019

Weber, A., & Harrison, T. M. (2019). Reducing toxic stress in the NICU to improve infant outcomes. *Nursing Outlook*, *67*(2), 169–189. https://doi.org/10.1016/j.outlook.2018.11.002

Weber, A. M., Harrison, T. M., & Steward, D. K. (2018). Expanding regulation theory with oxytocin: A psychoneurobiological model for infant development. *Nursing Research*, *67*(2), 133–145. https://doi.org/10.1097/NNR.0000000000000261

Section II

The Science and the Soul of Trauma-Informed Care in the NICU

4

The Science

Anyone who thinks science is trying to make human life easier or more pleasant is utterly mistaken.
—Albert Einstein

The more we learn, the more we realize how much more there is to know. As the science that underpins early-life adversity and adverse childhood experiences grows, it becomes increasingly obvious that the current paradigm in neonatal intensive care must change. If we are indeed to "do no harm," healthcare professionals, educators, and society at large must address the widespread nature of infant medical trauma and its implications for public health.

Understanding the biological processes associated with early-life adversity is a first step in changing the paradigm. Agorastos et al. (2019) present the top 10 neurobiological allostatic pathways associated with adverse early-life experiences and the subsequent sequelae. Adverse early-life experiences lead to disruptions, dysregulation, and perturbations of the developing human during critical and sensitive periods of development. Individual vulnerabilities such as genetic background, fetal programming, timing, duration, and intensity of the stressor, coupled with varied coping strategies and social supports all have implications for the long-term biopsychological effects of early-life adversity, medical, and childhood trauma on infants and families (Exhibit 4.1; Agorastos et al., 2019).

Relevant for humanity at large, this conceptual model (Exhibit 4.1) transcends the clinical setting. Families and professionals alike are subject to the neurobiological pathways highlighted in the work of Agorastos et al. (2019). Fragmented, unpredictable patterns of maternal care, aberrant rhythms of early-life sensory input, and other social determinants of health (Figure 4.1) influence the developmental trajectory and maturation of cognitive and emotional brain circuits (Blaze et al., 2015; Chen & Baram, 2016; Glynn & Baram, 2019; Weber et al., 2018). Addressing this global problem requires courage, compassion, commitment, and equipoise. Section II presents the science and soul of caring for hospitalized infants and families in crisis.

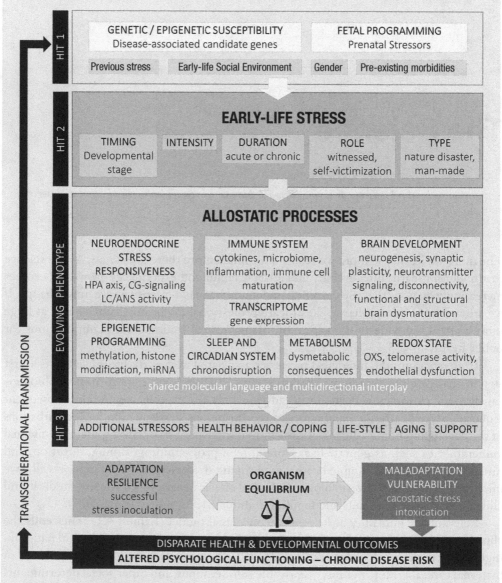

EXHIBIT 4.1 CONCEPTUAL MODEL OF DEVELOPMENTAL TRAJECTORIES OF EARLY-LIFE STRESS

CG, chorionic gonadotropin; HPA, hypothalamic–pituitary–adrenal; LC/ANS, locus ceruleus/autonomic nervous system; OXS, oxidative stress.

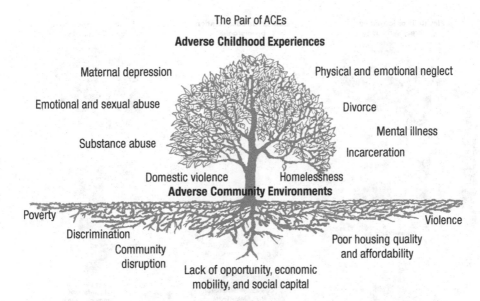

The Pair of ACEs

Adverse Childhood Experiences

Maternal depression

Physical and emotional neglect

Emotional and sexual abuse

Divorce

Mental illness

Substance abuse

Incarceration

Domestic violence   Homelessness
Adverse Community Environments

Poverty

Violence

Discrimination
Community
disruption

Poor housing quality
and affordability

Lack of opportunity, economic
mobility, and social capital

Figure 4.1 The pair of ACES: Adverse childhood experiences and adverse community events.

Source: With permission from Building Resilient Communities Collaborative and Networks.

THE NEUROENDOCRINE–IMMUNE NETWORK

Efforts to better understand the mechanisms underlying the link between early-life adversity and adult morbidity recognizes this relationship is nonlinear, complex, and interconnected across several biologic systems (Nusslock & Miller, 2016). Neuroprotective care for hospitalized infants isn't just about the brain as an isolated entity but involves everything that impacts the brain. Experiences that elicit a stress response or an immune response have significant implications for the developing brain, particularly during critical and sensitive periods of development.

Research suggests early-life adversity amplifies bidirectional communication between peripheral inflammation and neural circuitry responsible for the threat and reward system, as well as executive control (Nusslock & Miller, 2016). These adverse experiences sensitize the cortico-amygdala region in the brain responsible for threat detection and response, as well as systemic immune cells responsible for the propagation of inflammation (Figure 4.2). In the setting of chronic perceived threat during early life, low-grade inflammation, both centrally and peripherally, is established as an adaptive strategy to enhance threat vigilance (Nusslock & Miler, 2016). Unfortunately, this adaptation becomes maladaptive and even destructive over time.

Activation of the stress response system, mediated by both the hypothalamic–pituitary–adrenal (HPA) axis and the sympathetic nervous system (SNS), elicits a neuroendocrine and acute inflammatory response. Systemic immune activation increases microglial reactivity in the brain, promoting phagocytosis and the production of pro-inflammatory mediators

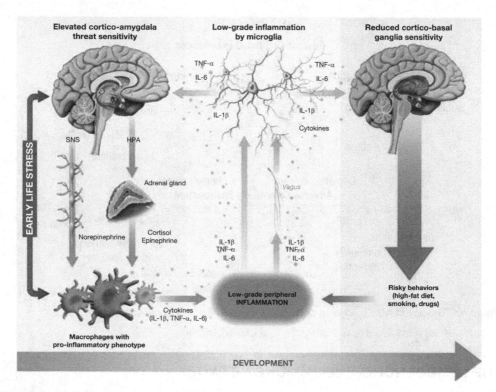

Figure 4.2 Depiction of neuroimmune-network hypothesis.

Illustration by Chi-Chun Liu and Qingyang Chen.
HPA, hypothalamic–pituitary–adrenal; IL, interleukin; SNS, sympathetic nervous system; TNF, tumor necrosis factor.
Source: Nusslock, R., & Miller, G. E. (2016). Early-life adversity and physical and emotional health across the lifespan: A neuro-immune network hypothesis. *Biological Psychiatry, 80*(1), 23–32. doi: 10.1016/j.biopsych.2015.05.017 Reprinted with permission from Elsevier.

that can damage developing brain structures (Danese & Lewis, 2017). Specific regions of the developing brain that are particularly vulnerable to stress include the limbic structures responsible for memory, learning, and emotion regulation, as well as the prefrontal cortex, critical for executive functioning and higher cognition (Berens et al., 2017).

A recent study comparing the cerebrospinal fluid (CSF) of preterm infants with full-term infants revealed a higher profile of inflammatory markers in the CSF of the preterm infant cohort (Boardman et al., 2018). Immune dysregulation undermines the developmental maturation of oligodendrocytes, the myelin-producing glial cells in the central nervous system. The subsequent hypomyelination increases susceptibility of the developing brain to white matter injury (Boardman et al., 2018). Accumulating evidence highlights aberrant connectivity within functional brain networks and white matter tracts that underlies neurodevelopmental impairment frequently associated with the preterm infant population (Rogers et al., 2018).

Chronic activation of the HPA axis induces HPA dysregulation and can lead to oxidative stress and cytotoxicity. Chronic elevation of inflammatory mediators, as a consequence of ongoing stress, contributes to low-level immunosuppression and perturbations to the infant's microbiome and gut microbiota increasing susceptibility to confounding disease, injury, and compromised neurodevelopmental outcomes (Berens et al. 2017; Cong et al., 2015). Hebb's Law (1949)—"neurons that fire together, wire together"—is the backdrop for the self-perpetuating cycle that evolves from a chronically activated neuroendocrine-immune (NEI) network (Figure 4.2). With a lowered stress threshold as a result of chronic perceived threat, cross-sensitization between the SNS and the HPA axis amplifies ongoing subclinical inflammation creating a positive-feedback loop through the neuro-immune network (Nusslock & Miller, 2016; Figure 4.2).

Understanding the physiology of the NEI network opens the door for innovative preventive strategies to mitigate the experience of toxic stress in the NICU and beyond. Admission to the NICU is stressful and traumatic in and of itself. The cascade of events associated with activation of the stress response system are superimposed onto the infant's existing medical and/or surgical condition. Neuroplasticity is the ability of the brain to reorganize and adjust through various neural processes (such as synaptogenesis, pruning, and myelination) in response to environmental conditions, genetic influences, and experiences. Although we have often looked upon neuroplasticity as an oasis of hope, plasticity is a double-edged sword. The brain can adapt to either positive or negative stimuli; what may be adaptive in the short term may actually become maladaptive over time (Johnson et al., 2013; Montirosso & Provenzi, 2015).

EPIGENETICS AND EARLY-LIFE ADVERSITY

Epigenetics is the science of chemical modifications to gene expression without altering the genetic code or the DNA. The epigenome acts as an interface between the DNA and the environment, which includes the experiences of the individual, and confers variation and uniqueness based on this dynamic interplay (Montirosso & Provenzi, 2015; Sweatt & Tamminga, 2016). Think of the genes as the hardware of the computer and the epigenetics as the software; epigenetic mechanisms control how the gene is expressed (Lester et al., 2016). Regulatory mechanisms for epigenetic transcription include histone tail modification, DNA methylation, and noncoding RNA molecules (microRNAs; Montirosso & Provenzi, 2015; Sweatt & Tamminga, 2016). For more information on epigenetics, see the Reader Resources at the end of this chapter.

DNA methylation (Figure 4.3) is the most studied epigenetic mechanism and involves the transfer of a methyl group at specific cytosine–phosphate–guanine sites in transcriptional relevant regions of the DNA strand (Everson et al., 2019; Montirosso et al., 2016; Moore et al., 2013). DNA methylation is a major epigenetic factor influencing gene activities and is essential for regulating tissue-specific gene expression (Moore et al., 2013). Multiple studies have shown a link between DNA methylation and early-life stress (Lux, 2018; Provenzi et al., 2015). Early-life stress activates the HPA axis and initiates epigenetic modifications of stress-related and stressor specific sensory networks (Lux, 2018).

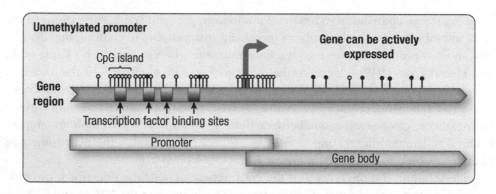

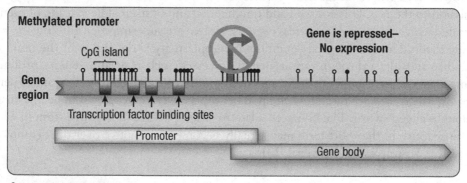

⎧ = Unmethylated CpG site
⎧ = Methylated CpG site

Figure 4.3 Role of promoter region DNA methylation on gene expression. Upper panel depicts a gene promoter with unmethylated CpG dinucleotides (*open circles*), allowing access to transcription binding sites and the opportunity for gene expression. Lower panel depicts methylated CpG dinucleotides (*filled circles*), which would block transcription factor binding and thus repress gene expression.

CpG, cytosine–phosphate–guanine.
Source: Lester, B. M., Conradt, E., & Marsit, C. (2016). Introduction to the special section on epigenetics. *Child Development*, *87*(1), 29–37. doi: 10.1111/cdev.12489 Reprinted with permission from John Wiley and Sons.

NICU-related stress has been connected to epigenetic modifications in preterm infants (Provenzi & Montirosso, 2015). Fumagalli et al. (2018) conducted a longitudinal study on a cohort of very preterm infants cared for in the NICU to assess the effects of NICU-related stress on methylation of the serotonin transporter gene *SLC6A4*. The study revealed a clear association between NICU-related stress and methylation of this serotonin transporter gene. In addition, infants with higher levels of *SLC6A4* methylation at discharge also had reduced brain volumes in their anterior temporal lobes at hospital discharge (Fumagalli et al., 2018). At 12-months corrected age, these infants demonstrated suboptimal performance on the Personal–Social scale of the Griffith Mental Development Scales (Fumagalli et al., 2018). The authors concluded that adverse experiences in the NICU influence epigenetic modifications that contribute to long-lasting programming of the socio-emotional development of very preterm infants (Fumagalli et al., 2018).

Serotonin is a neurotransmitter that is associated with feelings of well-being and happiness (along with other more complex functions). The *SLC6A4* gene encodes for a protein that is integral in the transmission of serotonin from the synaptic space into presynaptic neurons (Sosnowski et al., 2017). Decreased production of serotonin by methylation of the *SLC6A4* gene has been implicated in alterations of the serotonergic modulation of the HPA axis and neuropsychiatric disorders (Sosnowski et al., 2017). For more information on serotonin see the Reader Resources at the end of this chapter.

Provenzi et al. (2019) followed a cohort of very preterm and full-term infants over a period of 6 years. Blood samples were collected to assess *SLC6A4* methylation at birth and then again at discharge in the preterm cohort (Provenzi et al., 2019). At age 4.5 years, the emotional regulation of both groups was assessed. Controlling for adverse experiences between the period of discharge to age 4.5 years, the researchers concluded that *SLC6A4* methylation, as a consequence of NICU pain-related stress, contributed to long-lasting programming of anger regulation in preterm children (Provenzi et al., 2019).

Epigenetic regulation and modification underlies developmental programming of socio-emotional health and stress adaptation leading to an increased risk for mental illness and adult-onset disease (Lester et al. 2015; Montirosso & Provenzi, 2015). In addition to NICU-related stress, research now confirms that prenatal maternal psychosocial stress influences fetal HPA axis physiology via epigenetic pathways (Palma-Gudiel et al., 2015; Sosnowski et al., 2018). The epigenetic pathway is a hypermethylation of *NR3C1*, the gene that encodes glucocorticoid receptors to bind with glucocorticoid (Sosnowski et al., 2018). This increased methylation alters gene expression thereby limiting the individual's capacity to adapt to stress (Lester et al., 2015; Lux, 2018; Mulligan et al., 2012; Sosnowski et al. 2018). Similar to findings related to methylation of SLC6A4, higher mean DNA methylation of NR3C1 was significantly associated with compromised social-emotional development at 6 and 18 months of age (Folger et al. 2019).

Psychosocial factors and experiences early in life influence an infant's developmental trajectory through epigenetic changes that impact a wide range of psychobiological functions and phenotypic developmental outcomes (Provenzi et al., 2018). Understanding epigenetic vulnerability of the hospitalized infant to psychosocial adversity opens up new ways of interacting, supporting and protecting the hospitalized infant and family. The goal of behavioral epigenetics is to provide clinicians with a better understanding of the biological mechanisms underlying environmental exposures, both adverse and protective, to inform clinical practice and early interventions for at-risk infants and children (Provenzi et al., 2018).

THE ENERGY COSTS OF TRAUMATIC STRESS IN THE NICU

Every biological action, interaction, response, and function requires energy derived from mitochondria at the cellular level—without energy, there is no life (Picard et al. 2018).

Mitochondria play a key role in metabolic homeostasis due to their central role in energy production; but they also have a prominent role in apoptosis, control of calcium ion levels, steroid synthesis, heme synthesis, innate immune response, and metabolic cell signaling (Shaughnessy et al., 2014). Stress adaptation is dependent upon mitochondrial integrity to supply energy at the molecular, epigenetic, cellular, subcellular, and systemic levels to support and sustain a stress response. Essentially, mitochondria provide both the energy and subcellular signaling necessary to enable and direct stress adaptation (Picard et al. 2018).

The mitochondrion is the only subcellular organelle that has its own genome that encodes proteins essential for electron flow through the respiratory chain (also called the electron transport chain; Picard et al., 2018). This respiratory chain consumes oxygen channeling high-energy molecules through a series of reactions to create energy. The stored energy powers various mitochondrial functions that support growth, healing, and other complex processes to facilitate adaptation of the individual to their environment (Picard et al., 2018).

The stress response, or allostasis, requires energy to enable adaptation. Mitochondria sustain life and enable stress adaptation (Figure 4.4). In Figure 4.4, (A) depicts how, powered by solar energy, plants produce oxygen and food substrates (carbohydrates, lipids), which are used within mitochondria to power oxidative phosphorylation and adenosine triphosphate (ATP) synthesis. In this process, mitochondria release carbon dioxide and water, the substrates required by plants, thus sustaining the cycle of life. Part B shows how stressors interact with information contained within the organism, such as genetically encoded biological data, memories of past events, and the current psycho/physiological state reflected by molecular, neuroendocrine, immune, and metabolic factors. Together, these generate unique adaptive stress responses and behaviors. Without energy, stressors

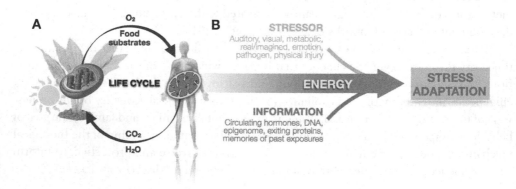

Figure 4.4 Mitochondria and stress adaptation.

Source: Picard, M., McEwen, B. S., Epel, E. S., & Sandi, C. (2018). An energetic view of stress: Focus on mitochondria. *Frontiers in Neuroendocrinology, 49*, 72–85. doi: 10.1016/j.yfrne.2018.01.001 Reprinted with permission from Elsevier.

would have no effect on the organism. But in the presence of heat and chemical energy, stressors and information interact in meaningful ways to enable stress adaptation. (Picard et al., 2018).

In living organisms, energy is present as heat and as chemical energy in the form of ATP and other chemical intermediates. Chemical reactions from ATP synthesis are responsible for thermoregulation in newborns and a whole host of other critical functions, including the stress response (Picard et al., 2018). Allostasis involves widespread energy-demanding physiological changes that range from basic maintenance of vital functions, to dealing with routine daily stressors, all the way to permanently adapting to chronic stress—all these energy demands are largely met by the work of the mitochondria (Picard et al., 2018). Acute and chronic stressors, including psychological stress, influence mitochondrial integrity and chronic stress can lead to maladaptive mitochondrial changes or mitochondrial allostatic load (MAL; Figure 4.5; Picard & McEwen, 2018).

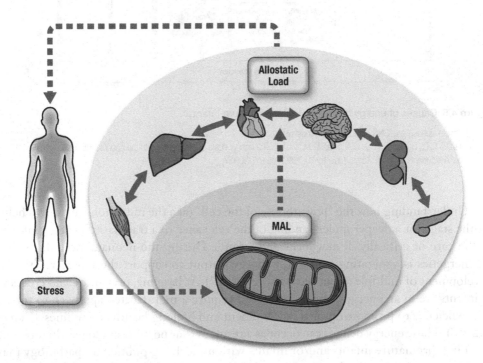

Figure 4.5 Model of mitochondrial allostatic load as a source of systemic allostatic load. *MAL* is defined as the dysregulation of mitochondrial functions resulting from the structural and functional changes that mitochondria undergo in response to stressors.

MAL, mitochondrial allostatic load.

Source: Picard, M., & McEwen, B. S. (2018). Psychological stress and mitochondria: A conceptual framework. *Psychosomatic Medicine*, *80*(2), 126–140. doi: 10.1097/PSY.0000000000000544 Reprinted with permission from Wolters Kluwer Health, Inc.

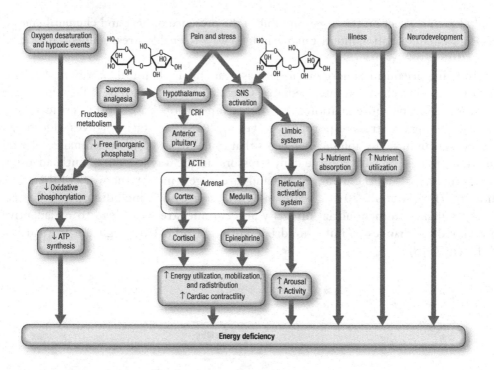

Figure 4.6 Causes of energy deficiency in the premature infant.

ATP, adenosine triphosphate; SNS, sympathetic nervous system.
Source: Tan, J. B. C., Boskovic, D. S., & Angeles, D. M. (2018). The energy costs of prematurity and the neonatal intensive care unit (NICU) experience. *Antioxidants, 7*(3), 37. https://doi.org/10.3390/antiox7030037

Understanding how the "powerhouse of the cell" (aka the mitochondria) works helps set the stage for a deeper understanding of the relevance of a trauma-informed approach to the care of critically ill newborns and infants. During the neonatal period, cellular bioenergetics is generating its highest energy output to support the rapid growth and development of multiple organ systems (Ten, 2017). At baseline, premature and critically ill infants are in an energy-deficient state and require a multifaceted approach to rectify this deficiency to promote optimal development and lifelong health and wellness (Tan et al. 2018). These energy deficits can occur as a result of four possible etiologies (Figure 4.6).

First, premature infants and/or infants with underlying pulmonary pathology may experience frequent episodes of apnea and/or oxygen desaturation, which compromises energy production at the mitochondrial level. Reduced tissue oxygenation decreases oxidative phosphorylation by aerobic respiration thereby reducing ATP synthesis (Tan et al., 2018). Oxygen desaturation and hypoxic events impose an allostatic load on the mitochondria impeding its ability to respond to the demand and, as you can see in Figure 4.6, impacts systemic allostatic load and overload (Picard & McEwen, 2018). This process escalates physiologic energy demands, underscored by any psychological

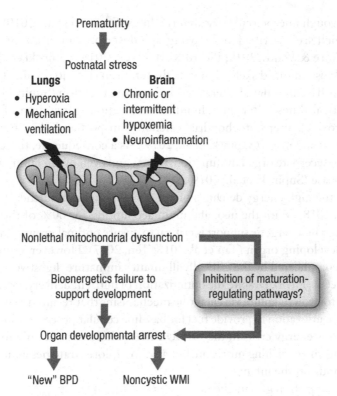

Figure 4.7 Hypothetical mitochondria-driven mechanisms for postnatal developmental failure of lungs and cerebral white matter in premature infants.

BPD, bronchopulmonary dysplasia; WMI, white matter injury.
Source: Ten, V. S. (2017). Mitochondrial dysfunction in alveolar and white matter developmental failure in premature infants. *Pediatric Research, 81*(2), 286–292. doi: 10.1038/pr.2016.216 Reprinted with permission from Springer Nature.

stress the infant may be experiencing, and can initiate a pathologic inflammatory or oxidative stress-induced cascade, both of which lead to poor outcomes (Di Fiore & Vento, 2019; Picard & McEwen, 2018).

Second, stressful stimuli and painful procedures reduce energy stores through ATP degradation as a consequence of the infant's behavioral and physiologic responses to pain (i.e., crying, grimacing, flailing, tachycardia; Tan et al., 2018). These behavioral and physiologic responses of the infant to stress and pain burn calories that may have been used for growth, healing, and development. The negative impact of stress on the developing infant cannot be overstated. Sublethal, exogenous stress arrests organ maturation via mitochondrial dysfunction (Ten, 2017). The pathway for mitochondrial dysfunction is similar and exemplified in Figure 4.7.

Third, critical illness alters metabolic function by decreasing the rate of absorption and utilization of nutrients while increasing metabolic demand through the activation and release of pro-inflammatory cytokines which further deplete energy stores (Tan et al., 2018). Other mitochondrially mediated (or energy mediated) critical care disease processes include sepsis through microcirculatory abnormalities (Supinski et al., 2019), lung disease (examples of which are described in the paragraph describing intermittent hypoxia and Figure 4.7; Di Fiore & Vento, 2019; Picard & McEwen, 2018; Supinski et al., 2019; Ten, 2017), critical illness-induced skeletal muscle dysfunction (Dassios et al., 2018; Supinski et al., 2019), as well as modulated alterations in immune function (Supinski et al., 2019). Disease and critical illness alter mitochondrial respiration, generation of free radicals (including superoxide), alter mitochondrial calcium transport and concentrations, affect apoptotic pathways and more (Supinski et al., 2019). As a consequence, these pathophysiologic processes exacerbate organ dysfunction, injury, and even organ failure in the setting of illness and disease (Supinski et al., 2019).

And, finally, the high energy demands of the developing brain further deplete energy stores (Tan et al. 2018). With the neonatal brain accounting for 60% of the infant's total metabolism, proper bioenergetic support is critical to ensure optimal growth and maturation of this actively developing organ (Tan et al. 2018; Ten, 2017). However, ensuring optimal energy stores is complicated by the critically ill infant's immature digestive and absorptive capabilities (Tan et al., 2018). Despite the optimization of nutrient delivery, many critically ill infants succumb to growth failure via catabolic mechanisms that result in tissue breakdown and energy storage utilization to provide fuel for baseline cellular processes (Tan et al., 2018).

Addressing this energy crisis in the NICU invites clinicians not only to explore new ways of enhancing and enriching nutrition, but also to explore strategies aimed at reducing the energy demands on the infant.

Energy-reducing strategies include:

- Skin-to-skin care,
- Responsive caregiving,
- Reducing and eliminating the experience of maternal separation,
- Protecting sleep,
- Ensuring optimal postural support,
- Facilitating breastfeeding and infant-driven eating experiences,
- Maintaining an environment that is nurturing and conducive to healing, rest, and recovery for hospitalized infants.

With regard to the nonpharmacologic management of procedural pain, caution is warranted with the use of oral sucrose. In two randomized controlled studies examining the effects of sucrose on pain and biochemical markers of ATP degradation, the researchers discovered a significant increase in ATP utilization and oxidative stress in preterm infants treated with sucrose (Angeles et al., 2015; Asmerom et al., 2013). Additional research is needed, and the prudent use of sucrose is indicated to minimize any potential adverse sequalae. Stevens et al. (2018) demonstrated that 0.1 mL of a 24% sucrose solution is the minimally effective dose to treat pain associated with a single heel lance in infants ranging between 24 and 42 weeks' gestational age.

SUMMARY

The structural regions of the brain and body that grow the fastest are the most metabolically active and most susceptible to the negative effects of early-life adversity (Hodel, 2018; Tan et al. 2018). Early-life adversity, mediated by toxic, traumatic stress, activates central, peripheral, cellular, and epigenetic processes in an effort to adapt to the stressor. These adaptations may become maladaptive over time, derailing healthy development and increasing the individual's risk for physiologic and psychologic pathology.

The HPA axis is functionally responsive to stress signals as early as 22 weeks' gestation (Howland et al., 2017). Chronic stress induces derangements in the NEI network, influences epigenetic modifications that undermine socioemotional development, and escalates energy demands on the critically ill infant that result in MAL and overload. These biological processes exacerbate pathophysiologic processes and contribute to infant morbidity and mortality.

The most potent activator of the stress response system in infants is maternal separation (Doom & Gunner, 2013). Parents are the most potent regulators of HPA axis reactivity. Understanding the dynamic interplay between these biological processes is critical for the delivery of safe, quality care (Koss & Gunner, 2018).

READER RESOURCES

Epigenetics

Epigenetics: Nature vs. nurture: www.youtube.com/watch?v=k50yMwEOWGU

Epigenetics 2—DNA methylation and bisulfite sequencing: www.youtube.com/watch?v=5NEoqa-k3xM

Garvan Institute. *Epigenetics basics:* www.youtube.com/watch?v=hgYMgNrr7mQ

Serotonin

2-minute neuroscience: Serotonin: www.youtube.com/watch?v=Xkl_x6wC0Lg

REFERENCES

Agorastos, A., Pervanidou, P., Chrousos, G. P., & Baker, D. G. (2019). Developmental trajectories of early life stress and trauma: A narrative review on neurobiological aspects beyond stress system dysregulation. *Frontiers in Psychiatry, 10*(118), 1–25. https://doi.org/10.3389/fpsyt.2019.00118

Angeles, D. M., Asmerom, Y., Boskovic, D. S., Slater, L., Bacot-Carter, S., Bahjri, K., Mukasa, J., Holden, M., & Fayard, E. (2015). Oral sucrose for heel lance enhances adenosine triphosphate use in preterm neonates with respiratory distress. *SAGE Open Medicine, 3*, 2050312115611431. https://doi.org/10.1177/2050312115611431

Asmerom, Y., Slater, L., Boskovic, D. S., Bahjri, K., Holden, M. S., Phillips, R., Deming, D., Ash-wal, S., Fayard, E., & Angeles, D. M. (2013). Oral sucrose for heel lance increases adenosine triphosphate use and oxidative stress in preterm neonates. *Journal of Pediatrics*, *163*(1), 29–35. https://doi.org/10.1016/j.jpeds.2012.12.088

Berens, A. E., Jensen, S. K. G., & Nelson, C. A., III (2017). Biological embedding of childhood adversity: From physiological mechanisms to clinical implications. *BMC Medicine*, *15*(1), 135. https://doi.org/10.1186/s12916-017-0895-4

Blaze, J., Asok, A., & Roth, T. L. (2015). The long-term impact of adverse caregiving environments on epigenetic modifications and telomeres. *Frontiers in Behavioral Neuroscience*, *9*(79), 1–12. https://doi.org/10.3389/fnbeh.2015.00079

Boardman, J. P., Ireland, G., Sullivan, G., Patky, R., Fleiss, B., Gressens, P., & Miron, V. (2018). The cerebrospinal fluid inflammatory response to preterm birth. *Frontiers in Physiology*, *9*, 1299. https://doi.org/10.3389/fphys.2018.01299

Chen, Y., & Baram, T. Z. (2016). Toward understanding how early-life stress reprograms cognitive and emotional brain networks. *Neuropsychopharmacology*, *41*(1), 197–206. https://doi.org/10.1038/npp.2015.181

Cong, X., Henderson, W. A., Graf, J., & McGrath, J. M. (2015). Early life experience and gut micro-biome: The brain-gut-microbiota signaling system. *Advances in Neonatal Care*, *15*(5), 314–323. https://doi.org/10.1097/ANC.0000000000000191

Danese, A., & Lewis, S. J. (2017). Psychoneuroimmunology of early-life stress: The hidden wounds of childhood trauma? *Neuropsychopharmacology Reviews*, *42*, 99–114. https://doi.org/10.1038/npp.2016.198

Dassios, T., Kaltsogianni, O., Krokidis, M., Hickey, A., & Greenough, A. (2018). Deltoid muscle morphometry as an index of impaired skeletal muscularity in neonatal intensive care. *European Journal of Pediatrics*, *177*(4), 507–512. https://doi.org/10.1007/s00431-018-3090-5

Di Fiore, J. M., & Vento, M. (2019). Intermittent hypoxemia and oxidative stress in preterm infants. *Respiratory Physiology & Neurobiology*, *266*, 121–129. https://doi.org/10.1016/j.resp.2019.05.006

Doom, J. R., & Gunner, M. R. (2013). Stress physiology and developmental psychopathology: Past, present and future. *Developmental Psychopathology*, *25*(4 Pt. 2), 1359–1373. https://doi.org/10.1017/S0954579413000667

Everson, T. M., Marsit, C. J., O'Shea, M., Burt, A., Hermetz, K., Carter, B. S., Helderman, J., Hofheimer, J. A., McGowan, E. C., Neal, C. R., Pastyrnak, S. L., Smith, L. M., Soliman, A., DellaGrotta, S. A., Dansereau, L. M., Padbury, J. F., & Lester, B. M. (2019). Epigenome-wide analysis identifies genes and pathways linked to neurobehavioral variation in preterm infants. *Scientific Reports*, *9*(1), 6322. https://doi.org/10.1038/s41598-019-42654-4

Folger, A. T., Ding, L., Ji, H., Yolton, K., Ammerman, R. T., Van Ginkel, J. B., & Bowers, K. (2019). Neonatal NR3C1 methylation and social-emotional development at 6 and 18 months of age. *Frontiers in Behavioral Neuroscience*, *13*, 14. https://doi.org/10.3389/fnbeh.2019.00014

Fumagalli, M., Provenzi, L., De Carli, P., Dessimone, F., Sirgiovanni, I., Giorda, R., Cinnante, C., Squarcina, L., Pozzoli, U., Triulzi, F., Brambilla, P., Borgatti, R., Mosca, F., & Montirosso, R. (2018). From early stress to 12-month development in very preterm infants: Preliminary findings on epigenetic mechanisms and brain growth. *PLoS One*, *13*(1), e0190602. https://doi.org/10.1371/journal.pone.0190602

Glynn, L. M., & Baram, T. Z. (2019). The influence of unpredictable, fragmented parental signals on the developing brain. *Frontiers in Neuroendocrinology*, *53*, 100736. https://doi.org/10.1016/j.yfrne.2019.01.002

Hebb, D. O. (1949). *The organization of behavior*. Wiley & Sons.

Hodel, A. S. (2018). Rapid infant prefrontal cortex development and sensitivity to early environmental experience. *Developmental Review, 48*, 113–144. https://doi.org/10.1016/j.dr.2018.02.003

Howland, M. A., Sandman, C. A., & Glynn, L. M. (2017). Developmental origins of the human hypothalamic–pituitary–adrenal axis. *Expert Review of Endocrinology & Metabolism, 12*(5), 321–339. https://doi.org/10.1080/17446651.2017.1356222

Johnson, S. B., Riley, A. W., Granger, D. A., & Riis, J. (2013). The science of early toxic stress for pediatric practice and advocacy. *Pediatrics, 131*(2), 319–327. https://doi.org/10.1542/peds.2012-0469

Koss, K. J., & Gunnar, M. R. (2018). Annual research review: Early adversity, the HPA axis, and child psychopathology. *Journal of Child Psychology & Psychiatry, 59*(4), 327–346. https://doi.org/10.1111/jcpp.12784

Lester, B. M., Conradt, E., & Marsit, C. (2016). Introduction to the special section on epigenetics. *Child Development, 87*(1), 29–37. https://doi.org/10.1111/cdev.12489

Lester, B. M., Marsit, C. J., Giarraputo, J., Hawes, K., LaGasse, L. L., & Padbury, J. F. (2015). Neurobehavior related to epigenetic differences in preterm infants. *Epigenomics, 7*(7), 1123–1136. https://doi.org/10.2217/epi.15.63

Lux, V. (2018). Epigenetic programming effects of early life stress: A dual-activation hypothesis. *Current Genomics, 19*(8), 638–652. https://doi.org/10.2174/1389202919666180307151358

Montirosso, R., & Provenzi, L. (2015). Implications of epigenetics and stress regulation on research and developmental care of preterm infants. *Journal of Obstetric, Gynecologic & Neonatal Nursing, 44*(2), 174–182. https://doi.org/10.1111/1552-6909.12559

Montirosso, R., Provenzi, L., Giorda, R., Fumagalli, M., Morandi, F., Sirgiovanni, I., Pozzoli, U., Grunau, R., Oberlander, T. F., Mosca, F., & Borgatti, R. (2016). SLC6A4 promoter region methylation and socio-emotional stress response in very preterm and full-term infants. *Epigenomics, 8*(7), 895–907. https://doi.org/10.2217/epi-2016-0010

Moore, L. D., Thuc, L., & Fan, G. (2013). DNA methylation and its basic function. *Neuropsychopharmacology, 38*(1), 23–38. https://doi.org/10.1038/npp.2012.112

Mulligan, C. J., D'Errico, N. C., Stees, J., & Hughes, D. A. (2012). Methylation changes in NR3C1 in newborns associated with maternal prenatal stress exposure and newborn birth weight. *Epigenetics, 7*(8), 853–857. https://doi.org/10.4161/epi.21180

Nusslock, R., & Miller, G. E. (2016). Early-life adversity and physical and emotional health across the lifespan: A neuro-immune network hypothesis. *Biological Psychiatry, 80*(1), 23–32. https://doi.org/10.1016/j.biopsych.2015.05.017

Palma-Guidiel, H., Cordova-Palomera, A., Eixarch, E., Deaschle, M., & Fananas, L. (2015). Maternal psychosocial stress during pregnancy alters the epigenetic signature of the glucocorticoid receptor gene promoter in their offspring: A meta-analysis. *Epigenetics, 10*(10), 893–902. https://doi.org/10.1080/15592294.2015.1088630

Picard, M., & McEwen, B. S. (2018). Psychological stress and mitochondria: A conceptual framework. *Psychosomatic Medicine, 80*(2), 126–140. https://doi.org/10.1097/PSY.0000000000000544

Picard, M., McEwen, B. S., Epel, E. S., & Sandi, C. (2018). An energetic view of stress: Focus on mitochondria. *Frontiers in Neuroendocrinology, 49*, 72–85. https://doi.org/10.1016/j.yfrne.2018.01.001

Provenzi, L., Brambilla, M., Borgatti, R., & Montirosso, R. (2018). Methodological challenges in developmental human behavioral epigenetics: Insights into study design. *Frontiers in Behavioral Neuroscience, 12*, 286. https://doi.org/10.3389/fnbeh.2018.00286

Provenzi, L., Fumagalli, M., Scotto di Minico, G., Giorda, R., Morandi, F., Sirgiovanni, I., Schiavolin, P., Mosca, F., Borgatti, & Montirosso, R. (2019). Pain-related increase in serotonin transporter gene methylation associates with emotional regulation in 4.5-year-old preterm-born children. *Acta Paediatrica*, *109*, 1166–1174. https://doi.org/10.1111/apa.15077

Provenzi, L., Fumagalli, M., Sirgiovanni, I., Giorda, R., Pozzoli, U., Morandi, F., Beri, S., Menozzi, G., Mosca, F., Borgatti, R., & Montirosso, R. (2015). Pain-related stress during neonatal intensive care unit stay and SLC6A4 methylation in very preterm infants. *Frontiers in Behavioral Neuroscience*, *9*, 99. https://doi.org/10.3389/fnbeh.2015.00099

Provenzi, L., & Montirosso, R. (2015). "Epigenethics" in the neonatal intensive care unit: Conveying complexity in health care for preterm children. *JAMA Pediatrics*, *169*(7), 617–618. https://doi.org/10.1001/jamapediatrics.2015.43

Rogers, C. E., Lean, R. E., Wheelock, M. D., & Smyser, C. D. (2018). Aberrant structural and functional connectivity and neurodevelopmental impairment in preterm children. *Journal of Neurodevelopmental Disorders*, *10*(1), 1–13. https://doi.org/10.1186/s11689-018-9253-x

Shaughnessy, D. T., McAllister, K., Worth, L., Haugen, A. C., Meyer, J. N., Domann, F. E., Van Houten, B., Mostoslavsky, R., Bultman, S. J., Baccarelli, A. A., Begley, T. J., Sobol, R. W., Hirschey, M. D., Ideker, T., Santos, J. H., Copeland, W. C., Tice, R. R., Balshaw, D. M., Tyson, F. L. (2014). Mitochondria, energetics, epigenetics, and cellular responses to stress. *Environmental Health Perspectives*, *122*(12), 1271–1278. https://doi.org/10.1289/ehp.1408418

Sosnowski, D. W., Booth, C., York, T. P., Amstadter, A. B., & Kliewer, W. (2018). Maternal prenatal stress and infant DNA methylation: A systematic review. *Developmental Psychobiology*, *60*(2), 127–139. https://doi.org/10.1002/dev.21604

Stevens, B., Yamada, J., Campbell-Yeo, M., Gibbins, S., Harrison, D., Dionne, K., Taddio, A., McNair, C., Willan, A., Ballantyne, M., Widger, K. M., Sidani, S., Estabrooks, C., Synnes, A., Squires, J., Victor, C., & Riahi, S. (2018). The minimally effective does of sucrose for procedural pain relief in neonates: A randomized controlled trial. *BMC Pediatrics*, *18*, 85. https://doi.org/10.1186/s12887-018-1026-x

Supinski, G. S., Schroder, E. A., & Callahan, L. A. (2019). Mitochondria and critical illness. *Chest*, *157*, 310–322. https://doi.org/10.1016/j.chest.2019.08.2182

Sweatt, J. D., & Tamminga, C. A. (2016). An epigenomics approach to individual differences and its translation to neuropsychiatric conditions. *Dialogues in Clinical Neuroscience*, *18*(3), 289–298.

Tan, J. B. C., Boskovic, D. S., & Angeles, D. M. (2018). The energy costs of prematurity and the neonatal intensive care unit (NICU) experience. *Antioxidants*, *7*(3), 37. https://doi.org/10.3390/antiox7030037

Ten, V. S. (2017). Mitochondrial dysfunction in alveolar and white matter developmental failure in premature infants. *Pediatric Research*, *81*(2), 286–292. https://doi.org/10.1038/pr.2016.216

Weber, A., Harrison, T. M., Steward, D., & Ludington-Hoe, S. (2018). Paid family leave to enhance the health outcomes of preterm infants. *Policy, Politics & Nursing Practice*, *19*(1–2), 11–28. https://doi.org/10.1177/1527154418791821

5

The Soul

The intuitive mind is a sacred gift and the rational mind is a faithful servant. We have created a society that honors the servant and has forgotten the gift.
—Albert Einstein

What is the intuitive mind? To me, the intuitive mind involves our inner wisdom, our soul if you like, speaking to us (if we dare to listen), guiding our decisions and our actions. Our intuition, informed by our expert knowledge, has the power to heal and transcend the experience of disease. The goal of nursing is not only to promote good health, but to enable our patients, their families, and even our colleagues to flourish (Allmark, 2017).

"As a nurse, our purpose is clear. We are hand holders, healers, and heart menders" (Soloman, 2019, p. 5). Our heart-centered actions bring us to that human-to-human interface where we are invited to truly "see" the person behind the diagnosis. In "seeing" them, we embrace the true nature of nursing as healing. This shift cannot happen unless we change the language and praxis of nursing to integrate the transpersonal and spiritual dimensions of nursing work into day-to-day practice. Words have power and meaning, and the language nurses use can reduce nursing practice to a series of tasks performed on bodies efficiently and objectively (Dahlke & Hunter, 2020). Language can perpetuate a sense of powerlessness or empowerment as nurses choose to embody the full breadth of a caring-healing paradigm balancing science with soul.

THE SCIENCE OF HUMAN CARING

Take a deep renewing breath. Fall into your heart; open your heart to this now, this breath of life. Listen quietly to your silent inner voice; why are you here? Why are you in nursing?
—Watson (2018)

With over 4 million nurses in the United States alone, nursing represents a formidable voice for change in healthcare. In her recent publication *Unitary Caring Science: The Philosophy and Praxis of Nursing* (2018), Dr. Jean Watson writes, "It is incumbent upon the discipline of nursing to give credible voice to another view of science, another view of human caring, healing, [and] health as part of the sacred circle of life" (pp. xviii–xix). Watson invites nursing and healthcare professionals to invert the existing paradigm in healthcare and embrace a praxis of unitary caring science. Shifting from a focus on treatment and cure to caring and healing, from a medical–clinicalized view of humanity to reverential respect for one humanity, is a return to home for the science and art of nursing (Watson, 2018). Nursing praxis, guided by a moral imperative to serve the whole person, reminds us that the patient and all of us are greater than the sum of our parts. As nurses, we manage the human experience of disease, honoring and preserving the dignity and integrity of the whole person.

As the profession of nursing continues to evolve, we must not lose our core identity. Anchoring ourselves to clinical paradigms devoid of an understanding of our shared humanity diminishes the noble profession of nursing. If our value rests on technical prowess, documentation efficiency, or task mastery, we reduce the art and science of nursing to that of skilled technicians that can be easily subsumed under other disciplines (Watson, 2018). Nursing must mature and embrace the primacy of human caring as a serious moral, ethical, ontological, and epistemological praxis that must not be taken for granted (Watson, 2018).

By retracing the theoretical underpinnings of nursing, from Nightingale to Newman, from Rogers to Watson and so many more, we embrace a whole-person unitary transformative worldview of nursing and operationalize this holistic view in our everyday caring encounters. Newman's theory of health as expanding consciousness becomes tangible through the adoption of caring partnerships and establishing these partnerships as critical nursing interventions. This approach to care enables the nurse to identify and empathize with the patient, thereby helping the patient and the family to find meaning in their difficult situation (Endo, 2017). When this approach to care is successfully implemented both the nurse and the family unit grow and gain higher levels of consciousness and insight through their shared care experience.

In caring for critically ill infants and their families, we help them to live wholly, to live through their disease, through the crisis, and through the trauma, not just to survive the experience but to thrive and to flourish. This aspect of caring demands we connect with unitary caring science, an evolved worldview of one humanity, one heart, and one world (Watson, 2018). And *the how* is easier than you think. The how is guided by your breath, your healing presence, as you realign with your inner wisdom and transmute the experience of care from "doing to" to "being with" the patient, the family, your colleagues.

Adopting a trauma-informed paradigm brings us closer to our higher self, our healing self, our compassionate and courageous self. Watson's 10 caritas processes (Box 5.1) are the road map used to facilitate our transformation and the transformation of the care experience.

BOX 5.1 TEN CARITAS PROCESSES

1. Practice loving-kindness to self and others.
2. Be authentically present to enable faith, hope, and the inner-subjective life world of oneself and others.
3. Foster one's own spiritual practices.
4. Develop trusting interpersonal caring relationships.
5. Forgive and show empathy to self and others.
6. Use all ways of knowing.
7. Engage in genuine teaching–learning experiences.
8. Create a caring–healing environment for all involved.
9. Value humanity.
10. Embrace the unknowns and miracles in life.

Source: Wei, H., & Watson, J. (2019). Healthcare interprofessional team members' perspectives on human caring: A directed content analysis study. *International Journal of Nursing Science*, *6*(1), 17–23. doi: 10.1016/j.ijnss.2018.12.001

Practice Loving-Kindness to Self and Others

What is the practice of loving-kindness? *Metta bhavana*, or loving-kindness, originates from the Buddhist tradition and is described as unconditional, inclusive love with wisdom. It is one of the four sublime virtues or immeasurables, which include loving-kindness as well as compassion, empathic joy, and equanimity. The definition of *loving-kindness* is tender and benevolent affection. Studies have shown practicing loving-kindness meditation preserves telomere length (a measure of aging and a biomarker of toxic stress), elicits positive emotions, and effectively treats chronic pain (Graser & Stangier, 2018; Le Nguyen et al., 2019; Shalev et al., 2013; Zeng et al., 2015), which suggests there is a fundamental benefit of loving-kindness within a healing paradigm.

The meditation practice aimed at cultivating *metta*, or benevolence, focuses on intention, an intention for happiness and well-being for self and others. It encourages us to embrace an attitude of friendliness toward what we are experiencing in any given moment, regardless of how difficult that may seem. The mantra for loving-kindness is "may I be happy, may I be well, may I be safe, may I be with ease."

In the clinical setting or during challenging situations, repeating this mantra over and over can bring a sense of calm and well-being. This mantra is also incorporated into the practice of loving-kindness meditation, which begins with blessing the self by repeating the mantra phrase over and over in a quiet and comfortable space until a sense of peace and ease is experienced. Once a sense of self-ease is achieved, the mantra is then directed toward others, "may you be happy, may you be well, may you be safe, may you be at ease."

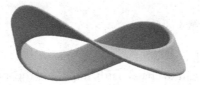

Figure 5.1 Möbius strip—a loop with only one side and only one boundary.

It may be challenging at first to find the time to practice loving-kindness meditation. I challenge you to shift your perspective. It's not about finding the time but creating the time and space to begin a loving-kindness meditation practice. Set your alarm clock 15 minutes earlier in the morning and use those 15 minutes to create your practice. As this practice becomes part of your daily life, you will experience a deepened sense of connection and compassion with yourself and with others. Resources for meditation and fostering loving-kindness are available at the end of this chapter.

Be Authentically Present

The core ingredients of authentic presence are thought to include self-awareness, courage, transparency, and confidence (Steckler et al., 2016). Miller and Cutshall (2012) define healing presence as *the condition of being consciously and compassionately in the present moment with another or with others, believing in and affirming their potential for wholeness, wherever they are in life*. Authentic presence creates a sacred, transpersonal caring moment (Norman et al., 2016). In this moment the patient and healthcare professional are truly tuned in to each other, experiencing a deep human connection (Norman et al., 2016). This oneness creates something similar to a Möbius strip (Figure 5.1), when one practices authentic presence in the caring moment, a shared interface emerges where the two become one.

Neither the developing infant nor the environment exist in isolation, but rather intersect at this shared surface. In care interactions, there are not two separate surfaces bumping against each other or two separate surfaces with an intervening "space," but a single, continuous, looped structure which is both organism and environment (M. Coughlin et al., 2009, p. 2204).

The challenge to practicing authentic presence in the clinical setting is often the culture. Healthcare cultures focused on productivity, checklists, and organizational metrics devoid of human connection undermine the provision of holistic nursing care. The nurse and clinician must ensure each and every care encounter is transformed into caring moments where authentic presence can flourish. One strategy I find very helpful is the practice of GRACE prior to any care encounter. This acronym (Figure 5.2), created by Joan Halifax PhD, a Buddhist teacher and Zen priest, was developed to help nurses stay open to the patient's experience, stay centered in the presence of suffering, and to cultivate and express compassion (Halifax, 2014). Resources for cultivating an authentic presence are available at the end of this chapter.

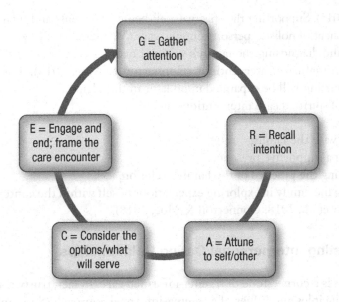

Figure 5.2 GRACE.

Source: Halifax, J. (2014). G.R.A.C.E. for nurses: Cultivating compassion in nurse/patient interactions. *Journal of Nursing Education and Practice, 4*(1), 121–128. https://doi.org/10.5430/jnep.v4n1p121

Foster Spiritual Practices

> [H]umans cannot be treated as objects, … humans cannot be separated from self, other, nature, and the larger universe. The caring–healing paradigm is located within a cosmology that is both metaphysical and transcendent with the co-evolving human in the universe. The context calls for a sense of reverence and sacredness with regard to life and all living things.
> —Watson (1997)

Spirituality is not the same as religiosity, although the two are not mutually exclusive. Spirituality is the essence of being human; it is what gives meaning and purpose to one's life, regardless of faith (Burkhardt & Nagai-Jacobson, 2016). Fostering spiritual practices for oneself enables one to be attuned to the spiritual needs of others. An individual's spirituality is expressed through interpersonal relationships, personal practices, and beliefs (Alemdar et al., 2018). Attending to the spiritual needs of mothers in the NICU significantly reduced (p <.05) maternal stress levels (Alemdar et al., 2018). Acknowledging the spiritual needs of the family in crisis is a crucial dimension of a holistic and comprehensive plan of care in the NICU.

Challenges to fostering spiritual practices include inadequate staffing, cultural differences, high workload, and a lack of education (Riahi et al., 2018). Spiritual well-being (religious or existential) and spiritual care perceptions are directly correlated with spiritual care practice

(Azarsa et al., 2015). Supporting the spiritual well-being of patients and their families is an essential component of holistic, person-centered care (Mamier et al., 2019).

Assessing and diagnosing the family's spiritual needs guides the nurse in identifying appropriate spiritual care interventions (Connerton & Moe, 2018). The construct of spirituality in nursing will be expanded upon later in this chapter.

Examples of spiritual care interventions include:

- Praying with the family,
- Offering a supportive presence,
- Facilitating the practice of the family's religion,
- Assisting the family in exploring expectations of self within the context of the crisis (Alemdar et al., 2018; Connerton & Moe, 2018).

Develop Trusting Interpersonal Caring Relationships

Trustworthiness is a cornerstone of trauma-informed care. In fact, trustworthiness is one of the stated principles and values of a trauma-informed approach (Substance Abuse and Mental Health Services Administration, 2014).

The four pillars of trust are:

- Consistency
- Communication
- Competence
- Caring

Together, these pillars convey a sense of reliability or reliance on the character, ability, and strength of an individual, a profession, and/or an organization or institution. Within the context of caring science, trusting relationships also exhibit respect, love, moral commitment, inner harmony, authentic presence, and caring consciousness (Watson, 2008). Developing trusting interpersonal caring relationships requires authenticity and loving-kindness to create a sense of safety and security that makes one feel seen in moments of vulnerability.

What does a trusting, caring interpersonal relationship look like? Acting from a place of love and compassion fosters healing for self and others. Shifting from a separatist perspective of "you and me" to "we and us" builds the rapport necessary for connection; we are in this moment together. Making eye contact, providing verbal validation of the presenting concern(s) and responding to the person's pre-verbal, behavioral, or verbal cues consistently and reliably builds trust.

Forgive and Show Empathy

This caritas process invites us to acknowledge positive and negative feelings from a non-judgmental perspective. It's easy to accept and/or experience positive emotions from our self and from others. Truth be told, we look forward to these types of experiences as they feed the ego. The challenge begins when we encounter or experience negative emotions. In these challenging moments we are invited to transcend our ego.

Extensive research links forgiveness to better health outcomes (O'Beirne et al., 2020; Racine et al., 2019). Many chronic pain patients have difficulty with forgiveness. Negative emotions (such as anger) increase allostatic load on the body and alter modulation of neural inputs, which increase pain perception (O'Beirne et al., 2020). Patients who participated in a forgiveness intervention reported lower levels of sensory pain, believed to be a consequence of emotional and cognitive processes that influence the sensory qualities of perceived pain (O'Beirne et al., 2020; Racine et al., 2019).

When we can accept ourselves and others as we are—imperfect beings doing the very best we can in any given moment—we open our hearts to empathy and compassion. Both are the gateway to forgiveness—forgiveness of self and others. The traumas of childhood become the dramas of adulthood and forgiveness is the key that frees us all from our trauma stories enabling us to cultivate resilience (Kelly, 2018). Resources for practicing self-compassion are available at the end of this chapter.

Use All Ways of Knowing

Four fundamental patterns of knowing in nursing were described by Carper (1978) and include empirics, or the science of nursing; aesthetics, or the art of nursing; personal knowledge, which includes experiential, interpersonal and intuitive knowing; and ethics, or the moral dimensions of nursing (Carper, 1978). Our patterns of knowing in nursing have expanded well beyond Carper's original four. Nursing science in the current century embraces the metaphysical as well as embodied physical and empirical ways of knowing (Watson, 2018).

Watson (2018) describes "all ways of knowing" to include personal, intuitive, empirical, aesthetic, ethical, experimental, technical, metaphysical, and spiritual knowing and learning (Table 5.1). Examples of expanded ways of knowing include the work of Constantinides (2019) and the concept of compassionate knowing grounded by intentional presence, as well as the work of Willis et al. (2019), who defined the concept of spiritual knowing as a pattern of knowing unique to the discipline of nursing.

Applying all ways of knowing to clinical nursing practice acknowledges nursing as an evolved, moral–ethical, scientific discipline, distinct from conventional biomedical science, aligned with unitary caring science (Watson, 2018).

Engage in Transpersonal Teaching–Learning Experiences

Reciprocal teaching–learning experiences are relational in nature and guided by love and respect (Wei & Watson, 2019). This caritas process reminds us true learning is not a passive act, but an exchange that builds a meaningful and trusting rapport between teacher and learner; it's a "heart-to-heart dialogue" (Wei & Watson, 2019). In the wise words of

Table 5.1 **Definitions**

Personal knowing	A knowing accumulated from our life experiences gained through observation, reflection, and self-actualization
Intuitive knowing	Unconscious reasoning or knowing within; pattern recognition; gut instinct
Empirical knowing	Knowledge from research and objective facts
Aesthetic knowing	Knowing through an integration of other ways of knowing that expand our understanding of a phenomenon; the "aha" moment of a new insight or perspective
Ethical knowing	A knowing that arises from our moral code; a knowing of right and wrong based on our obligation to protect and respect human life
Experimental knowing	A knowing that comes from trying different approaches
Technical knowing	Knowing acquired through skill development and technology
Metaphysical and spiritual knowing and learning	A knowing gained from a search for meaning in the world that embraces concepts such as being/becoming, universality, spirituality, time and space

Maya Angelou, *people won't remember what you did, they won't remember what you said, but they will remember how you made them feel.*

Examples of transpersonal teaching–learning experiences include both formal and informal encounters. These encounters integrate knowledge, skills, and facts with mental support, encouragement, and reassurance. Human caring and relational accountability are fundamental to transform the teaching-learning process from a task-driven event to a reciprocal, respectful experience (Wei & Watson, 2019).

Create a Caring–Healing Environment

The core measures for trauma-informed care identify three components of a healing environment—the physical, human, and organizational dimensions (Table 5.2; M. Coughlin, 2014, 2016; M. Coughlin et al., 2009). Wei and Watson (2019) reiterate and expand upon these attributes for a caring–healing environment within the context of unitary caring science. A true healing environment cannot be created in isolation but must reflect and integrate body, mind, and soul; it is the place where body, mind, and soul rest and become restored (Wei & Watson, 2019).

In a recent study, Williams et al. (2018), uncovered five themes related to the NICU environment described as either stressful or helpful to NICU parents. These themes included the quality of communication with the healthcare team, the team's bedside manner, feeling alienated from their infant's care, support from other NICU parents and

Table 5.2 Attributes and Criteria for the Healing Environment Core Measure

The physical environment is a soothing, spacious, and aesthetically pleasing space that is conducive to rest, healing, and establishing therapeutic relationships.	1. Sensory input is age-appropriate; dose and duration of sensory input are guided by the infant's behavioral and physiological responses.
	2. The space safely accommodates the provision of quality clinical care, 24-hour parental presence, and privacy.
	3. The design of the space honors the holistic and human dimensions of those whoinhabit it, integrates stress-reducing strategies, and facilitates social and therapeutic interactions for patients, families, and professionals.
The human environment emanates teamwork, mindfulness, and caring.	1. The interprofessional team exhibits shared responsibility in problem-solving and decision-making to formulate holistic plans for patient care; team members assume complementary roles that facilitate cooperation.
	2. Team members support each other in "always doing the right thing" for the patient, the family, and the staff.
	3. All verbal, written, and behavioral communication is respectful, complete, and patient-centered; there is zero tolerance for behaviors that compromise safety and/or undermine respectful relationships.
The organizational environment reflects a just culture committed to quality and safety.	1. Core measures for age-appropriate care provide the standard of care for all patient- care encounters and are reviewed/revised annually to reflect the latest evidence-based best practices.
	2. Practice standards are integrated into the annual performance evaluation across all disciplines and professionals who interface with the neonatal/infant population.
	3. A just-culture framework ensures balanced accountability at the individual and organizational level for continuous learning, quality improvement, and patient safety.

Source: Reprinted with permission from Caring Essentials Collaborative, LLC.

families, and the physical environment and regulations of the NICU (Williams et al., 2018). Understanding parental perspectives and their experiences in the NICU setting provides context for opportunities to improve and create a truly caring–healing environment for patients, families, and ourselves. What can you do to create an environment that is more healing for your patients and their families?

Value Humanity

Axiology is the study of values. Dr. Watson introduces axiology as a starting point to re-examine the moral values associated with caring, compassion, love, truth, beauty, and unity in nursing and healthcare at large (Watson, 2018). This caritas process invites us to transform how we engage with our patients to reflect these moral values and create sacred acts even during the most mundane of tasks.

Reverentially assisting with basic needs respects and sustains human dignity. This caritas process requires authentic presence, loving-kindness, and trustworthiness. When applied to a care encounter, it is the tenderness with which we greet the patient and the patience we practice when we wait those few minutes for the patient to acknowledge our presence; it is how we afford the patient a sense of modesty as we gently remove the diaper and slowly replace it with a clean one, reassuring them and inviting them to guide the care encounter; this is how we create sacred acts out of the most mundane tasks.

Embrace the Miracles in Life

This caritas process invites clinicians to embrace the unknown and be open to miracles. Despite the advances in healthcare and technology, science does not hold all the answers. Being open to the unknown and the notion that we share a universal connection enables us to connect to something larger than ourselves and sustain hope and belief for our patients and ourselves (Ponte & Schafer, 2013; Wei & Watson, 2019). This caritas process acknowledges the mystery surrounding life itself.

"Recognizing the mysteries and miracles in everyday life is the true key to understanding this caritas process" (Sitzman & Watson, 2018, p. 183). Practicing this process builds on a foundation of loving-kindness, authentic presence, spiritual well-being, and marveling at the miracle of life. This process invites you to cultivate an awareness that miracles are all around us. Each life is a miracle and in caring for one human being, whether it be yourself or others, you are caring for all of humanity.

> *There are only two ways to live your life. One is as though nothing is a miracle. The other is as though everything is a miracle.*
> —Albert Einstein

QUANTUM PHYSICS AND CONSCIOUSNESS

Nightingale's vision of nursing came to fruition in 2020 as the world celebrated the year of the nurse and midwife. Dr. Jean Watson and other preeminent nursing scholars and theorists have coalesced nursing's disciplinary discourse into a mature body of knowledge. Nursing science is a distinct caring–healing discipline grounded by a unitary worldview that recognizes nursing phenomena as unified wholeness, evolving consciousness, oneness, and caring.

> *We are entering a quantum universe that we cannot ignore … if we are to survive.*
> —Watson (2018)

Consciousness defines our existence. It involves a subjective awareness of phenomenal experiences associated with our inner and outer worlds. It is our sense of self and encompasses our feelings, choices, memories, thoughts, language. When we meditate, consciousness includes those inner generated images we perceive in our mind's eye. But, despite what we know about consciousness, what consciousness actually is remains largely unknown (Hameroff & Penrose, 2014)

Although the study of consciousness has traditionally been the realm of philosophers, recently, neuroscientists, biologists, and physicists have begun to explore this unchartered territory (Li et al., 2019). Physicists have put forth a theory linking quantum aspects of brain activity to consciousness, demonstrating experimentally that intentions activate the cerebral cortex and other neural correlates of consciousness (Beck & Eccles, 1992; Hameroff & Penrose, 2014). These *neural correlates of consciousness*, however, don't answer the whole question about consciousness, which physicists refer to as the *hard problem* (Keppler & Shani, 2020). The "hard problem" is understanding how matter (e.g., the brain) is capable of having subjective experiences (Hunt & Schooler, 2019).

In Figure 5.3, each triangle represents a pyramidal cell, and the ascending lines extending from the top of the triangles are apical dendrites. Light spots (*arrowheads*), which are transported along apical dendrites with different colors, represent different kinds of psychons that could give rise to unique experiences. The dendrites cluster automatically while

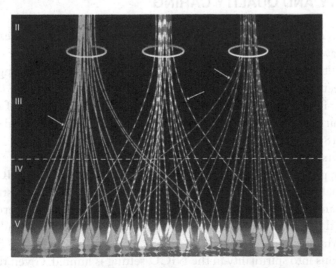

Figure 5.3 Schematic diagram of dendrons and psychons of layer V pyramidal cells.

Source: Reprinted with permission from Nancy International Ltd, Subsidiary of AME Publishing Company.

ascending to the superficial layer of the cortex to configure dendrons (*circles*) according to the different psychons they transmit. In addition, pyramidal cells are divided into different groups based on the distinct conscious experiences that they process (Li et al., 2019).

The gap between the physical (our physical selves and our physical world) and the phenomenal (our subjective experiences) requires a bridge and quantum physics appears to be that bridge (Keppler & Shani, 2020; Li et al., 2019; Ponte & Schafer, 2013). Research into this quantum realm has given us insight into our own consciousness and its connection with the consciousness of the cosmos. This cosmic consciousness, also known as the *zero-point field* or the *ubiquitous field of consciousness*, is hypothesized as an inherently sentient medium (Keppler, 2018, 2020). This construct is supported through the work of a specialized branch of physics called stochastic electrodynamics (Keppler, 2018, 2020; Keppler & Shani, 2020; Ponte & Schafer, 2013).

In Margaret Newman's theory of *health as expanding consciousness*, we understand health is an expression of life and not simply the absence of disease (Bateman & Merryfeather, 2014; Newman, 1997). As we embrace the majesty and mystery of life, the goal of nursing is to guide the patient and their family in a process of pattern recognition that facilitates self-discovery, growth, and expanded consciousness (Bateman & Merryfeather, 2014; Newman, 1997). Nursing as a discipline makes room for the science and the soul. Instead of searching for the answers to disease at the cellular and molecular level, we explore more complex, nonphysical, nonlocal models to explain and understand human phenomena (Watson, 2020). This holistic perspective opens the door to a grander understanding and a higher level of abstraction as we tap into a spiritual science and a science of consciousness (Watson, 2020).

SPIRITUALITY AND QUALITY CARING

If consciousness defines our existence, spirituality is its essence, giving meaning and purpose to life (Hawthorne & Gordon, 2019). Religion is one expression of spirituality but does not define the construct. Caring for the human spirit, through caring relationships and interconnectedness, is a quintessential aspect of quality nursing care (Hawthorne & Gordon, 2019). However, in clinical practice, nurses perceive a variety of barriers to the provision of spiritual care (Box 5.2; Hawthorne & Gordon, 2019; Mamier et al., 2019; Riahi et al., 2018).

The benefits of providing spiritual nursing care impact both nurse and patient. As reported earlier, providing spiritual care interventions to mothers in the NICU statistically reduced maternal stress levels (Alemdar et al., 2018). However, in a recent study examining the prevalence and correlates of providing spiritual care, NICU nurses were least likely to provide spiritual care interventions when compared to their pediatric and adult nursing counterparts (Mamier et al., 2019).

Investigations into spirituality in the NICU setting is limited. Given that spirituality allows a human being to find meaning and purpose in life, the experience of the NICU

BOX 5.2 PERCEIVED BARRIERS TO PROVIDING SPIRITUAL CARE

Lack of education
Time constraints
Low priority
Confusion about boundaries
Belief that spirituality is a private topic
Staffing deficits
Cultural differences
Workload
Lack of management support
Lack of awareness of spiritual needs

for parents and staff can, at best, be described as traumatic (M. Coughlin, 2016; Sade-ghi et al., 2016). Life-threatening illness and the associated bearing witness to the family in crisis is often accompanied by contemplation of fundamental spiritual and existential questions (Caitlin et al., 2001).

Brelsford et al. (2016) found that NICU parents' religious and spiritual beliefs affected their coping capacity and family cohesion. Specifically, parents with negative spiritual coping, described as feelings of abandonment or anger with a higher power, tended to experience higher levels of denial and lower levels of feeling connected to their family (Brelsford et al., 2016). Parents who utilized positive religious coping (such as prayer) also used negative religious coping while in the NICU, which speaks to the multilevel aspects of stress and processing grief and loss associated with the desired pregnancy outcome (Brelsford et al., 2016).

Addressing spirituality and spiritual needs in the NICU for the infant, the family, and staff is critical. However, this key domain of the human experience is often overlooked in environments that prioritize bureaucratic, time-pressured, and institutional demands over holistic human caring endeavors (Caldeira & Hall, 2012; K. Coughlin et al., 2017; Watson, 2020). The spiritual well-being and spiritual intelligence of nurses has a beneficial effect on families and staff (Azarsa et al., 2015). Religious and spiritual views can be a source of support (Brelsford & Doheny, 2016). Spirituality is a unique aspect of the human experience that is capable of transforming trauma from a place of isolation, fear, and despair, to one of connectedness, courage, and joy.

READER RESOURCES

Authentic Presence

How to cultivate authentic presence: www.linkedin.com/pulse/how-cultivate-authentic-presence-chyonne-kreltszheim

Loving Kindness and Meditation

The Center for Contemplative Mind in Society: www.contemplativemind.org/practices/tree/loving-kindness

How to practice loving kindness meditation: www.verywellmind.com/how-to-practice-loving-kindness-meditation-3144786

Insight Meditation Center: www.insightmeditationcenter.org/books-by-gil-fronsdal

Meditation for compassion: www.headspace.com/meditation/compassion

Self-Compassion

The power of self-compassion: www.youtube.com/watch?v=BTQP7XzDxjI

REFERENCES

Alemdar, D. K., Ozdemir, F. K., & Tufekci, F. G. (2018). The effect of spiritual care on stress levels of mothers in NICU. *Western Journal of Nursing Research*, 40(7), 997–1011. https://doi.org/10.1177/0193945916686775

Allmark, P. (2017). Aristotle for nurses. *Nursing Philosophy*, 18(3), e12141. https://doi.org/10.1111/nup.12141

Azarsa, T., Davoodi, A., Khorami Markani, A., Gahramanian, A., & Vargaeei, A. (2015). Spiritual wellbeing, attitude toward spiritual care and its relationship with spiritual care competence among critical care nurses. *Journal of Caring Science*, 4(4), 309–320. https://doi.org/10.15171/jcs.2015.031

Bateman, G. C., & Merryfeather, L. (2014). Newman's theory of health as expanding consciousness: A personal evolution. *Nursing Science Quarterly*, 27(1), 57–61. https://doi.org/10.1177/0894318413509725

Beck, F., & Eccles, J. C. (1992). Quantum aspects of brain activity and the role of consciousness. *Proceedings of the National Academy of Sciences of the United States of America*, 89(23), 11357–11361. https://doi.org/10.1073/pnas.89.23.11357

Brelsford, G. M., & Doheny, K. K. (2016). Religious and spiritual journeys: Brief reflections from mothers and fathers in a neonatal intensive care unit (NICU). *Pastoral Psychology*, 65(1), 79–87. https://doi.org/10.1007/s11089-015-0673-1

Brelsford, G. M., Ramirez, J., Veneman, K., Doheny, K. K. (2016). Sacred spaces: Religious and secular coping and family relationships in the neonatal intensive care unit. *Advances in Neonatal Care*, 16(4), 315–322. https://doi.org/10.1097/ANC.0000000000000263

Burjkhardt, M. A., & Nagai-Jacobson, M. G. (2016). Spirituality and health. In Dossey, B. M. & Keegan, L. (Eds.), *Holistic nursing, a handbook for practice* (6th ed., pp. 135–162). Jones & Bartlett Learning.

Caitlin, E. A., Guillemin, J. H., Thiel, M. M., Hammond, S., Wang, M. L., & O'Donnell, J. (2001). Spiritual and religious components of patient care in the neonatal intensive unit: Sacred themes and a secular setting. *Journal of Perinatology, 21*(7), 426–430. https://doi.org/10.1038/sj.jp.7210600

Caldeira, S., & Hall, J. (2012). Spiritual leadership and spiritual care in neonatology. *Journal of Nursing Management, 20*(8), 1069–1075. https://doi.org/10.1111/jonm.12034

Carper, B. A. (1978). Fundamental patterns of knowing in nursing. *Advances in Nursing Science, 1*(1), 13–23. https://doi.org/10.1097/00012272-197810000-00004

Connerton, C. S., & Moe, C. S. (2018). The essence of spiritual care. *Creative Nursing, 24*(1), 36–41. https://doi.org/10.1891/1078-4535.24.1.36

Constantinides, S. M. (2019). Compassionate knowing: Building a concept grounded in Watson's theory of caring science. *Nursing Science Quarterly, 32*(3), 219–225. https://doi.org/10.1177/0894318419845386

Coughlin, K., Mackley, A., Kwadu, R., Shanks, V., Sturtz, W., Munson, D., & Guillen, U. (2017). Characterization of spirituality in maternal-child caregivers. *Journal of palliative Medicine, 20*(9), 994–997. https://doi.org/10.1089/jpm.2016.0361

Coughlin, M. (2014). *Transformative nursing in the NICU: Trauma-informed, age-appropriate care.* Springer Publishing Company.

Coughlin, M. (2016). *Trauma-informed care in the NICU: Evidenced-based practice guidelines for neonatal clinicians.* Springer Publishing Company.

Coughlin, M., Gibbins, S., & Hoath, S. (2009). Core measures for developmentally supportive care in neonatal intensive care units: Theory, precedence and practice. *Journal of Advanced Nursing, 65*(10), 2239–2248. https://doi.org/10.1111/j.1365-2648.2009.05052.x

Dahlke, S., & Hunter, K. F. (2020). How nurses' use of language creates meaning about healthcare users and nursing practice. *Nursing Inquiry, 27*, e12346. https://doi.org/10.1111/nin.12346

Endo, E. (2017). Margaret Newman's theory of health as expanding consciousness and a nursing intervention from a unitary perspective. *Asia-Pacific Journal of Oncology Nursing, 4*(1), 50–52. https://doi.org/10.4103/2347-5625.199076

Graser, J., & Stangier, U. (2018). Compassion and loving-kindness meditation: An overview and prospects for the application in clinical samples. *Harvard Review of Psychiatry, 26*(4), 201–215. https://doi.org/10.1097/HRP.0000000000000192

Halifax, J. (2014). G.R.A.C.E. for nurses: Cultivating compassion in nurse/patient interactions. *Journal of Nursing Education and Practice, 4*(1), 121–128. https://doi.org/10.5430/jnep.v4n1p121

Hameroff, S., & Penrose, R. (2014). Consciousness in the universe: A review of the "Orch OR" theory. *Physics of Life Reviews, 11*(1), 39–78. https://doi.org/10.1016/j.plrev.2013.08.002

Hawthorne, D. M., & Gordon, S. C. (2019). Invisibility of spiritual nursing care in clinical practice. *Journal of Holistic Nursing, 38*, 147–155. https://doi.org/10.1177/0898010119889704

Hunt, T., & Schooler, J. W. (2019). The easy part of the hard problem: A resonance theory of consciousness. *Frontiers in Human Neuroscience, 13*, 378. https://doi.org/10.3389/fnhum.2019.00378

Kelly IV, J. D. (2018). Forgiveness: A key resiliency builder. *Clinical Orthopaedics and Related Research, 476*(2), 203–204. https://doi.org/10.1007/s11999.0000000000000024

Keppler, J. (2018). The role of the brain in conscious processes: A new way of looking at the neural correlates of consciousness. *Frontiers in Psychology, 9*, 1346. https://doi.org/10.3389/fpsyg.2018.01346

Keppler, J. (2020). The common basis of memory and consciousness: Understanding the brain as a write-read head interacting with an omnipresent background field. *Frontiers in Psychology, 10,* 2968. https://doi.org/10.3389/fpsyg.2019.02968

Keppler, J., & Shani, I. (2020). Cosmopsychism and consciousness research: A fresh view on the causal mechanisms underlying phenomenal states. *Frontiers in Psychology, 11,* 371. https://doi.org/10.3389/fpsyg.2020.00371

Le Nguyen, K. D., Lin, J., Algoe, S. B., Brantley, M. M., Kim, S. L., Brantley, J., Salzberg, S., & Fredrickson, B. L. (2019). Loving-kindness meditation slows biological aging in novices: Evidence from a 12-week randomized controlled trial. *Psychoneuroendocrinology, 108,* 20–27. https://doi.org/10.1016/j.psyneuen.2019.05.020

Li, T., Tang, H., Zhu, J., & Zhang, J. H. (2019). The finer scale of consciousness: Quantum theory. *Annals of Translational Medicine, 7*(20), 585. https://doi.org/10.21037/atm.2019.09.09

Mamier, I., Johnston Taylor, E., & Wehtje Winslow, B. (2019). Nurse spiritual care: Prevalence and correlates. *Western Journal of Nursing Research, 41*(4), 537–554. https://doi.org/10.1177/0193945918776328

Miller, J. E., & Cutshall, S. C. (2012). *The art of being a healing presence.* Willowgreen Publishing.

Newman, M. A. (1997). Evolution of the theory of health as expanding consciousness. *Nursing Science Quarterly, 10*(1), 22–25. https://doi.org/10.1177/089431849701000109

Norman, V., Rossillo, K., & Skelton, K. (2016). Creating healing environments through the theory of caring. *AORN Journal, 104*(5), 401–409. https://doi.org/10.1016/j.aorn.2016.09.006

O'Beirne, S., Katsimigos, A.-M., & Harmon, D. (2020). Forgiveness and chronic pain: A systematic review. *Irish Journal of Medical Science.* https://doi.org/10.1007/s11845-020-02200-y

Ponte, D. V., & Schafer, L. (2013). Carl Gustav Jung, quantum physics and the spiritual mind: A mystical vision of the twenty-first century. *Behavioral Sciences, 3*(4), 601–618. https://doi.org/10.3390/bs3040601

Racine, A. G., Recine, L., & Paldon, T. (2019). How people forgive: A systematic review of nurse-authored qualitative research. *Journal of Holistic Nursing, 38,* 233–251. https://doi.org/10.1177/0898010119828080

Riahi, S., Goudarzi, F., Hasanvand, S., Abdollahzadeh, H., Ebrahimzadeh, F., & Dadvari, Z. (2018). Assessing the effect of spiritual intelligence training on spiritual care competency in critical care nurses. *Journal of Medicine and Life, 11*(4), 346–354. https://doi.org/10.25122/jml-2018-0056

Sadeghi, N., Hasanpour, M., Heidarzadeh, M., Alamolhoda, A., & Waldman, E. (2016). Spiritual needs of families with bereavement and loss of an infant in the neonatal intensive care unit: A qualitative study. *Journal of Pain and Symptom Management, 52*(1), 35–42. https://doi.org/10.1016/j.jpainsymman.2015.12.344

Shalev, I., Entringer, S., Wadhwa, P. D., Wolkowitz, O. M., Puterman, E., Lin, J., & Epel, E. S. (2013). Stress and telomere biology: A lifespan perspective. *Psychoneuroendocrinology, 38*(9), 1835–1842. https://doi.org/10.1016/j.psyneuen.2013.03.010

Sitzman, K., & Watson, J. (2018). The tenth caritas process: Open to mystery and allow miracles to enter. In K. Sitzman & J. Watson (Eds.), *Caring science, mindful practice: Implementing Watson's human caring science* (2nd ed., pp. 183–194). Springer Publishing Company.

Solomon, J. (2019). *The one and done workbook: From idea to implementation.* Author.

Steckler, N. A., Rawlins, D. B., Williamson, P. R., & Suchman, A. L. (2016). Preparing to lead change: An innovative curriculum integrating theory, group skills and authentic presence. *Healthcare*, *4*(4), 247–251. https://doi.org/10.1016/j.hjdsi.2015.10.005

Substance Abuse and Mental Health Services Administration. (2014). *SAMHSA's concept of trauma and guidance for a trauma-informed approach*. Substance Abuse and Mental Health Services Administration.

Watson, J. (1997). The theory of human caring: Retrospective and prospective. *Nursing Science Quarterly*, *10*(1), 49–52. https://doi.org/10.1177/089431849701000114

Watson, J. (2008). *Nursing: The philosophy and science of caring* (Rev. ed.). University Press of Colorado.

Watson, J. (2018). *Unitary caring science: The philosophy and praxis of nursing*. University Press of Colorado.

Watson, J. (2020). Nursing's global covenant with humanity—Unitary caring science as sacred activism. *Journal of Advanced Nursing*, *76*(2), 699–704. https://doi.org/10.1111/jan.13934

Wei, H., & Watson, J. (2019). Healthcare interprofessional team members' perspectives on human caring: A directed content analysis study. *International Journal of Nursing Science*, *6*(1), 17–23. https://doi.org/10.1016/j.ijnss.2018.12.001

Williams, K. G., Patel, K. T., Stausmire, J. M., Bridges, C., Mathis, M. W., & Barkin, J. L. (2018). The neonatal intensive care unit: Environmental stressors and supports. *International Journal of Environmental Research and Public Health*, *15*(1), 60. https://doi.org/10.3390/ijerph15010060

Willis, D. G., & Leone-Sheehan, D. M. (2019). Spiritual knowing: Another pattern of knowing in the discipline. *Advances in Nursing Science*, *42*(1), 58–68. https://doi.org/10.1097/ANS.0000000000000236

Zeng, X., Chiu, C. P., Wang, R., Oei, T. P., & Leung, F. Y. (2015). The effect of loving-kindness meditation on positive emotions: A meta-analytic review. *Frontiers in Psychology*, *6*, 1693. https://doi.org/10.3389/fpsyg.2015.01693

Section III

Core Measures for Trauma-Informed, Age-Appropriate Care

6

The Healing Environment

It is often thought that medicine is the curative process ... medicine ... assists nature to remove the obstruction, but does nothing more ... nursing has to ... put the patient in the best condition for nature to act upon him.
  —Nightingale (1859)

A healing environment is designed to support and stimulate the inherent healing capacity of the body, mind, and soul. This chapter presents the latest research and evidence-based best practices related to the healing environment for the hospitalized infant, the family, and the healthcare professional.

WHAT IS THE HEALING ENVIRONMENT?

The Samueli Institute coined the term *optimal healing environment* and proposed a whole-system, healing-focused framework for delivering care (Firth et al., 2015; Sakallaris et al., 2015). The framework includes people in relationships, their health creating and healing behaviors, and the surrounding physical environment (Firth et al., 2015). This framework supports and stimulates salutogenesis.

Salutogenesis is the opposite of pathogenesis, or the biologic mechanism that leads to disease. Salutogenesis is about understanding the origins of positive health; the *salutary* or health-promoting factors that contribute to health and wellness (d'Alessio, 2019; Fries, 2020; Sakallaris et al., 2015; Silva et al., 2018). These health-promoting factors create an optimal healing environment (Figure 6.1; Silva et al., 2018).

The components of an optimal healing environment, according to Jonas and Chez (2004), encompass:

1. The conscious development of intention, awareness, expectations, and a belief in healing.

2. The adoption of transformative self-care practices that facilitate personal cohesion and the experience of wholeness and well-being.
3. The cultivation of techniques that foster healing presence grounded in compassion, love, and an awareness of our universal interconnectivity.
4. The development of listening and communication skills that foster trust and a bond between healthcare professional and patient.
5. The instruction and practice of health-promoting behaviors that influence a lifestyle choice for self-healing.
6. The responsible adoption of integrative medicine that supports healing processes.
7. The physical space where healing is practiced.

Fries (2020) defines health as a lifelong, multidimensional adaptive process comprised of intersecting biological, psychological, social, environmental, and spiritual systems. This definition aligns with the principles of nursing science founded by Florence Nightingale 150 years ago. Nightingale professed it is the nurse who must put the patient in the best position for nature to heal and described core elements constituting a total healing environment, encompassing both internal and external dimensions of the environment (Dossey et al., 2005).

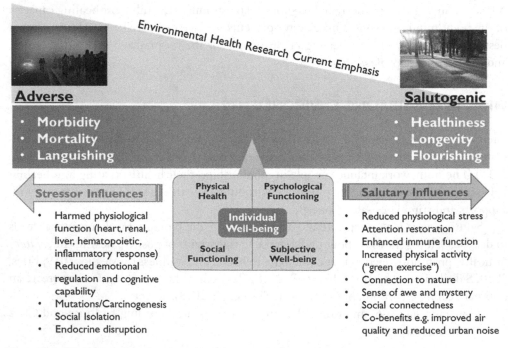

Figure 6.1 Continuum of environmental health research: from adverse to salutogenic.

Source: Reprinted with permission from Silva, R., Rogers, K., & Buckley, T. J. (2018). Advancing environmental epidemiology to assess the beneficial influence of the natural environment on human health and well-being. *Environmental Science & Technology, 52*(17), 9545–9555. doi: 10.1021/acs.est.8b01781

> **BOX 6.1** CORE ELEMENTS OF NIGHTINGALE'S INTERNAL HEALING ENVIRONMENT
>
> Internal environment
>
> - Engages body–mind–spirit wholeness.
> - Fosters healing relationships and partnerships.
> - Promotes self-care and health-promoting and health-sustaining behaviors.
> - Engages with and is affected by the elements of the external healing environment.
>
> *Source:* Dossey, B. M., Selanders, L. C., Beck, D.-M., & Attewell, A. (2005). *Florence Nightingale today: Healing, leadership, global action.* American Nurses Association.

The internal dimensions of a healing environment are grounded in ethics, philosophy, and epistemology to create transpersonal caring moments comprised of intentionality, authenticity, and healing presence (Box 6.1; Dossey et al., 2005; Watson, 2018). The external dimensions (Table 6.1), also grounded in science, reflect the caring actions that are an extension of the internal environment and necessary to ensure healing *...how to put the constitution in such a state as that it will have no disease, or that it can recover from disease, takes a higher place* (Dossey et al., 2005; Nightingale, 1859).

Nightingale focused on health and the maintenance of a state of health and wellness. She referred to disease as a body's response to repair itself. Aaron Antonovsky, the father of salutogenesis, agrees with Nightingale's perspective and argued understanding and treating disease is not the most effective way to produce healthy populations (Fries, 2020). We are not either sick or healthy; sickness and wellness are interrelated dimensions of the human experience reflected along a continuum (Figure 6.2; Fries, 2020).

Shifting from a pathogenic or disease oriented focus to a salutogenic or health and wellness focus requires a reorientation not only toward disease prevention, but toward health promotion and health maintenance (Fries, 2020; Silva et al., 2018). The ideal healing environment understands the unitary ontology of health and sickness (Fries, 2020; Watson, 2018). Healing environments go beyond the aesthetics of the space and are designed to support the engagement of its occupants internally, interpersonally, and behaviorally (Sakallaris et al., 2015).

Nature plays a critical role in creating an environment that reduces stress, fosters healing, and awakens us to our connectedness with the world (Sakallaris et al., 2015; Silva et al., 2018; Watson, 2018). A growing body of research highlights the health benefits of human contact with nature (Table 6.2; Frumkin et al., 2017). Natural environments encompass any outdoor space that retains noticeable elements of nature, ranging from pristine wilderness to urban green and/or blue spaces including green infrastructure (Frumkin et al.,

Table 6.1 **Core Elements of Nightingale's External Healing Environment**

External Environment	
Bed and bedding	• Promote proper cleanliness • Use correct bed, height, mattress, bedding, etc.
Cleanliness (rooms and walls)	• Dust free; odor free • Orderliness of space
Cleanliness (personal)	• Proper bathing and skin care of patient and nurse • Proper handwashing techniques (patient and nurse)
Food	• Proper portions and types of food • Proper presentation of food
Health of houses	• Provide pure air, pure water, efficient drainage, and light
Light	• Provide a room with light, windows, and a view • These are essential to health and recovery
Noise	• Avoid noise and useless activity such as clanking, loud conversations with or among caregivers • Speak clearly for patient to hear without having to strain • Avoid surprising the patient
Petty management	• Ensure patient privacy, rest, a quiet room, and instructions for the person managing the patient
Variety	• Provide flowers, plants, and avoid those with fragrances • Be aware of the effects of the mind on the body • Help patient vary their painful thoughts • Use soothing colors • Be aware of the positive effect of certain music on the sick
Ventilation and warming	• Provide pure air within and without; open windows, regulate room temperature • Avoid odiferous disinfectants and sprays

Source: Dossey, B. M., Selanders, L. C., Beck, D.-M., & Attewell, A. (2005). *Florence Nightingale today: Healing, leadership, global action.* American Nurses Association.

2017; Silva et al., 2018). Contact with nature can be viewed across a spectrum (Figure 6.3; Frumkin et al., 2017).

Experiences with nature are informed by the spacial scale of the nature encounter (a potted plant or a wilderness adventure), the proximity (looking through a window or holding nature in hand), the sensory experience (sights, sounds, smell, etc.), the activities embodied by

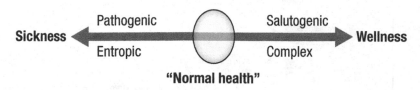

Figure 6.2 Antonovsky's continuum model for health.

Source: Fries, C. J. (2020). Healing health care: From sick care towards salutogenic healing systems. *Social Theory & Health, 18*(1), 16–32. Reprinted with permission from Springer Publishing Company.

Table 6.2 Summary of Evidence-Based Health Benefits of Human Contact With Nature

Physical Health	Emotional Health	Behavioral Health
• Improved postoperative recovery • Improved pain control • Improved immune function • Improved birth outcomes • Reduced obesity • Improved congestive heart failure • Reduced diabetes • Reduced mortality • Lower blood pressure • Improved general health in adults, cancer survivors and children	• Greater happiness, well-being and life satisfaction • Increased prosocial behavior and social connectedness • Reduced stress • Better sleep	• Improved mental health • Reduced depression and anxiety • Reduced aggression • Reduced ADHD symptoms • Improved child development (cognitive and motor)

ADHD, attention deficit hyperactivity disorder.
Source: Frumkin, H., Bratman, G. N., Breslow, S. J., Cochran, B., Kahn Jr., P. H., Lawler, J. J., Levin, P. S., Tandon, P. S., Varanasi, U., Wolf, K. L., & Wood, S. A. (2017). Nature contact and human health: A research agenda. *Environmental Health Perspectives, 125*(7), 1–18. doi: 10.1289/EHP1663

nature contact (hiking or hospitalization), and the level of an individual's awareness of nature (mindfulness or level of consciousness; Frumkin et al., 2017; Silva et al., 2018).

Summary

Healing transcends the idea of cure as a holistic and transformative process leading to an existential awakening regardless of the presence or absence of disease (Firth et al., 2015). Evidence-based, healing spaces, including the NICU, improve patient safety and make patients, families, and staff environments healthier (O'Callaghan et al., 2019). A trauma-informed healing environment supports this transformative process promoting cohesion of mind, body, and soul in coherence with nature and the natural world while optimizing health and wellness.

We can only be healthy if the environment in which we live is also healthy.

—Jerald L. Schnoor

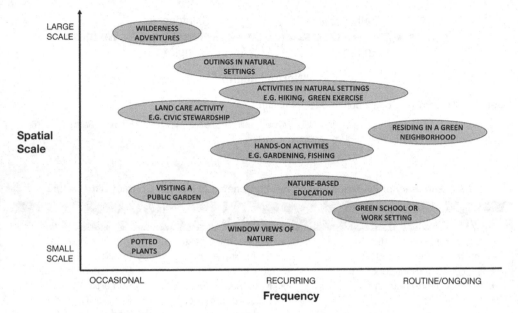

Figure 6.3 A spectrum of the forms of contact with nature.

Source: Reprinted with permission from Frumkin, H., Bratman, G. N., Breslow, S. J., Cochran, B., Kahn Jr., P. H., Lawler, J. J., Levin, P. S., Tandon, P. S., Varanasi, U., Wolf, K. L., & Wood, S. A. (2017). Nature contact and human health: A research agenda. *Environmental Health Perspectives, 125*(7), 1–18. doi: 10.1289/EHP1663

THE HEALING ENVIRONMENT AND THE CLINICIAN

The nurse work environment encompasses physical, human, and organizational characteristics that either facilitate or constrain professional nursing practice (Smith, 2018). A healthy work environment is safe, empowering, and satisfying, impacting the nurse's psychological health, job satisfaction, retention, workplace interpersonal relationships, job performance, and productivity (Table 6.3; Wei et al., 2018). Optimizing the nurse work environment is a cost-effective strategy to improve patient and nurse outcomes and reduce nurse turnover (Smith, 2018; Wei et al., 2018). Challenges to establishing a healthy, healing work environment for nurses include the physical layout, the human dimensions of the environment, and the organization's willingness to invest in creating sustainable, supportive healing spaces.

Physical Layout

With regard to the physical layout, NICU designs are changing and evolving, transitioning from open bay floor plans to single-family rooms (SFR) with nurses describing benefits to both layouts (Doede et al., 2018). In a systematic review (O'Callaghan et al., 2019), staff satisfaction scores were notably higher for the SFR design (Box 6.2). Additionally, once the

Table 6.3 **Attributes and Examples for the Healing Environment Core Measure**

Healing Environment Core Measure	
Attributes	**Examples**
1. The physical environment is a soothing, spacious, and aesthetically pleasing healing space conducive to rest, growth, and establishing connectedness	*Infant:* Sensory input is age-appropriate and aligned with best-practice recommendations; the space comfortably accommodates the 24-hour presence of the infant's family. *Family:* The design honors the holistic and human needs of its inhabitants integrating stress-reducing elements (nature, art, music) and ensuring personal space, privacy, and community access. *Staff:* The physical layout supports efficiency in workflow, provides protected space for staff rest and recovery, promotes collaboration and community, and ensures optimal spacial dimensions at each bedside for safe care delivery.
2. The human environment emanates compassion, authenticity and healing intention while preserving the natural world and practicing environmental stewardship	*Infant:* The infant's repertoire of pre-verbal communication (behavioral and physiologic) is recognized, acknowledged, and guides caring encounters. *Family:* Parental presence and partnerships are a system-wide priority; parents enjoy unrestricted access to their infant. *Staff:* The interprofessional team is collaborative and respectful. There is zero tolerance for behaviors that undermine safety, compromise respectful relationships, or threaten the environment (internally, interpersonally, and externally).
3. The organizational environment reflects a commitment to healing spaces and experiences that align with a trauma-informed approach while fostering ecological sustainability in support for a healthy planet	*Infant:* The core measures for trauma-informed care provide the evidence-based standard for all patient encounters. *Family:* Families have access to physical, emotional, financial, and spiritual resources to support them through their hospital experience. Care is coordinated during the hospital stay and through the post discharge experience. *Staff:* The organization ensures staff have appropriate resources to support their holistic health and well-being while on duty to include, but not limited to, clean and restful locations to take respite, access to healthy nourishment around the clock, dedicated staff nap areas, etc. In addition, staff participate in a system-wide process to support planet health.

Source: Reprinted with permission from Caring Essentials Collaborative, LLC.

staff had transitioned to the SFR, they reported better communication, a reduced sense of isolation, and decreased noise, fatigue, and stress (O'Callaghan et al., 2019).

Noise levels are reported to be lower in the SFR layout. However, noisiness remains a challenge for NICU clinicians (Doede et al., 2018). The complex nature of the acoustic environment in the NICU causes stress and disrupts the clinician's workflow and

BOX 6.2 HIGHER STAFF SATISFACTION SCORES ASSOCIATED WITH THE SINGLE FAMILY ROOM (SFR) NICU DESIGN

- Quality of the physical/work environment
- Patient care
- Job quality
- Health and safety
- Security
- Interaction with technology

SFR, single-family rooms.
Source: Adapted from O'Callaghan, N., Dee, A., & Philip, R. K. (2019). Evidence-based design for neonatal units: A systematic review. *Maternal Health, Neonatology and Perinatology, 5*(6). https://doi.org/10.1186/s40748-019-0101-0

concentration (Hasagawa et al., 2020). Three categories of noise have been identified as annoying and disruptive to clinicians in the NICU (Table 6.4). In the research examining evidence-based hospital design, the recurring outcomes associated with the built environment revolve around staff job satisfaction and patient's stress reduction and satisfaction (Brambilla et al., 2019). Involving nurses and families in the design, as the primary inhabitants of the space next to the patient, is paramount to ensure a design that benefits all (Doede & Trinkoff, 2020).

Human Dimensions

Human aspects of the work environment that undermine healing can be debilitating to the nurse, compromise the quality of patient care, and undercut the organization's bottom line. Lateral violence, also called horizontal violence, workplace bullying, or incivility, is pervasive in the nursing literature (Bambi et al., 2019; Myers et al., 2016; Parker et al., 2016; Pfeifer & Vessey, 2017). The prevalence of workplace incivility/bullying has not changed in more than 20 years, with rates ranging from 67.5% to 90.4% (Bambi et al., 2018; Chatziioannidis et al., 2018; Crawford et al., 2019). Five overarching themes contribute to the phenomenon of lateral violence or bullying (Figure 6.4; Crawford et al., 2019).

   This destructive "eat our young" rite of passage in nursing is often condoned within organizational cultures, structures and practices that contribute to negative socialization experiences and uncivil workplaces (Crawford et al., 2019; Edmonson & Zelonka, 2019). The quality of leadership and leading by intimidation and fear, contribute to a bullying culture (Edmonson & Zelonka, 2019; Kaiser, 2017). Workplace bullying is associated with higher burnout and higher nurse turnover with many nurses leaving the profession

Table 6.4 Noise Categories Described as Disruptive and Stressful in the NICU

Facility Noise	Human Speech/ Activity Noise	Alarm Noise
• Rolling medical carts/service carts • HVAC systems • Unit doors opening/closing • Patient room doors opening/closing • Privacy curtain tracks • Hand sanitizers • Cabinets opening/closing • Falling/dropping objects • Sinks • Footsteps • Exterior noise	• Staff conversations • Visitor conversations • Visitor sounds (e.g., footfall) • Patient sounds (e.g., crying) • Emergency procedures/events	• Alarms on medical equipment • Paging systems • Telephone ringing/ conversations

HVAC, heating, ventilation, and air conditioning.
Source: Adapted from Hasegawa, Y., Ryherd, E., Ryan, C. S., & Darcy-Mahoney, A. (2020). Examining the utility of perceptual noise categorization in pediatric and neonatal hospital units. *Health Environments Research Design Journal.* https://doi.org/10.001177/1937586720911216

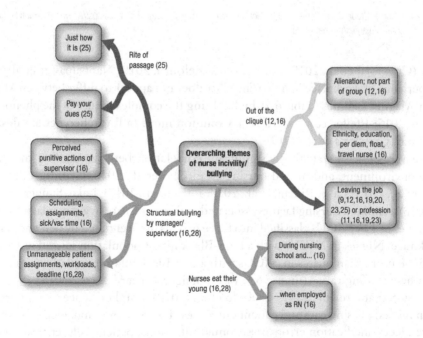

Figure 6.4 Themes of nurse-to-nurse lateral violence/incivility/bullying. The reference numbers indicate the citations for each theme discussed in the original publication.

Source: Crawford, C. L., Chu, F., Judson, L. H., Cuenca, E., Jadalla, A. A., Tze-Polp, L., Kawar, L. N., Runnels, C., & Garvida Jr., R. (2019). An integrative review of nurse-to-nurse incivility, hostility, and workplace violence: A GPS for nurse leaders. *Nursing Administration Quarterly,* 43(2), 138–156. doi: 10.1097/NAQ.0000000000000338 Reprinted with permission from Wolters Kluwer Health, Inc.

Table 6.5 **The Five Components of the Magnet® Model and the Forces of Magnetism**

Components	Forces
Transformational leadership	• Quality of nursing leadership • Management style
Structural empowerment	• Organizational structure • Personnel policies and programs • Community and the healthcare organization • Image of nursing • Professional development
Exemplary professional practice	• Professional models of care • Consultation and resources • Autonomy • Nurses as teachers • Interdisciplinary relationships
New knowledge, innovation, and improvements	• Quality improvement
Empirical quality results	• Quality of care

Source: American Nurses Credentialing Center. (n.d.). *Magnet model—Creating a Magnet culture.* https://www.nursingworld.org/organizational-programs/magnet/magnet-model

entirely (Crawford et al., 2019; Edmonson & Zelonka, 2019; Nantsupawat et al., 2017). The experience of workplace bullying/incivility does not appear to differ between Magnet® and non-Magnet facilities (Table 6.5), highlighting the complex nature of the phenomenon (Hickson, 2015; Pfeifer & Vessey, 2017). Common nurse bully archetypes are described in Table 6.6 (Crawford et al., 2019).

Research shows a statistically significant correlation between staffing the nursing practice environment, and missed nursing care (Cho et al., 2020; Griffiths et al., 2018; Hessels et al., 2015; Lake, Riman, et al., 2020; Lake et al., 2017). Lake, Staiger, Edwards, et al. (2018) examined nursing factors associated with missed care in a secondary analysis of 1,037 nurses in 134 NICUs classified into three groups differentiated by percent of infants of Black race. Nurses in NICUs with a high-Black infant population missed nursing care nearly 50% more than nurses in NICUs with a low-Black infant population as a result of poorer nurse staffing ratios (Figure 6.5; Lake, Staiger, Edwards, et al., 2018).

In a systematic review, Recio-Saucedo et al. (2018) found evidence to support a link between missed nursing care and patient outcomes. The outcomes included an increase in pressure ulcers, medication errors, nosocomial infections, patient falls, critical incidents, 30-day hospital readmission and mortality. In the NICU, missed nursing care is common (Box 6.3). Parents report less satisfaction with care and treatment in NICUs with more missed nursing care (Lake, Smith, et al., 2020). Nursing workload, a dimension of the nurse work environment, is significantly associated with missed nursing care in the NICU (Tubbs-Cooley et al., 2019).

Table 6.6 Common Nurse Bully Archetypes

The *super nurse*	Is often more experienced or specialized than most and communicates a sense of superiority through an elitist attitude, condescending manner, and "corrective comments."
The *resentful nurse*	Develops and holds grudges, encourages others to "gang up" on the transgressor, and tends to create drama that can permeate the work environment.
The *PGR nurse*	Uses PGR to bully other nurses, and is often quick to take offense to a neutral remark.
The *backstabbing nurse*	Is "two-faced," cultivating friendships that they then betray, using information as a weapon to enhance their power.
The *green-with-envy nurse*	Expresses bitterness to those who have what they do not: looks, status, personality, possessions. Their victims often do not realize they are a target.
The *cliquish nurse*	Uses exclusion as a means of aggression, showing favoritism to some while ignoring others.

PGR, put-downs, gossip, and rumors.

Source: Crawford, C. L., Chu, F., Judson, L. H., Cuenca, E., Jadalla, A. A., Tze-Polp, L., Kawar, L. N., Runnels, C., & Garvida Jr., R. (2019). An integrative review of nurse-to-nurse incivility, hostility, and workplace violence: A GPS for nurse leaders. *Nursing Administration Quarterly, 43*(2), 138–156. doi: 10.1097/NAQ.0000000000000338 Reprinted with permission from Wolters Kluwer Health, Inc.

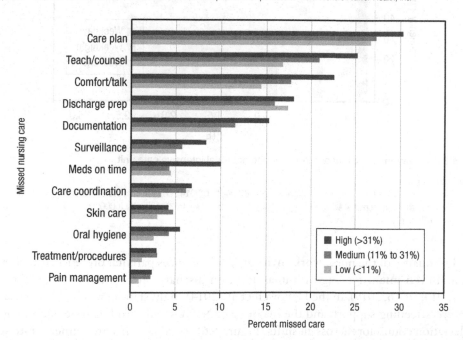

Figure 6.5 Distribution of missed care by hospital concentration of Black very low birthweight infants.

Source: Lake, E. T., Staiger, D., Edwards, E. M., Smith, J. G., & Rogowski, J. A. (2018). Nursing care disparities in neonatal intensive care units. *Health Services Research, 53*(Suppl. 1), 3007–3026. https://doi.org/10.1111/1475-6773.12762 Reprinted with permission from John Wiley and Sons.

BOX 6.3 MOST FREQUENTLY MISSED NURSING CARE IN THE NICU

- Teaching and counseling families
- Comforting and talking with patients
- Supporting breastfeeding
- Discharge preparation

Source: Adapted from Lake, E. T., Smith, J. G., Staiger, D. O., Hatfield, L. A., Cramer, E., Kalisch, B. J., & Rogowski, J. A. (2020). Parent satisfaction with care and treatment relates to missed nursing care in neonatal intensive care units. *Frontiers in Pediatrics, 8,* 74. https://doi .org/10.3389/fped.2020.00074

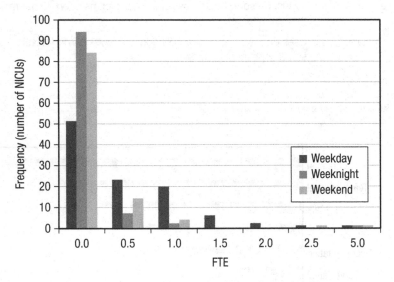

Figure 6.6 Lactation consultant availability in the neonatal intensive care unit.

FTE, full-time equivalent.
Source: Hallowell, S. G., Spatz, D. L., Hanlon, A. L., Rogowski, J. A., & Lake, E. T. (2014). Characteristics of the NICU work environment associated with breastfeeding support. *Advances in Neonatal Care, 14*(4), 290–300. doi: 10.1097/ANC.0000000000000102 Reprinted with permission from Wolters Kluwer Health, Inc.

The quality of the nurse work environment influences parental presence, breastfeeding, and even infant feeding of human milk on discharge from the NICU (Hallowell et al., 2014, 2016, 2019). In the Hallowell et al. (2014) study, staffing was highly correlated with breastfeeding support, and the majority of NICUs had zero full-time equivalencies for lactation counselors across all shifts (Figure 6.6). Administrative investments into staff nursing ratios along with positive nurse work environments resulted in a greater number of very low birth weight infants discharged home on a human milk diet (Hallowell et al., 2016). Additionally, NICUs with positive work environments report a higher number of parents present in the NICU (Hallowell et al., 2019). The attributes of the work environment that fostered parental presence and supported breastfeeding included an effective nurse manager, sufficient staffing and adequate resources (Hallowell et al., 2014, 2019).

Teamwork is crucial to creating and sustaining a healing environment which can be derailed by an unhealthy work environment. The quality of teamwork is linked to the quality and safety of health care delivery (Rosen et al., 2018). Effective teams not only ensure patient safety but also create positive, engaging, and resilient workplaces. Higher levels of teamwork are associated with higher levels of staff engagement (Rosen et al., 2018). Core competencies for building successful teams are described in Table 6.7 (Rosen et al., 2018).

Organizational Environment

To make economically sound investments in healthcare, organizations must invest not only in the necessary materials, technology, and design, but in the people who actually do the work. Nurse staffing ratios in the NICU are generally driven by infant acuity and as such, according to the American Academy of Pediatrics/American College of Obstetricians and Gynecologists guidelines, understaffing in NICUs is pervasive (Rogowski et al., 2015). Staffing patterns in the NICU must encompass not only infant acuity but staff nurse education, experience, certification, and the availability of other providers to ensure that optimal safe, quality care is rendered (Rogowski et al., 2015).

Gender hierarchies and inequalities between nursing and medicine undermine nurse autonomy and invalidate the intangible dimensions of nursing practice (Galbany-Estragues & Comas-d'Argemir, 2017). Creating healing environments begins with healing intention at the organizational and system level. Investing in a safe, healthy, and healing environment for clinicians ensures a healthy return on investment in the way of quality outcomes for patients, staff, and the organization at large (Sakallaris et al., 2016).

EVIDENCE-BASED STRATEGIES TO SUPPORT A HEALING ENVIRONMENT FOR CLINICIANS

Optimal healing environments for clinicians must include respite areas for clinicians to rest and refresh themselves. Comfortable, aesthetically pleasing, accessible staff-designated spaces for meals and rest must be available (Nejati, Shepley, et al., 2016). Breaks and meals should be protected time to afford the clinician the opportunity to recover and rejuvenate (Nejati et al., 2016a).

The perceived importance of break areas by staff impact job health, satisfaction, and retention, as well as job performance and the quality of patient care (Figures 6.7–6.9; Nejati, Shepley, et al. 2016). Respite areas that include access to nature have significantly higher restorative potential (Nejati et al., 2016b). As mentioned in Chapter 10, hospitals should ensure clinicians have dedicated spaces to nap to optimize performance and mitigate safety hazards related to shift work (Geiger Brown et al., 2016; Li et al., 2019).

Table 6.7 Teamwork Competency Frameworks for Healthcare Professionals

Framework	Competencies	Definition or Examples of Associated KSAs
Core competencies for interprofessional collaborative practice	Interprofessional practice values	Work with individuals of other professions to maintain a climate of mutual respect and shared values
	Roles/responsibilities	Use knowledge of own role and other professions to appropriately assess and address the health care needs of patients to promote/advance health of populations
	Interprofessional communication	Communicate with patients, families, communities, and professionals in a responsive and responsible manner that supports a team approach to the promotion and maintenance of health and the prevention and treatment of disease
	Teams and teamwork	Apply relationship-building values and principles of team dynamics to perform effectively in different roles to plan, deliver, and evaluate patient/population centered care, population health programs, and policies (11 subcompetencies)
Nontechnical skills in healthcare competency framework	Communication	Uses language clearly, organizes information, ensures shared understanding
	Team working and interprofessional skills	Exchanges relevant information within the team, focuses on the patient and their care when conflict arises, values team input
	Personal behaviors	Displays personal attributes of compassion, integrity and honesty, applies critical self-appraisal, welcomes feedback on performance, identifies when stress may pose a risk, recognizes fatigue, and considers appropriate actions to negate risk
	Analytical skills	Gathers and analyses information to support risk awareness, changes trajectory-facing significant risks, identifies options, re-evaluates based on situational awareness
TeamSTEPPS framework	Team structure	Identifies multiteam system components that must work together to ensure safety
	Communication	Structured process by which information is clearly and accurately exchanged among team members

(continued)

Table 6.7 Teamwork Competency Frameworks for Healthcare Professionals *(continued)*

Framework	Competencies	Definition or Examples of Associated KSAs
	Leadership	Ability to maximize the activities of team members by ensuring that team actions are understood, changes in information are shared, and team members have the necessary resources
	Situation monitoring	Process of actively scanning and assessing situational elements to gain information or understanding or to maintain awareness to support team functioning
	Mutual support	Ability to anticipate and support team members' needs through accurate knowledge about their responsibilities and workload

KSAs, Knowledge, skills, and attitudes.
Source: Rosen, M. A., DiazGranados, D., Dietz, A. S., Benishek, L. E., Thompson, D., Pronovost, P. J., & Weaver, S. J. (2018). Teamwork in healthcare: Key discoveries enabling safer, high-quality care. *American Psychologist, 73*(4), 433–450. doi: 10.1037/amp0000298 Reprinted with permission from American Psychological Association.

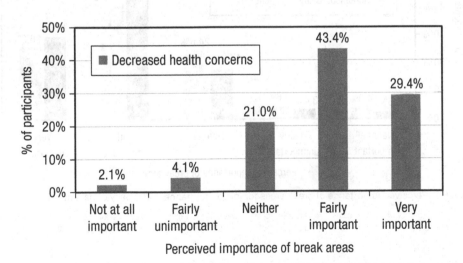

Figure 6.7 Perceived importance of break areas for job-related health concerns.

Source: Nejati, A., Shepley, M., Rodiek, S., Lee, C., & Varni, J. (2016). Restorative design features for hospital staff break areas: A multi-method study. *Health Environments Research Design Journal, 9*(2), 16–35. doi: 10.1177/1937586715592632 Reprinted with permission from John Wiley and Sons.

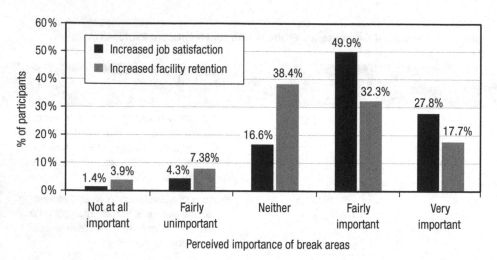

Figure 6.8 Perceived importance of break areas for staff satisfaction and retention.

Source: Nejati, A., Shepley, M., Rodiek, S., Lee, C., & Varni, J. (2016). Restorative design features for hospital staff break areas: A multi-method study. *Health Environments Research Design Journal, 9*(2), 16–35. doi: 10.1177/1937586715592632 Reprinted with permission from John Wiley and Sons.

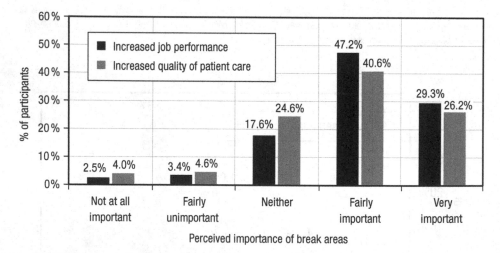

Figure 6.9 Perceived importance of break areas for job performance and quality of patient care.

Source: Nejati, A., Shepley, M., Rodiek, S., Lee, C., & Varni, J. (2016). Restorative design features for hospital staff break areas: A multi-method study. *Health Environments Research Design Journal, 9*(2), 16–35. doi: 10.1177/1937586715592632 Reprinted with permission from John Wiley and Sons.

Oppressive work environments because of organizational hierarchies, power differentials, and a lack of control over nursing practice, contribute to lateral violence, bullying, and incivility (Woodward, 2020). To improve job satisfaction and retention, while reducing lateral violence among nurses, a cultural shift promoting structural empowerment is needed (Box 6.4; Fragkos et al., 2020; Woodward, 2020). Structural empowerment restores the locus of control for nursing practice to nursing. Organizational

---

BOX 6.4 BENEFITS OF STRUCTURAL EMPOWERMENT

Increased staff self-efficacy
High motivation
Increased autonomy
Decreased job-related stress
Increased job satisfaction
Overall positive organizational and individual well-being

Sources: Adapted from Fragkos, K. C., Makrykosta, P., & Frangos, C. C. (2020). Structural empowerment is a strong predictor of organizational commitment in nurses: A systematic review and meta-analysis. *Journal of Advanced Nursing*, 76(4), 939–962. https://doi.org/10.1111/jan.14289; Goedhart, N. S., van Oostveen, C. J., & Vermeulen, H. (2017). The effect of structural empowerment of nurses on quality outcomes in hospitals: A scoping review. *Journal of Nursing Management*, 25(3), 194–206.

---

culture is the key to creating transformational healthcare and begins with transparent management, transformational leadership, and staff empowerment.

Strategies to prevent workplace incivility are listed in Box 6.5 (Bambi et al., 2017). In addition, personal techniques that may be adopted by the individual to counteract bullying are presented in Table 6.8 (Bambi et al., 2017).

BOX 6.5 STRATEGIES TO PREVENT WORKPLACE INCIVILITY, LATERAL VIOLENCE, AND BULLYING IN THE PROFESSIONAL NURSE'S COMMUNITY

- Increase awareness of workplace incivility, lateral violence, and bullying among nurses, managers, and administrators
- Perform informative and educational campaigns to implement prevention
- Provide nurses with assertive communication and conflict management skills to face bullying
- Require/cultivate leadership styles centered on authentic relationships
- Implement zero tolerance strategies toward every kind of abuse
- Create codes of conduct defining acceptable and unacceptable behaviors, disruptive behaviors and the management processes of inappropriate behaviors
- Exploration of appropriate legislation

Source: Adapted from Bambi, S., Guazzini, A., De Felippis, C., Lucchini, A., & Rasero, L. (2017). Preventing workplace incivility, lateral violence and bullying between nurses. A narrative literature review. *Acta Biomedica*, 88(Suppl. 5), 39–47. doi: 10.23750/abm.v88i5-S.6838

Table 6.8 **Suggested Personal Techniques to Counteract Bullying**

Techniques	Behaviors
Verbal	• Express feelings to perpetrator, asking them to stop bullying. • Appease the person. • Understand the perpetrator's anger. • Maintain a calm attitude. • Provide memories in a careful way. • Communicate face-to-face. • Mirror behavior of the perpetrator. • Talk about the incident to a colleague. • Talk about the incident with the perpetrator's boss. • Talk about the incident with human resources. • Talk about the incident with a professional association.
Nonverbal techniques	• Maintain eye contact with the perpetrator. • Increase physical distance from the perpetrator. • Use touch as appropriate. • Use surrounding space limitations to calm person.
Writing about the incident	• Document the date and time of the incident. • Share the write-up with the perpetrator asking them to stop the negative behavior. • Maintain a record of future events to share with leadership (retain copies for self).

Source: Adapted from Bambi, S., Guazzini, A., De Felippis, C., Lucchini, A., & Rasero, L. (2017). Preventing workplace incivility, lateral violence and bullying between nurses. A narrative literature review. *Acta Biomedica, 88*(Suppl. 5), 39–47. doi: 10.23750/abm.v88i5-S.6838

Leadership has a pivotal role in mitigating workplace incivility. As compelling role models, leaders influence organizational culture and climate through their actions and their leadership style (Table 6.9; Kaiser, 2017). The transformational leadership style creates a more positive interpersonal workplace environment through staff and team empowerment. Combining organizational, leadership, and individual strategies to address horizontal violence are effective in changing organizational culture (Table 6.10; Parker et al., 2016).

NICU staffing patterns must reflect patient acuity, nurse education and experience, specialty certification, the availability of other providers, as well as an understanding of nurse workload to ensure the provision of safe, quality patient care (Rogowski et al., 2013, 2015; Sherenian et al., 2013; Tubbs-Cooley et al., 2019). Nursing workloads have increased over the past decade while work environments have deteriorated (Lake, Staiger, Cramer, et al., 2018). Organizations and nurse leaders must analyze and measure the multiple domains of workload, which include the physical layout and work processes in order to optimize job performance and gain a keener sense of staffing needs (Tubbs-Cooley et al., 2019).

Table 6.9 Summary of Behavioral Leadership Styles

Transformational leadership	• Involves identifying a need for change, creating and instilling a vision in the group, and assisting followers to exceed their abilities in order to attain the vision • Leaders have a vested, personal interest in helping followers reach their fullest potential • Focus on interpersonal relationships between leader and follower • Team members are engaged, highly motivated, and fully empowered
Autocratic leadership	• Traditional style of leadership emphasizing hierarchy and power differentials • Little job control or decision-making by subordinates • Emphasizes task completion over interpersonal relationships, viewing people merely as instruments to perform task-defined work • Minimal communication and interaction occurs between the leader and the subordinates
Democratic leadership	• Leader seeks input from the group members and considers their feedback in making decisions • Encourages the expression of ideas from members, solicits discussion, and weighs all the information to make the best possible decision • Empowers members and supports teamwork • Members and leaders are treated as equals; power differentials are unimportant
Laissez-faire leadership	• Passive/avoidant leadership style • Leader is "hands off" and uninvolved with organizational members • Leader provides little direction to employees
Transactional leadership	• Emphasis on management aspects of leadership • Centered on control, organization, and short-term planning • Little attention is paid to interpersonal relationships except for the purpose of task-related work

Source: Kaiser, J. A. (2017). The relationship between leadership style and nurse-to-nurse incivility: Turning the lens inward. *Journal of Nursing Management, 25,* 110–118. doi: 10.1111/jonm.12447 Reprinted with permission from John Wiley and Sons.

Increasing exposure to nature strengthens the human immune system through exposure to biodiversity enriching our indigenous microbiota and reducing our risk for noncommunicable diseases (Figure 6.10; Haahtela et al., 2019). Nature contact is an effective, evidence-based strategy to support a healthy and healing micro-environment (Frumkin et al., 2017; Haahtela et al., 2019). Additional evidence-based benefits of the natural environment include its influence on promoting healthy behaviors, improving

Table 6.10 **Strategies to Mitigate Horizontal Violence**

Organizational Strategies	Leadership Strategies	Individual Strategies
Policies for disruptive behavior and zero tolerance for horizontal violence	Magnet® teams and champions	Education: "Lighting the Way"
Performance expectations	Education: leadership retreat	Cognitive rehearsal and scripting
American Nurses Credentialing Center's Magnet® Recognition Program journey and designation	Shared governance model	Peer evaluation and feedback
	Role modeling	Empowerment through shared governance
	Counseling for staff accountability and performance	Performance accountability

Source: Parker, K. M., Harrington, A., Smith, C. M., Sellers, K., & Millenbach, L. (2016). Creating a nurse-led culture to minimize horizontal violence in the acute care setting. *Journal for Nurses in Professional Development, 32*(2), 56–63. doi: 10.1097/NND.0000000000000224 Reprinted with permission from Wolters Kluwer Health, Inc.

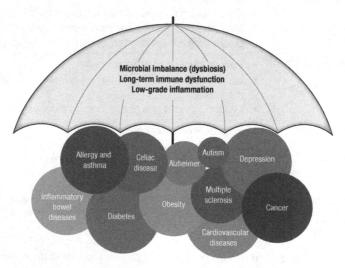

Figure 6.10 Several noncommunicable diseases have been suggested to share the same underlying risk factors.

Source: Haahtela, T., von Hertzen, L., Anto, J. M., Bai, C., Baigenzhin, A., Bateman, E. D., Behera, D., Bennoor, K., Camargos, P., Chavannes, N., Correia de Sousa, J., Cruz, A., Do Ceu Teixeira, M., Erhola, M., Furman, E., Gemicioglu, B., Gonzalez Diaz, S., Hellings, P. W., Jousilahti, P., . . . Billo, N. E. (2019). Helsinki by nature: The nature step to respiratory health. *Clinical and Translational Allergy, 9,* 57. https://doi.org/10.1186/s13601-019-0295-2

emotional and psychological responses to life stressors, and the feelings of awe and majesty inspired in the presence of nature, a truly healing space (refer to Chapter 4 and Chapter 9; Silva et al., 2018).

THE HEALING ENVIRONMENT AND THE FAMILY

The NICU environment, both physical and human, are repeatedly identified as stressors to the family in crisis (refer to Chapter 9). Limitations in space, the lack of accommodations, visiting restrictions, and continuous alarms inhibit parent—infant interactions contributing to feelings of separation, isolation, and fear (Fernandez Medina et al., 2019; Provenzi & Santoro, 2015; Twohig et al., 2016; Treherne et al., 2017). Williams et al. (2018) uncovered five themes identified by NICU mothers describing stressors associated with the NICU environment (Table 6.11).

Additional themes related to parent perceptions of closeness and separation have been described as a consequence of the NICU environment (Figure 6.11; Treherne et al., 2017).

A lack of privacy makes parent–infant interactions difficult, and during breastfeeding, mothers expressed feelings of self-consciousness (Fernandez Medina et al., 2019; Treherne et al., 2017). The busy, noisy and sometimes crowded environment distracts parents from engaging and interacting with their infant (Treherne et al., 2017). The medical equipment, particularly the incubator, has been described as a barrier to parent involvement in the care of their infant (Treherne et al., 2017).

Fathers and mothers in the NICU report different parental experiences. Mothers share feelings of marginalization and alienation and fathers express a need for information and practical support from nurses (De Bernardo et al., 2017; Provenzi & Santori, 2015; Provenzi et al., 2016). The built environment and the organizational culture of the NICU may contribute to these feelings. Welcoming, supportive environments that ensure consistent access to accurate information and appropriate resources can mitigate the emotional anguish of parents (Hall et al., 2017; Sacks & Peca, 2020).

Ethnic and racial disparities can additionally confound the healing environment (Barfield et al., 2019; Beck et al., 2020; Profit et al., 2017; Sigurdson et al., 2018, 2019). Structural racism is the totality of ways in which societies foster racial discrimination through mutually reinforcing systems and creates implicit bias (Bailey et al., 2017; Barfield et al., 2019). Healthcare is delivered within this context which contributes to disparate care and outcomes (Sigurdson et al., 2019). The physical environment is intimately linked to patient experience but is not a panacea. It can easily be derailed by a culture that does not open-heartedly embrace family presence in the NICU (Anaker et al., 2017; Heath, 2017).

The quality of care delivery in the NICU reflects the quality of the healing environment which varies greatly from NICU to NICU. Profit et al. (2017) report statistically significant variations in the quality of care both between and within NICUs. Very low birth weight infants cared for in NICUs with a high percentage of Black infants have higher

Table 6.11 Five Themes Describing the Environmental Stressors and Supports in the NICU

1. Communication with the medical staff	The lack of quality communication with nursing staff was a major stressor
2. Bedside manner of medical staff	Poor bedside manner (described as the attitude, professionalism, and manner of care expressed by nurses) was a stressor
3. Feeling alienated from infant cares	Women expressed feelings of exclusion from the process of care and felt unwelcomed in the NICU
4. Support from other NICU moms and families	Communicating with other mothers was a source of stress relief
5. NICU physical environment and regulations	The environment was considered either a stressor or highlight depending on the rules and regulations that were enforced as well as the availability of rest areas, bathrooms, and nourishment

Source: Williams, K. G., Patel. K. T., Stausmire, J. M., Bridges, C., Mathis, M. W., & Barkin, J. L. (2018). The neonatal intensive care unit: Environmental stressors and supports. *International Journal of Environmental Research and Public Health, 15*(1), 60. https://doi.org/10.3390/ijerph15010060

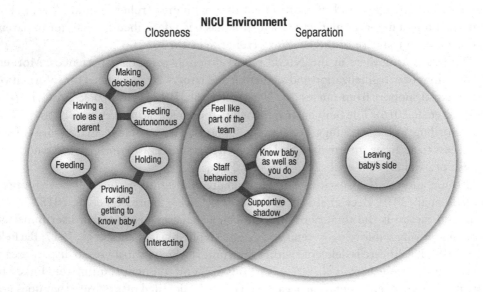

Figure 6.11 Themes of closeness and separation in the NICU from the parent perspective.

Source: Treherne, S. C., Feeley, N., Charbonneau, L., & Axelin, A. (2017). Parents' perspectives of closeness and separation with their preterm infants in the NICU. *Journal of Obstetric, Gynecologic & Neonatal Nursing, 46*, 737–747. doi: 10.1016/j.jogn.2017.07.005 Reprinted with permission from Elsevier.

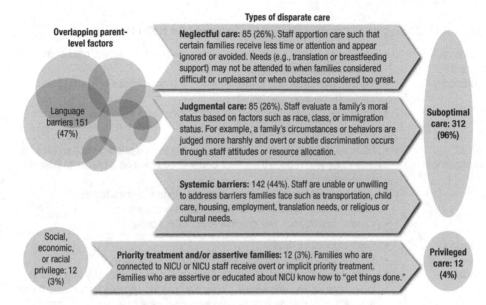

Figure 6.12 Types of disparate care in the NICU.

Source: Sigurdson, K., Morton, C., Mitchell, B., & Profit, J. (2018). Disparities in NICU quality of care: A qualitative study of family and clinician accounts. *Journal of Perinatology, 38*(5), 600–607. doi: 10.1038/s41372-018-0057-3 Reprinted with permission from Springer Nature.

rates of infection, poorer nurse–patient ratios, and infants and/or families are more likely to receive suboptimal care (Lake, Staiger, Edwards, et al., 2018; Sigurdson et al., 2018, 2019). Disparate care (Figure 6.12), categorized as neglectful, judgmental, and systemic barriers to care, is experienced by families across a variety of dimensions that includes but is not limited to race and/or ethnicity (Sigurdson et al., 2018).

A healing environment for NICU families begins with family presence and trusting relationships between parents and clinicians. Societal inequalities are mirrored in healthcare and threaten the vulnerable population served in the NICU (Sigurdson et al., 2018). Care environments that adopt and implement evidence-based best practices in family-centered care as the cornerstone of the healing environment will improve care for all.

EVIDENCE-BASED STRATEGIES TO SUPPORT A HEALING ENVIRONMENT FOR FAMILIES

The NICU space must be optimized to promote healing for families in crisis. Treherne et al. (2017) uncovered several best practice strategies that cultivate a healing environment in the NICU (Table 6.12). Hall et al. (2017) propose a paradigm shift moving from a limited scope of care exclusively focused on the infant's medical condition to an expanded view that encompasses the family in crisis. The term *newborn intensive parenting unit (NIPU)* was coined to reflect this paradigm shift (Figure 6.13; Hall et al., 2017).

Table 6.12 Strategies to Create a Healing Environment for NICU Parents

Promote parent autonomy	• Facilitate and encourage opportunities for parents to feed, hold and interact with their infant • Partner with parents and involve them in team discussions and decision-making • Empower parents, validate their role identity, and build their confidence and competence in caring for their infant
NICU environment	• Educate parents on the technology and how to work around it to care for their baby and reduce the effect of the equipment as a barrier to parent involvement • Adhere to light and sound recommendations to minimize this environmental stressor to families, infants and staff • Create care spaces that provide and protect privacy
Leaving the infant's bedside	• Create goodbye rituals • Ensure consistency in care delivery between clinicians • Collect parent contact info and offer to call parents with any changes in infant status; also encourage parents to call for updates (make sure there is an effective mechanism to take incoming calls to avoid exacerbating parent stress from being on hold or enduring multiple call transfers)

Source: Adapted from Treherne, S. C., Feeley, N., Charbonneau, L., & Axelin, A. (2017). Parents' perspectives of closeness and separation with their preterm infants in the NICU. *Journal of Obstetric, Gynecologic & Neonatal Nursing, 46,* 737–747. doi: 10.1016/j.jogn.2017.07.005

The NIPU landscape affords parents sleeping accommodations and amenities that support parental comfort (Box 6.6) and promotes prolonged parental presence and active involvement in the care of their infant (Hall et al., 2017). In-facility resources are just one aspect of the healing environment for NICU families. Social systems support, to include improved maternity leave policies and reliable hospital access through childcare and transportation resources, may increase parental presence in the NICU creating a healing environment for the parents and the infant (Lewis et al., 2019)

A systematic review and meta-analysis of studies between 2004 and 2018 found SFR NICUs facilitate greater parental presence, parent participation in infant care, and a higher rate of skin-to-skin care and exclusive breastfeeding compared to the open ward floor plan (van Veenendaal et al., 2019). Feeley et al. (2020) investigated the association of NICU stress, symptoms of depression, perceptions of nurse–parent support and family-centered care, sleep disturbances, breastfeeding self-efficacy, and readiness for discharge in mothers whose infants were cared for in an open ward versus a unit with pods and SFR. Mothers in the pod/SFR group reported significantly lower NICU stress, greater respect from staff, and spent significantly more time at their infant's bedside (Feeley et al., 2020).

Promoting parent-infant closeness is the quintessential healing milieu. Buil et al. (2020) investigated the use of the supported diagonal flexion position (SDF; Figure 6.14) for skin-to-skin care and mother-infant communication. The SDF position promoted more maternal vocalizations to the infant and mothers spent more time gazing and smiling at

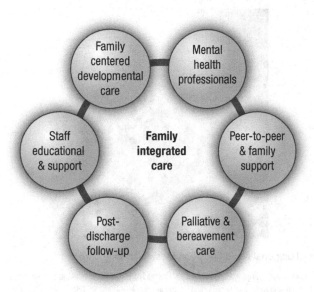

Figure 6.13 Components of comprehensive family support in the NIPU.

NIPU, newborn intensive parenting unit.
Source: Adapted from Hall, S. L., Hynan, M. T., Phillips, R., Lassen, S., Craig, J. W., Goyer, E., Hatfield, R. F., & Cohen, H. (2017). The neonatal intensive parenting unit: An introduction. *Journal of Perinatology, 37*(12), 1259–1264. https://doi.org/10.1038/jp.2017.108 Reprinted with permission from Springer Nature.

BOX 6.6 NIPU AMENITIES

- Provision of meals
- Bathrooms and showers
- Laundry facilities
- Access to computers and WiFi
- Kitchens where families can store and prepare meals
- Lounge space where families can gather for peer-to-peer support and educational sessions

Source: Hall, S. L., Hynan, M. T., Phillips, R., Lassen, S., Craig, J. W., Goyer, E., Hatfield, R. F., & Cohen, H. (2017). The neonatal intensive parenting unit: An introduction. *Journal of Perinatology, 37*(12), 1259–1264. https://doi.org/10.1038/jp.2017.108

their infant's face than mother's holding in the traditional vertical skin-to-skin orientation (Buil et al., 2020).

Promoting parent–infant closeness and minimizing separation are key to a healing environment for families (Feeley et al., 2016). Physical contact, presence at the bedside, parent

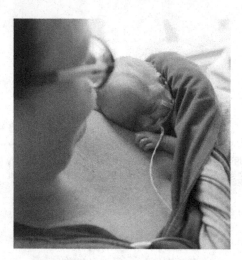

Figure 6.14 Supported diagonal flexion position for skin-to-skin care.

Source: Buil, A., Sankey, C., Caeymaex, L., Apter, G., Gratier, M., & Devouche, E. (2020). Fostering mother-very preterm infant communication during skin-to-skin contact through a modified positioning. *Early Human Development, 141*, 104939. https://doi.org/10.1016/j .earlhumdev.2019.104939 Reprinted with permission from Elsevier.

caregiving, skin-to-skin care, and just being together as a family can transcend the trauma experience for NICU parents and families. The use of technologies to support communication, such as text messaging parents with clinical updates, and the use of video technology to enhance visual access and connection to the infant has received favorable feedback from parents and clinicians (Globus et al., 2016; Le Bris et al., 2020). With an open-heart and innovative open-mind, nurses can create a truly healing environment for the family in crisis.

THE HEALING ENVIRONMENT AND THE INFANT

The healing environment for the hospitalized infant is one where the infant has continuous access to their parents, pain and stress are managed and mitigated consistently and reliably, sleep is protected, and care encounters are guided by the infant's behavioral state, communication, and comfort. The physical environment must be conducive to rest and recovery, with light and sound levels within the recommended ranges and other sensory inputs guided by the infant's response to the stimulation. Despite these requirements, hospitalized infants are often exposed to neurotoxic chemicals from medical equipment, aberrant lighting, excessive sounds, and restricted social interactions that alter their neurobehavioral health and developmental trajectory (Santos et al., 2015).

The physical, psychosocial, and clinical environment of the NICU are sources of toxic stress for the critically ill infant; examples of these stressors are listed in Table 6.13 (Weber & Harrison, 2019). The newborn period is a sensitive and critical time for brain growth and development. Exposure to toxic stressors during this vulnerable period has lifelong implications. Deprivation of positive sensory stimuli and an overabundance of

Table 6.13 **Examples of Environmental Stressors in the NICU**

Physical Environment	Psychosocial Environment	Clinical Environment
• Bright lighting • Loud noises • Noxious smells • Negative oral tastes and experiences	• Maternal separation • Lack of developmentallysupportive social interactions • Noncontingent caregiver responses to infant cues	• Clinical procedures necessary for the health and safety of the infant • Time constraints and rationed care

negative stimuli induce systemic, physiologic derangements with short-term and long-term consequences for the physical and emotional well-being of the hospitalized infant (Weber & Harrison, 2019).

Cheong et al. (2020) review four environmental exposures linked to long-term neurodevelopmental outcomes of preterm infants (Box 6.7). Although infants who received formula diets demonstrated better linear growth than infants on a donor breast milk diet, formula intake was associated with a twofold increased risk of developing necrotizing enterocolitis (Quigley et al., 2018). Painful procedures and pain-related stress are associated with alterations in brain development (refer to Chapter 9). Excessive noise, high-frequency sounds, and exposure to ototoxic medications damage cochlear development leading to hearing impairments and also compromised language development (Cheong et al., 2020; Liszka et al., 2019). SFR design has shown to decrease noise pollution in the NICU (Cheong et al., 2020; Joshi et al., 2018); however, concerns have been raised regarding the potential social and auditory isolation the infant may experience when parents are not consistently present in the SFR NICU (Jobe, 2017; Pineda et al., 2017).

The quality of developmental care, defined by an optimal environment, protection of sleep, management of pain and stress, supportive caregiving, and family presence, is

---

BOX 6.7 EARLY ENVIRONMENTAL EXPOSURES IN THE NICU IMPACTING NEURODEVELOPMENTAL OUTCOMES IN PRETERM INFANTS

1. Breast milk and breastfeeding
2. Noise, pain, and the hospital environment
3. Developmental care
4. Parenting and parent mental health

Source: Adapted from Cheong, J. L. Y., Burnett, A. C., Treyvaud, K., & Spittle, A. J. (2020). Early environment and long-term outcomes of preterm infants. *Journal of Neural Transmissions,* *127*(1), 1–8. doi: 10.1007/s00702-019-02121-w

associated with short-term and long-term outcomes (Cheong et al., 2020; Montirosso et al., 2017). Kangaroo care (aka skin-to-skin care) is associated with lower mortality, lower risk of neonatal infections and hospitalizations, and more exclusive breastfeeding (Cheong et al., 2020). Parenting and parent mental health have an enduring influence on infant and child development. Understanding the vulnerability of the family in crisis to depression, acute stress disorder, and posttraumatic stress disorder invites clinicians and institutions serving this fragile population to create infrastructural processes and resources to optimize parent and family well-being.

The NICU environment also influences and alters the infant's microbiome (Hartz et al., 2015; Younge et al., 2018). Changes in the infant's microbiome are associated with parental skin contact, diet (breast milk versus formula), environmental surfaces, nursing workspaces, caregiving equipment, clinician skin contact, and antibiotic use (Hartz et al., 2015). Early-life perturbations to the preterm infant's gut microbiota have been reported as a consequence of hospitalization and exposure to antibiotics (Gasparrini et al., 2019; Hartz et al., 2015). The collateral damage associated with these perturbations correlate with chronic metabolic and immune disorders later in life to include allergies, psoriasis, adiposity, diabetes, and inflammatory bowel disease (Figure 6.15; Gasparrini et al., 2019). Antibiotic stewardship as well as the adoption of best practices to optimize the infant's microbiome to support the proliferation of commensal bacteria is critical for the health and well-being of this vulnerable population (Gasparrini et al., 2019; Hartz et al., 2015; Pammi et al., 2017; Younge et al., 2018).

EVIDENCE-BASED STRATEGIES TO SUPPORT A HEALING ENVIRONMENT FOR INFANTS

Optimal characteristics of the built healing environment for hospitalized infants includes access to nature, music, art, and natural light, reduced crowding, reduced noise, and soft, cyclical, and user-controlled artificial lighting (Gaminiesfahani et al., 2020). The quintessential healing environment for the hospitalized infant, however, is in the arms of the parent in skin-to-skin contact.

Skin-to-skin care is an effective, evidence-based intervention that reduces newborn morbidity and mortality and has significant stress-reducing effects on physiologic stress outcomes compared with incubator care (Pados et al., 2020). In a retrospective study of infants between the ages of 24 and 28 weeks of gestation, researchers examined the onset and dose-dependent effect of skin-to-skin care (Casper et al., 2018). The study concluded that early, regular, and prolonged skin-to-skin care in the extremely preterm infant was associated with a reduced risk of bronchopulmonary dysplasia (BPD) development, cholestasis, and nosocomial infection (Casper et al., 2018).

Skin-to-skin care promotes early initiation of breastfeeding (Mekonnen et al., 2019), improves weight gain (Evereklian & Posmontier, 2017), and improves cardiac output and cerebral perfusion, while decreasing pulmonary vascular resistance (Sehgal et al., 2020). In addition, skin-to-skin care can shape the infant's microbiome, reducing the prevalence

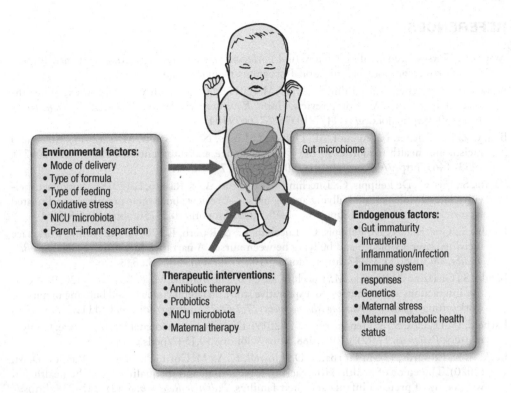

Figure 6.15 Factors determining the composition of gut microbiota in the preterm infant.

Source: Staude, B., Oehmke, F., Lauer, T., Behnke, J., Gopel, W., Schloter, M., Schultz, H., Krauss-Etschmann, S., & Ehrhardt, H. (2018). The microbiome and preterm birth: A change in paradigm with profound implications for pathophysiological concepts and novel therapeutic strategies. *BioMed Research International.* https://doi.org/10.1155/2018/7218187

of pathogenic organisms, such as *Pseudomonas* and *Neisseria,* and enhancing the presence of commensal bacteria (Biagi et al., 2018; Hendricks-Munoz et al., 2015). Beyond the preterm infant population, the practice of skin-to-skin care for hospitalized infants has extended beyond the NICU. The practice has shown to be safe and feasible for infants with surgical needs as well as infants with complex cardiac conditions cared for in cardiac care ICUs (Kelley-Quon et al., 2019; Lisanti et al., 2020).

Parent presence, participation in caregiving, and infant-holding experiences during hospitalization are associated with improved neurodevelopmental outcomes at 4 and 5 years of age (Pineda et al., 2018). Developmental care interventions mediated by maternal voice improve physiologic and behavioral stability in preterm infants (Filipa et al., 2017) and language skill acquisition at 36 months of age (Montirosso et al., 2016). Evidence-based strategies to create a healing environment for the infant begins with acknowledging the infant as a whole person, responding to the infant's physical, emotional, and spiritual needs.

A person is a person, no matter how small.
—Dr. Seuss, *Horton Hears a Who*

REFERENCES

American Nurses Credentialing Center. (n.d.). *Magnet model—Creating a Magnet culture.* https://www.nursingworld.org/organizational-programs/magnet/magnet-model

Anaker, A., Heylighen, A., Nordin, S., & Elf, M. (2017). Design quality in the context of healthcare environments: A scoping review. *Health Environments Research & Design Journal, 10*(4), 136–150. https://doi.org/10.1177/1937586716679404

Bailey, Z. D., Krieger, N., Agenor, M., Graves, J., Linos, N., & Bassett, M. T. (2017). Structural racism and health inequities in the USA: Evidence and interventions. *Lancet, 389*(10077), 1453–1463. https://doi.org/10.1016/S0140-6736(17)30569-X

Bambi, S., Foa, C., De Felippis, C., Lucchini, A., Guazzini, A., & Rasero, L. (2018). Workplace incivility, lateral violence and bullying among nurses. A review about their prevalence and related factors. *Acta Biomedica, 89*(Suppl. 6), 51–79. https://doi.org/10.23750/abm.v89i6-S.7461

Bambi, S., Guazzini, A., De Felippis, C., Lucchini, A., & Rasero, L. (2017). Preventing workplace incivility, lateral violence and bullying between nurses. A narrative literature review. *Acta Biomedica, 88*(Suppl. 5), 39–47. https://doi.org/10.23750/abm.v88i5-S.6838

Bambi, S., Guazzini, A., Piredda, M., Lucchini, A., Grazia de Marinis, M., & Rasero, L. (2019). Negative interactions among nurses: An explorative study on lateral violence and bullying in nursing work settings. *Journal of Nursing Management, 27,* 749–757. https://doi.org/10.1111/jonm.12738

Barfield, W. D., Cox, S., & Henderson, Z. T. (2019). Disparities in neonatal intensive care: Context matters. *Pediatrics, 144*(2), e20191688. https://doi.org/10.1542/peds.2019-1688

Beck, A. F., Edwards, E. M., Horbar, J. D., Howell, E. A., McCormick, M. C., & Pursley, D. M. (2020). The color of health: How racism, segregation, and inequality affect the health and well-being of preterm infants and their families. *Pediatric Research, 87*(2), 227–234. https://doi.org/10.1038/s41390-019-0513-6

Biagi, E., Aceti, A., Quercia, S., Beghetti, I., Rampelli, S., Turroni, S., Soverini, M., Zambrini, A. V., Faldella, G., Candela, M., Corvaglia, L., & Brigidi, P. (2018). Microbial community dynamics in mother's milk and infant's mouth and gut in moderately preterm infants. *Frontiers in Microbiology, 9,* 2512. https://doi.org/10.3389/fmicb.2018.02512

Brambilla, A., Rebecchi, A., & Capolongo, S. (2019). Evidence based hospital design. A literature review of the recent publications about the EBD impact of built environment on hospital occupants' and organizational outcomes. *Annali de Igiene, 31*(2), 165–180. https://doi.org/10.7416/ai.2019.2269

Buil, A., Sankey, C., Caeymaex, L., Apter, G., Gratier, M., & Devouche, E. (2020). Fostering mother-very preterm infant communication during skin-to-skin contact through a modified positioning. *Early Human Development, 141,* 104939. https://doi.org/10.1016/j.earlhumdev.2019.104939

Casper, C., Sarapuk, I., & Pavlyshyn, H. (2018). Regular and prolonged skin-to-skin contact improves short-term outcomes for very preterm infants: A dose-dependent intervention. *Archives de Pediatrie, 25*(8), 469–475. https://doi.org/10.1016/j.arcped.2018.09.008

Chatziioannidis, I., Bascialla, F. G., Chatzivalsama, P., Vouzas, F., & Mitsiakos, G. (2018). Prevalence causes and mental health impact of workplace bullying in the neonatal intensive care unit environment. *BMJ Open, 8*(2), e018766. https://doi.org/10.1136/bmjopen-2017-018766

Cheong, J. L. Y., Burnett, A. C., Treyvaud, K., & Spittle, A. J. (2020). Early environment and long-term outcomes of preterm infants. *Journal of Neural Transmissions, 127*(1), 1–8. https://doi.org/10.1007/s00702-019-02121-w

Cho, S-H., Lee, J-Y., You, S. J., Song, K. J., & Hong, K. J. (2020). Nurse staffing, nurses prioritization, missed care, quality of nursing care, and nurse outcomes. *International Journal of Nursing Practice, 26*(1), e12803. https://doi.org/10.1111/ijn.12803

Crawford, C. L., Chu, F., Judson, L. H., Cuenca, E., Jadalla, A. A., Tze-Polp, L., Kawar, L. N., Runnels, C., & Garvida Jr., R. (2019). An integrative review of nurse-to-nurse incivility, hostility, and workplace violence: A GPS for nurse leaders. *Nursing Administration Quarterly*, *43*(2), 138–156. https://doi.org/10.1097/NAQ.0000000000000338

d'Alessio, P. A. (2019). Salutogenesis and beyond. *Dermatologic Therapy*, *32*(1), e12783. https://doi.org/10.1111/dth.12783

De Bernardo, G., Svelto, M., Giordano, M., Sordino, D., & Riccitelli, M. (2017). Supporting parents in taking care of their infants admitted to a neonatal intensive care unit: A prospective cohort pilot study. *Italian Journal of Pediatrics*, *43*, 36. https://doi.org/10.1186/s13052-017-0352-1

Doede, M. & Trinkoff, A. M. (2020). Emotional work of neonatal nurses in a single-family room NICU. *Journal of Obstetric, Gynecologic & Neonatal Nursing*, pii: S0884-2175(20)30041-1. https://doi.org/10.1016/j.jogn.2020.03.001

Doede, M., Trinkoff, A. M., & Gurses, A. P. (2018). Neonatal intensive care unit layout and nurses' work. *Health Environments Research*, *11*(1), 101–118. https://doi.org/10.1177/1937586717713734

Dossey, B. M., Selanders, L. C., Beck, D.-M., & Attewell, A. (2005). *Florence Nightingale today: Healing, leadership, global action*. American Nurses Association.

Edmonson, C. & Zelonka, C. (2019). Our own worst enemies: The nurse bullying epidemic. *Nursing Administration Quarterly*, *43*(3), 274–279. https://doi.org/10.1097/NAQ.0000000000000353

Evereklian, M. & Posmontier, B. (2017). The impact of kangaroo care on premature infant weight gain. *Journal of Pediatric Nursing*, *34*, e10–e16. https://doi.org/10.1016/j.pedn.2017.02.006

Feeley, N., Genest, C., Niela-Vilen, H., Charbonneau, L., & Axelin, A. (2016). Parents and nurses balancing parent-infant closeness and separation: A qualitative study of NICU nurses' perceptions. *BMC Pediatrics*, *16*, 134. https://doi.org/10.1186/s12887-016-0663-1

Feeley, N., Robins, S., Genest, C., Stremler, R., Zelkowitz, P., & Charbonneau, L. (2020). A comparative study of mothers of infants hospitalized in an open ward neonatal intensive care unit and a combined pod and single family room design. *BMC Pediatrics*, *20*, 38. https://doi.org/10.1186/s12887-020-1929-1

Fernandez Medina, I. M., Fernandez-Sola, C., Lopez-Rodriguez, M. M., Hernandez-Padilla, J. M., Jimenez Lasserrotte, M. D. M. J., & Granero-Molina, J. (2019). Barriers to providing mothers' own milk to extremely preterm infants in the NICU. *Advances in Neonatal Care*, *19*(5), 349–360. https://doi.org/10.1097/ANC.0000000000000652

Filipa, M., Panza, C., Ferrari, F., Frassoldati, R., Kuhn, P., Balduzzi, S., & D'Amico, R. (2017). Systematic review of maternal voice interventions demonstrate increased stability in preterm infants. *Acta Paediatrica*, *106*(8), 1220–1229. https://doi.org/10.1111/apa.13832

Firth, K., Smith, K., Sakallaris, B. R., Bellanti, D. M., Crawford, C., & Avant, K. C. (2015). Healing, a concept analysis. *Global Advances in Health and Medicine*, *4*(6), 44–50. https://doi.org/10.7453/gahmj.2015.056

Fragkos, K. C., Makrykosta, P., & Frangos, C. C. (2020). Structural empowerment is a strong predictor of organizational commitment in nurses: A systematic review and meta-analysis. *Journal of Advanced Nursing*, *76*(4), 939–962. https://doi.org/10.1111/jan.14289

Fries, C. J. (2020). Healing health care: From sick care towards salutogenic healing systems. *Social Theory & Health*, *18*(1), 16–32. https://doi.org/10.1057/s41285-019-00103-2

Frumkin, H., Bratman, G. N., Breslow, S. J., Cochran, B., Kahn Jr., P. H., Lawler, J. J., Levin, P. S., Tandon, P. S., Varanasi, U., Wolf, K. L., & Wood, S. A. (2017). Nature contact and human health: A research agenda. *Environmental Health Perspectives*, *125*(7), 1–18. https://doi.org/10.1289/EHP1663

Galbany-Estragues, P. & Comas-d'Argemir, D. (2017). Care, autonomy, and gender in nursing practice: A historical study of nurses' experiences. *Journal of Nursing Research*, *25*(5), 361–357. https://doi.org/10.1097/JNR.0000000000000184

Gaminiesfahani, H., Lozanovska, M., & Tucker, R. (2020). A scoping review of the impact on children of the built environment design characteristics of healing spaces. *Health Environments Research & Design Journal*, 1937586720903845. https://doi.org/10.1177/1937586720903845

Gasparrini, A. J., Wang, B., Sun, X., Kennedy, E. A., Hernandez-Leyva, A., Ndao, I. M., Tarr, P. I., Warner, B. B., & Dantas, G. (2019). Metagenomic signatures of early life hospitalization and antibiotic treatment in the infant gut microbiota and resistome persist long after discharge. *Nature Microbiology*, *4*(12), 2285–2297. https://doi.org/10.1038/s41564-019-0550-2

Geiger Brown, J., Sagherian, K., Zhu, S., Wieroniey, M., Blair, L., Warren, J., Hinds, P., & Szeles, R. (2016). Napping on the night shift: A two-hospital implementation project. *American Journal of Nursing*, *116*(5), 26–33. https://doi.org/10.1097/01.NAJ.0000482953.88608.80

Globus, O., Leibovitch, L., Maayan-Metzger, A., Schushan-Eissen, I., Morag, I., Mazkereth, R., Glasser, S., Kaplan, G., & Strauss, T. (2016). The use of short message services (SMS) to provide medical updating to parents in the NICU. *Journal of Perinatology*, *36*(9), 739–743. https://doi.org/10.1038/jp.2016.83

Goedhart, N. S., van Oostveen, C. J., & Vermeulen, H. (2017). The effect of structural empowerment of nurses on quality outcomes in hospitals: A scoping review. *Journal of Nursing Management*, *25*(3), 194–206.

Griffiths, P., Recio-Saucedo, A., Dall'Ora, C., Briggs, J., Maruotti, A., Meredith, P., Smith, G. B., Ball, J.; the Missed Care Study Group. (2018). The association between nurse staffing and omissions in nursing care: A systematic review. *Journal of Advanced Nursing*, *74*(7), 1474–1487. https://doi.org/10.1111/jan.13564

Haahtela, T., von Hertzen, L., Anto, J. M., Bai, C., Baigenzhin, A., Bateman, E. D., Behera, D., Bennoor, K., Camargos, P., Chavannes, N., Correia de Sousa, J., Cruz, A., Do Ceu Teixeira, M., Erhola, M., Furman, E., Gemicioglu, B., Gonzalez Diaz, S., Hellings, P. W., Jousilahti, P., … Billo, N. E. (2019). Helsinki by nature: The nature step to respiratory health. *Clinical and Translational Allergy*, *9*, 57. https://doi.org/10.1186/s13601-019-0295-2

Hall, S. L., Hynan, M. T., Phillips, R., Lassen, S., Craig, J. W., Goyer, E., Hatfield, R. F., & Cohen, H. (2017). The neonatal intensive parenting unit: An introduction. *Journal of Perinatology*, *37*(12), 1259–1264. https://doi.org/10.1038/jp.2017.108

Hallowell, S. G., Rogowski, J. A., & Lake, E. T. (2019). How nurse work environments relate to the presence of parents in neonatal intensive care. *Advances in Neonatal Care*, *19*(1), 65–72. https://doi.org/10.1097/ANC.0000000000000431

Hallowell, S. G., Rogowski, J. A., Spatz, D. L., Hanlon, A. L., Kenny, M., & Lake, E. T. (2016). Factors associated with infant feeding of human milk at discharge from neonatal intensive care: Cross-sectional analysis of nurse survey and infant outcomes data. *International Journal of Nursing Studies*, *53*, 190–203. https://doi.org/10.1016/j.ijnurstu.2015.09.016

Hallowell, S. G., Spatz, D. L., Hanlon, A. L., Rogowski, J. A., & Lake, E. T. (2014). Characteristics of the NICU work environment associated with breastfeeding support. *Advances in Neonatal Care*, *14*(4), 290–300. https://doi.org/10.1097/ANC.0000000000000102

Hartz, L. E., Bradshaw, W., & Brandon, D. H. (2015). Potential NICU environmental influences on the neonate's microbiome: A systematic review. *Advances in Neonatal Care*, *15*(5), 324–325. https://doi.org/10.1097/ANC.0000000000000220

Hasegawa, Y., Ryherd, E., Ryan, C. S., & Darcy-Mahoney, A. (2020). Examining the utility of perceptual noise categorization in pediatric and neonatal hospital units. *HERD: Health Environments Research & Design Journal*, *13*(4), 144–157. https://doi.org/10.1177/1937586720911216

Heath, S. (2017, May 15). *Does hospital environment, culture affect family engagement?* Patient Engagement HIT. https://patientengagementhit.com/news/does-hospital-environment-culture-affect-family-engagement

Hendricks-Munoz, K. D., Xu, J., Parikh, H. I., Xu, P., Fettweis, J. M., Kim, Y., Louie, M., Buck, G. A., Thacker, L. R., & Sheth, N. U. (2015). Skin-to-skin care and the development of the preterm infant oral microbiome. *American Journal of Perinatology*, *32*(13), 1205–1216. https://doi.org/10.1055/s-0035-1552941

Hessels, A. J., Flynn, L., Cimiotti, J. P., Cadmus, E., & Gershon, R. R. M. (2015). The impact of the nursing practice environment on missed nursing care. *Clinical Nursing Studies*, *3*(4), 60–65. https://doi.org/10.5430/cns.v3n4p60

Hickson, J. (2015). New nurses' perceptions of hostility and job satisfaction: Magnet versus non-Magnet. *Journal of Nursing Administration*, *45*(10 Suppl.), S36–S44. https://doi.org/10.1097/NNA.0000000000000251

Jobe, A. H. (2017). The single-family room neonatal intensive care unit—Critical for improving outcomes? *Journal of Pediatrics*, *185*, 10–12. https://doi.org/10.1016/j.jpeds.2017.02.046

Jonas, W. B., & Chez, R. A. (2004). Toward optimal healing environments in healthcare. *Journal of Complimentary and Alternative Medicine*, *10*(1), S1–S6. https://doi.org/10.1089/1075553042245818

Joshi, R., Straaten, H. V., Mortel, H. V., Long, X., Andriessen, P., & Pul, C. V. (2018). Does the architectural layout of a NICU affect alarm pressure? A comparative clinical audit of a single-family room and an open bay area NICU using a retrospective study design. *BMJ Open*, *8*(6), e022813. https://doi.org/10.1136/bmjopen-2018-022813

Kaiser, J. A. (2017). The relationship between leadership style and nurse-to-nurse incivility; turning the lens inward. *Journal of Nursing Management*, *25*, 110–118. https://doi.org/10.1111/jonm.12447

Kelley-Quon, L. I., Kenney, B. D., Bartman, T., Thomas, R., Robinson, V., Nwomeh, B. C., & Bapat, R. (2019). Safety and feasibility of skin-to-skin care for surgical infants: A quality improvement project. *Journal of Pediatric Surgery*, *54*(11), 2428–2434. https://doi.org/10.1016/j.jpedsurg.2019.02.016

Lake, E. T., de Cordova, P. B., Barton, S., Singh, S., Agosto, P. D., Ely, B., Roberts, K. E., & Aiken, L. H. (2017). Missed nursing care in pediatrics. *Hospital Pediatrics*, *7*(7), 378–384. https://doi.org/10.1542/hpeds.2016-0141

Lake, E. T., Riman, K. A., & Sloane, D. M. (2020). Improved work environments and staffing lead to less missed nursing care: A panel study. *Journal of Nursing Management*. https://doi.org/10.1111/jonm.12970

Lake, E. T., Smith, J. G., Staiger, D. O., Hatfield, L. A., Cramer, E., Kalisch, B. J., & Rogowski, J. A. (2020). Parent satisfaction with care and treatment relates to missed nursing care in neonatal intensive care units. *Frontiers in Pediatrics*, *8*, 74. https://doi.org/10.3389/fped.2020.00074

Lake, E. T., Staiger, D., Edwards, E. M., Smith, J. G., & Rogowski, J. A. (2018). Nursing care disparities in neonatal intensive care units. *Health Services Research*, *53*(Suppl. 1), 3007–3026. https://doi.org/10.1111/1475-6773.12762

Lake, E. T., Staiger, D. O., Cramer, E., Hatfield, L. A., Smith, J. G., Kalisch, B. J., & Rogowski, J. A. (2018). Association of patient acuity and missed nursing care in U.S. neonatal intensive care units. *Medical Care Research and Review*, 1077558718806743. https://doi.org/10.1177/1077558718806743

Le Bris, A., Mazille-Orfanos, N., Simonot, P., Luherne, M., Flamant, C., Gascoin, G., O'Laighin, G., Harte, R., & Pladys, P. (2020). Parents; and healthcare professionals' perceptions of the use of live video recording in neonatal units: A focus group discussion. *BMC Pediatrics*, *20*, 143. https://doi.org/10.1186/s12887-020-02041-9

Lewis, T. P., Andrews, K. G., Shenberger, E., Betancourt, T. S., Fink, G., Pereira, S., & McConnell, M. (2019). Caregiving can be costly: A qualitative study of barriers and facilitators to conducting kangaroo mother care in a US tertiary hospital neonatal intensive care unit. *BMC Pregnancy and Childbirth*, *19*, 227. https://doi.org/10.1186/s12884-019-2363-y

Li, H., Shao, Y., Xing, Z., Li, Y., Wang, S., Zhang, M., Ying, J., Shi, Y., & Sun, J. (2019). Napping on night-shifts among nursing staff: A mixed-methods systematic review. *Journal of Advanced Nursing*, *75*(2), 291–312. https://doi.org/10.1111/jan.13859

Lisanti, A., Buoni, A., Steigerwalt, M., Daly, M., McNelis, S., & Spatz, D. (2020). Kangaroo care for hospitalized infants with congenital heart disease. MCN, *The American Journal of Maternal/Child Nursing*, *45*(3), 163–168. https://doi.org/10.1097/NMC.0000000000000612

Liszka, L., Smith, J., Mathur, A., Schlaggar, B. L., Colditz, G., & Pineda, R. (2019). Differences in early auditory exposure across neonatal environments. *Early Human Development*, *136*, 27–32. https://doi.org/10.1016/j.earlhumdev.2019.07.001

Mekonnen, A. G., Yehualashet, S. S., & Bayleyegn, A. D. (2019). The effects of kangaroo mother care on the time to breastfeeding initiation among preterm and LBW infants: A meta-analysis of published studies. *International Breastfeeding Journal*, *14*, 12. https://doi.org/10.1186/s13006-019-0206-0

Montirosso, R., Giusti, L., Del Prete, A., Zanini, R., Bellu, R., Borgatti, R.; NEO-ACQUA Study Group. (2016). Language outcomes at 36 months in prematurely born children is associated with the quality of developmental care in NICUs. *Journal of Perinatology*, *36*(9), 768–774. https://doi.org/10.1038/jp.2016.57

Montirosso, R., Tronick, E., & Borgatti, R. (2017). Promoting neuroprotective care in neonatal intensive care units and preterm infant development: Insights from the neonatal adequate care for quality of life study. *Child Development Perspectives*, *11*(1), 9–15. https://doi.org/10.1111/cdep.12208

Myers, G., Cote-Arsenault, D., Worral, P., Rolland, R., Deppoliti, D., Duxbury, E., Stoecker, M., & Sellers, K. (2016). A cross-hospital exploration of nurses' experiences with horizontal violence. *Journal of Nursing Management*, *24*, 624–633. https://doi.org/10.1111/jonm.12365

Nantsupawat, A., Kunaviktikul, W., Nantsupawat, R., Wichaikhum, O.-A., Thienthong, H., & Poghosyn, L. (2017). Effects of nurse work environment on job dissatisfaction, burnout, intention to leave. *International Nursing Review*, *64*, 91–98. https://doi.org/10.1111/inr.12342

Nejati, A., Rodiek, S., & Shepley, M. (2016a). The implications of high-quality staff break areas for nurses' health, performance, job satisfaction and retention. *Journal of Nursing Management*, *24*(4), 512–523. https://doi.org/10.1111/jonm.12351

Nejati, A., Rodiek, S., & Shepley, M. (2016b). Using visual simulation to evaluate restorative qualities of access to nature in hospital staff break areas. *Landscape and Urban Planning*, *148*, 132–138. https://doi.org/10.1016/j.landurbplan.2015.12.012

Nejati, A., Shepley, M., Rodiek, S., Lee, C., & Varni, J. (2016). Restorative design features for hospital staff break areas: A multi-method study. *Health Environments Research Design Journal*, *9*(2), 16–35. https://doi.org/10.1177/1937586715592632

Nightingale, F. (1969). Notes on nursing: What it is and what it is not. Dover Publications.

O'Callaghan, N., Dee, A., & Philip, R. K. (2019). Evidence-based design for neonatal units: A systematic review. *Maternal Health, Neonatology and Perinatology*, *5*(6). https://doi.org/10.1186/s40748-019-0101-0

Pados, B. & Hess, F. (2020). Systematic review of the effects of skin-to-skin care on short-term physiologic stress outcomes in preterm infants in the neonatal intensive care unit. *Advances in Neonatal Care*, *20*(1), 48–58. https://doi.org/10.1097/ANC.0000000000000596

Pammi, M., O'Brien, J. L., Ajami, N. J., Wong, M. C., Versalovic, J., & Petrosino, J. F. (2017). Development of the cutaneous microbiome in the preterm infant: A prospective longitudinal study. *PLoS One*, *12*(4), e0176669. https://doi.org/10.1371/journal.pone.0176669

Parker, K. M., Harrington, A., Smith, C. M., Sellers, K., & Millenbach, L. (2016). Creating a nurse-led culture to minimize horizontal violence in the acute care setting. *Journal for Nurses in Professional Development, 32*(2), 56–63. https://doi.org/10.1097/NND.0000000000000224

Pfeifer, L. E. & Vessey, J. A. (2017). An integrative review of bullying and lateral violence among nurses in Magnet® organizations. *Policy, Politics, & Nursing Practice, 18*(3), 113–124. https://doi.org/10.1177/1527154418755802

Pineda, R., Bender, J., Hall, B., Shabosky, L., Annecca, A., & Smith, J. (2018). Parent participation in the neonatal intensive care unit: Predictors and relationships to neurobehavior and developmental outcomes. *Early Human Development, 117*, 32–38. https://doi.org/10.1016/j.earlhumdev.2017.12.008

Pineda, R., Durant, P., Mathur, A., Inder, T., Wallendorf, M., & Schlaggar, B. L. (2017). Auditory exposure in the neonatal intensive care unit: Room type and other predictors. *Journal of Pediatrics, 183*, 56–66. https://doi.org/10.1016/j.jpeds.2016.12.072

Profit, J., Gould, J. B., Bennett, M., Goldstein, B. A., Draper, D., Phibbs, C. S., & Lee, H. C. (2017). Racial/ethnic disparity in NICU quality of care delivery. *Pediatrics, 140*(3), e20170918. https://doi.org/10.1542/peds.2017-0918

Provenzi, L. & Santoro, E. (2015). The lived experience of fathers of preterm infants in the neonatal intensive care unit: A systematic review of qualitative studies. *Journal of Clinical Nursing, 24*(13–14), 1784–1794. https://doi.org/10.1111/jocn.12828

Provenzi, L., Barello, S., Fumagalli, M., Graffigna, G., Sirgiovanni, I., Savarese, M., & Montirosso, R. (2016). A comparison of maternal and paternal experiences of becoming parents of a very preterm infant. *Journal of Obstetric, Gynecologic & Neonatal Nursing, 45*(4), 528–541. https://doi.org/10.1016/j.jogn.2016.04.004

Quigley, M., Embleton, N. D., & McGuire, W. (2018). Formula versus donor breast milk for feeding preterm or low birth weight infants. *Cochrane Database of Systematic Reviews, 6*, 002971. https://doi.org/10.1002/14651858.CD002971.pub4

Recio-Saucedo, A., Dall'Ora, C., Maruotti, A., Ball, J., Briggs, J., Meredith, P., Redfern, O. C., Kovacs, C., Prytherch, D., Smith, G. B., & Griffiths, P. (2018). What impact does nursing care left undone have on patient outcomes? Review of the literature. *Journal of Clinical Nursing, 27*(11–12), 2248–2259. https://doi.org/10.1111/jocn.14058

Rogowski, J. A., Staiger, D., Patrick, T., Horbar, J., Kenny, M., & Lake, E. T. (2013). Nurse staffing and NICU infection rates. *JAMA Pediatrics, 167*(5), 444–450. https://doi.org/10.1001/jamapediatrics.2013.18

Rogowski, J. A., Staiger, D. O., Patrick, T. E., Horbar, J. D., Kenny, M. J., & Lake, E. T. (2015). Nurse staffing in neonatal intensive care units in the United States. *Research in Nursing and Health, 38*(5), 333–341. https://doi.org/10.1002/nur.21674

Rosen, M. A., DiazGranados, D., Dietz, A. S., Benishek, L. E., Thompson, D., Pronovost, P. J., & Weaver, S. J. (2018). Teamwork in healthcare: Key discoveries enabling safer, high-quality care. *American Psychologist, 73*(4), 433–450. https://doi.org/10.1037/amp0000298

Sacks, E. & Peca, E. (2020). Confronting the culture of care: A call to end disrespect, discrimination, and detainment of women and newborns in health facilities everywhere. *BMC Pregnancy and Childbirth, 20*(1), 249. https://doi.org/10.1186/s12884-020-02894-z

Sakallaris, B. R., MacAllister, L., Smith, K., & Mulvihill, D. L. (2016). The business case for optimal healing environments. *Global Advances in Health and Medicine, 5*(1), 94–102. https://doi.org/10.7453/gahmj.2015.097

Sakallaris, B. R., MacAllister, L., Voss, M., Smith, K., & Jonas, W. B. (2015). Optimal healing environments. *Global Advances in Health and Medicine, 4*(3), 40–45. https://doi.org/10.7453/gahmj.2015.043

Santos, J., Pearce, S. E., & Stroupstrup, A. (2015). Impact of hospital-based environmental exposures on neurodevelopmental outcomes of preterm infants. *Current Opinions in Pediatrics*, *27*(2), 254–260. https://doi.org/10.1097/MOP.0000000000000190

Sehgal, A., Nitzan, I., Jayawickreme, N., & Menahem, S. (2020). Impact of skin-to-skin parent-infant care on preterm circulatory physiology. *Journal of Pediatrics, pii*: S0022-3476(20)30395-4. https://doi.org/10.1016/j.jpeds.2020.03.041

Sherenian, M., Profit, J., Schmidt, B., Suh, S., Xiao, R., Zupancic, J.A., & DeMauro, S. B. (2013). Nurse-to-patient rations and neonatal outcomes: A brief systematic review. *Neonatology*, *104*(3), 179–183. https://doi.org/10.1159/000353458

Sigurdson, K., Mitchell, B., Liu, J., Morton, C., Gould, J. B., Lee, H. C., Capdarest-Arest, N., & Profit, J. (2019). Racial/ethnic disparities in neonatal intensive care: A systematic review. *Pediatrics*, *144*(2), e20183114. https://doi.org/10.1542/peds.2018-3114

Sigurdson, K., Morton, C., Mitchell, B., & Profit, J. (2018). Disparities in NICU quality of care: A qualitative study of family and clinician accounts. *Journal of Perinatology*, *38*(5), 600–607. https://doi.org/10.1038/s41372-018-0057-3

Silva, R., Rogers, K., & Buckley, T. J. (2018). Advancing environmental epidemiology to assess the beneficial influence of the natural environment on human health and well-being. *Environmental Science & Technology*, *52*(17), 9545–9555. https://doi.org/10.1021/acs.est.8b01781

Smith, J. G. (2018). The nurse work environment: Current and future challenges. *Journal of Applied Biobehavioral Research*, *23*, e12126. https://doi.org/10.1111/jabr.12126

Treherne, S. C., Feeley, N., Charbonneau, L., & Axelin, A. (2017). Parents' perspectives of closeness and separation with their preterm infants in the NICU. *Journal of Obstetric, Gynecologic & Neonatal Nursing*, *46*, 737–747. https://doi.org/10.1016/j.jogn.2017.07.005

Tubbs-Cooley, H. L., Mara, C. A., Carle, A. C., Mark, B. A., & Pickler, R. H. (2019). Association of nurse workload with missed nursing care in the neonatal intensive care unit. *JAMA Pediatrics*, *173*(1), 44–51. https://doi.org/10.1001/jamapediatrics.2018.3619

Twohig, A., Reulbach, U., Figuerdo, R., McCarthy, A., McNicholas, F., & Molloy, E. J. (2016). Supporting preterm infant attachment and socioemotional development in the neonatal intensive care unit: Staff perceptions. *Infant Mental Health*, *37*(2), 160–171. https://doi.org/10.1002/imhj.21556

van Veenendaal, N. R., Heideman, W. H., Limpens, J., van der Lee, J. H., van Goudoever, J. B., van Kempen, A. A. M. W., & van der Schoor, S. R. D. (2019). Hospitalising preterm infants in single family rooms versus open bay units: A systematic review and meta-analysis. *The Lancet Child & Adolescent Health*, *3*(3), 147–157. https://doi.org/10.1016/S2352-4642(18)30375-4

Watson, J. (2018). Unitary caring science: The philosophy and praxis of nursing. University Press of Colorado.

Weber, A., & Harrison, T. M. (2019). Reducing toxic stress in the NICU to improve infant outcomes. *Nursing Outlook*, *67*(2), 169–189. https://doi.org/10.1016/j.outlook.2018.11.002

Wei, H., Sewell, K. A., Woody, G., & Rose, M. A. (2018). The state of the science of nurse work environments in the United States: A systematic review. *International Journal of Nursing Science*, *5*(3), 287–300. https://doi.org/10.1016/j.ijnss.2018.04.010

Williams, K. G., Patel. K. T., Stausmire, J. M., Bridges, C., Mathis, M. W., & Barkin, J. L. (2018). The neonatal intensive care unit: Environmental stressors and supports. *International Journal of Environmental Research and Public Health*, *15*(1), 60. https://doi.org/10.3390/ijerph15010060

Woodward, K. F. (2020). Individual nurse empowerment: A concept analysis. *Nursing Forum*, *55*(2), 136–143. https://doi.org/10.1111/nuf.12407

Younge, N. E., Araujo-Perez, F., Brandon, D., & Seed, P. C. (2018). Early-life microbiota in hospitalized preterm and full-term infants. *Microbiome*, *6*, 98. https://doi.org/10.1186/s40168-018-0486-4

7

Compassionate Family Collaborative Care

Alone we can do so little; together we can do so much.
—Helen Keller

Partnering with parents and families in crisis hinges on the emotional intelligence and well-being of the clinician. It requires the clinician to cultivate personal wholeness in order to be able to give fully to others. You cannot give what you do not have. If you do not have compassion for your self, you will not be able to give compassion to others. If you are not able to forgive yourself, you are unable to forgive another.

Bearing witness to suffering takes its toll on one's capacity to love self and others (refer to Chapters 5 and 12) and impedes true, authentic collaboration. The attributes of compassionate family collaborative care (CFCC) include emotional well-being, self-efficacy, and communication with the infant, the family, and the clinician. This chapter presents the latest research and evidence-based best practices related to CFCC for the hospitalized infant, family, and healthcare professional.

WHAT IS COMPASSIONATE FAMILY COLLABORATIVE CARE?

CFCC begins with an understanding that everyone is doing their best in any given moment. This "best" is met with an open heart and a compassionate response. Compassion is the recognition of distress and suffering in another with a desire to respond. Kindness is compassion in action. Compassion without collaboration leads to inconsistency (Lown et al., 2016).

To collaborate is to work jointly, to cooperate with and willingly assist a group to achieve together. Collaboration without compassion produces technically correct results

BOX 7.1 PRINCIPLES OF COMPASSIONATE COLLABORATIVE CARE

1. Patients and family members are involved in health professional education and practice design in order to truly transform healthcare.
2. Healthcare professionals share information and strive to facilitate patient and family participation as their comfort allows, while honoring the preferences of patients and families who choose not to be so involved.
3. Compassion and collaboration involve attributes, values, and skills that can be taught, modeled, learned, and assessed and must be integrated into health professional education and practice at all levels and continuously reinforced.
4. The well-being of professional and family caregivers is critical to their ability to function effectively. Promotion of caregivers' resilience, and thus their ability to care for and heal others, must be proactively supported.
5. Leaders of healthcare and educational organizations and systems must create cultures and provide resources that support compassionate, collaborative care.

Source: Adapted from Lown, B. A., McIntosh, S., Gaines, M. E., McGuinn, K., & Hatem, D. (2016). Integrating compassionate collaborative care (the "Triple C") into health professional education to advance the Triple Aim of health care. *Academic Medicine, 91*(3), 310–316. doi: 10.1097/ACM.0000000000001077

but misses the mark in meeting the individual's emotional, spiritual, and psychosocial needs (Lown et al., 2016). Adapted from the principles of compassionate collaborative care (Box 7.1), CFCC prioritizes respectful caring relationships, emotional support, authentic communication, and shared empowerment (Lown et al., 2016; Pfaff & Markaki, 2017).

CFCC creates an environment where individuals thrive: patient, family, and professional. The definition of *thrive* is to grow and develop well; to flourish. Thriving is about coping with life's adversities and actively pursuing opportunities for growth and development (Feeney & Collins, 2015a). The idea of thriving through relationships is built on attachment theory and traditional social support theory, and encompasses five broad categories of well-being or thriving (Table 7.1; Feeney & Collins, 2015a, 2015b)

Thriving in the NICU is relevant for infants, families, and clinicians and is an integral component to successful collaboration. The five components of thriving (Table 7.1) underpin the quality of compassionate collaborative relationships. CFCC takes teamwork to the next level. Although both involve a group of people working together, compassionate collaborative teamwork forms the basis of person-centered, relationship-based, high-quality care.

Emotional well-being, self-efficacy, and effective, respectful communication are the hallmarks of CFCC for the patient, the family, and the professional. A CFCC model is

Table 7.1 **Components of Thriving**

Thriving Component	Examples
1. Hedonic well-being	Happiness, life satisfaction, subjective well-being, pleasant affect, healthy affective balance—ratio of positive to negative affect
2. Eudaimonic well-being	Having purpose and meaning in life, having and progressing toward meaningful life goals, mastery/efficacy, control, autonomy/self-determination, personal growth, movement toward full potential
3. Psychological well-being	Positive self-regard, self-acceptance, resilience/hardiness, optimism, absence (or reduced incidence) of mental health symptoms or disorders
4. Social well-being	Deep and meaningful human connections, positive interpersonal expectancies (including perceived available support), prosocial orientation, faith in others/humanity
5. Physical well-being	Physical fitness (healthy weight and activity levels), absence (or reduced incidence) of illness and disease, health status above expected baselines, longevity

Source: Feeney, B. C., & Collins, N. L. (2015b). Thriving through relationships. *Current Opinions in Psychology, 1,* 22–28. https://doi.org/10.1016/j.copsyc.2014.11.001 Reprinted with permission from Elsevier.

poised to upend a culture that suffers from low trust and limited collaboration (Maghsoudi et al., 2020). Communication, sharing information, and joint decision-making are core collaborative practices that promote transparency, create trust, and increase social sustainability.

Social sustainability involves creating an accessible, integrated, and equitable community that successfully meets individual and public health needs (Maghsoudi et al., 2020). High-performing collaborative teams integrate the concept of social sustainability to ensure equity and quality of health (Amoo et al., 2016). The World Health Organization Commission of Social Determinants of Health (SDH) emphasizes the importance of collaboration in addressing SDH.

SDH (Box 7.2) are environmental conditions in which people live, work, play, worship, and age that affect a wide range of health functioning and quality of life outcomes and risks. The 2030 Agenda for Sustainable Development adopted by the United Nations is a blueprint for global health and well-being framed by three interrelated pillars: environment, sociality, and economics (Khayatzadeh-Mahani et al., 2019). The Sustainable Development Goals (SDG; Box 7.3) provide a new way of addressing SDH through multisector collaboration.

BOX 7.2 SOCIAL DETERMINANTS OF HEALTH

- Economic stability
- Education
- Social and community context
- Health and healthcare
- Neighborhood and built environment

BOX 7.3 UNITED NATIONS' SUSTAINABLE DEVELOPMENT GOALS

1. No poverty
2. Zero hunger
3. Good health and well-being
4. Quality education
5. Gender equality
6. Clean water and sanitation
7. Clean energy
8. Decent work and economic growth
9. Industry, innovation, and infrastructure
10. Reduced inequalities
11. Sustainable cities and communities
12. Climate action
13. Life below the water
14. Life on land
15. Peace, justice, and strong institutions
16. Partnerships for the goals
17. Responsible consumption and production

Source: United Nations. Department of Economic and Social Affairs: Sustainable Development. (n.d.). *The 127 goals.* sdgs.un.org/goals

Multisector collaboration refers to partnerships among governmental, nonprofit, private and public organizations, community groups, and individuals who come together to solve problems that affect the community (Khayatzadeh-Mahani et al., 2019). Healthcare organizations are a linchpin for community and global health. Understanding the unique economic, social, and environmental factors that influence the health and well-being of the community served by a healthcare organization is core to social sustainability and a moral imperative (Kruk et al., 2018).

First, "do no harm" means healthcare professionals cannot turn their backs on the needs of the whole person, the family, and society at large if committed to quality and safety. The care of critically ill infants cannot be framed by admission and discharge, but must reflect an understanding of the continuum of need for families in crisis. Availability of responsive social support networks, mental health resources, transportation options, adequate nutrition, and shelter is life saving for the family in crisis and is the responsibility of each healthcare team member.

Family engagement is critical to quality care delivery in the NICU. It is linked with fewer adverse events, better patient management, fewer diagnostic tests, decreased use of health services, and shorter lengths of stay (Goodridge et al., 2018). Parents want to participate in the care of their infant, share decision-making, and crave honest, timely, comprehensive information regarding their infant's health and outcomes (Soltys et al., 2020; Umberger et al., 2018).

Summary

To ensure parent presence and engagement within the NICU, clinicians must understand and address the economic, social, spiritual, emotional, and environmental barriers faced by families in crisis. The needs of the infant and family extend beyond the baby's bed space. Perinatal and neonatal healthcare professionals are uniquely positioned to identify vulnerable populations and design comprehensive compassion-based strategies to address SDH and SDG during the NICU stay and beyond (Callister & Edwards, 2017; GBD 2016 SDG Collaborators, 2017).

COMPASSIONATE FAMILY COLLABORATIVE CARE AND THE CLINICIAN

One cannot practice what one does not practice. To enter into a CFCC model, healthcare systems and clinicians must be firmly grounded in the practice of collaboration. Effective nurse–physician collaboration is essential for improved patient outcomes (House & Havens, 2017). Improved outcomes include lower mortality rates, lower ICU readmission rates, and a decrease in healthcare-acquired conditions (Georgiou et al., 2017; Profit et al., 2017; Tawfik et al., 2017; C. D. Welch et al., 2017). Table 7.2 outlines the attributes of the Compassionate Family Collaborative Care Core Measure with examples.

Power differentials, gender issues, and reduced levels of nurse autonomy confound the capacity of healthcare professionals to collaborate authentically and lead to moral distress and burnout (Edwards et al., 2017; Karanikola et al., 2014; Migotto et al., 2019). The humanistic values of nursing have been implicated as a limiting factor to collaboration in a physician-dominated hierarchy (Brown et al., 2014). Differing perspectives, role competition, and turf issues have also been identified as contributing factors that limit collaboration between nurses and physicians (Brown et al., 2014).

Table 7.2 Attributes and Examples of the Compassionate Collaborative Care Core Measure

Attributes	Examples
1. Assessing and supporting emotional well-being is a priority.	*Infant:* Parents are the infant's primary caregivers; spending quality time in physical and emotional proximity with parents is a priority. *Family:* Emotional and psychological well-being of the family in crisis is assessed routinely; there is a process for appropriate referral, care, and support. Staff: Behaviors that reflect burnout and/or staff responses indicative of trauma exposure are responded to compassionately and in a timely manner.
2. Strategies to cultivate and maintain self-efficacy are mentored, supported, and validated.	*Infant:* Infant behavioral cues and developmental capabilities are nurtured in partnership with parents and clinicians over the hospital experience. *Family:* A formal parent education program is integrated into the NICU culture with opportunities for return demonstration to confirm competence and build confidence. *Staff:* Staff are mentored, coached,and supported in the adoption of new knowledge, skills, and attitudes to ensure the highest quality of care.
3. Communication is consistent, compassionate,and reciprocated with respectful active listening.	*Infant:* All infant caring encounters are guided by the infant's behavioral and physiological cues for readiness. *Family:* Parents are valued and respected partners in care; they receive compassionate, consistent information and collaborate in shared-decision-making. *Staff:* All staff receive compassionate communication training and exemplify the tenets of compassionate communication with their patients, the families, and each other.

Source: Reprinted with permission from Caring Essentials Collaborative, LLC.

Hierarchy and power differentials are major barriers to open communication and collaboration among healthcare professionals (Marcelin et al., 2019; Omura et al., 2018a, 2018b). Gender and cultural norms also influence the degree to which nurses participate in assertive communication and speaking up behaviors (Omura et al., 2018b). Assertive communication is requisite for patient safety; however, cultural norms of hierarchy and power constrain nurses' communication and consequently impair collaboration.

Migotto et al. (2019) present the results of a cross-sectional study examining the impact of gender on collaboration. The historical dominant–subservient relationship in the traditional male medical model has shifted with more women entering medicine and more men entering nursing. Migotto et al. (2019) uncover the unconscious gender bias in healthcare that pervades society at large. A decrease in collaboration was reported with male nurses versus female nurses when the unit was led by female physicians.

Adopting a CFCC model serves as a foundation to cultivate effective partnerships among clinicians, patients, families, organizational leadership, and communities (Lown et al., 2016). Clinician perceptions and mindset regarding parents as primary caregivers can undermine the adoption of family-centered care and compassionate family collaboration (Oude Maatman et al., 2020). Education on family-centered care and compassion training is key.

Perceived barriers to compassion have been described by Singh et al. (2018). Personal, workplace/systems and relational barriers between clinicians and their patients have been identified (Table 7.3; Singh et al., 2018). Understanding how these facilitators and barriers

Table 7.3 Barriers and Facilitators to Compassion

Category	Theme	Subthemes
Challenges to compassion	Personal challenges	• Egotistic caregiving • Individual differences in clinician innate virtues
	Relational challenges	• Conditional compassion: Stigmatization and prejudice toward patients • Conditional compassion: Perceived lack of patient and family receptivity to compassion
	Systemic challenges	• Competing system demands • Time constraints
	Maladaptive responses	• Treating challenges to compassion as excuses for not being compassionate
Facilitators to compassion	Personal facilitators	• Self-care • Contemplative practices • Personal experiences of suffering
	Relational facilitators	• Expressions of gratitude and positive feedback for clinician compassion • Sense of connection
	Systemic facilitators	• Compassionate organization and practice culture
	Adaptive responses	• Cultivating compassion through intentional action

Source: Singh, P., Raffin-Bouchal, S., McClement, S., Hack, T. F., Stajduhar, K., Hagen, N. A., Sinnarajah, A., Chochinov, H. M., & Sinclair, S. (2018). Healthcare providers' perspectives on perceived barriers and facilitators of compassion: Results from a grounded theory study. *Journal of Clinical Nursing, 27*(9–10), 2083–2097. doi: 10.1111/jocn.14357 Reprinted with permission from John Wiley & Son.

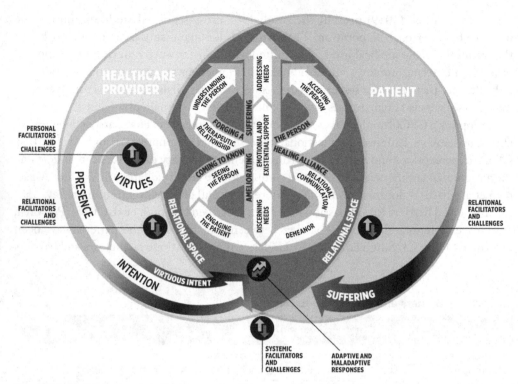

Figure 7.1 Facilitators and challenges to a healthcare provider compassion model.

Source: Singh, P., Raffin-Bouchal, S., McClement, S., Hack, T. F., Stajduhar, K., Hagen, N. A., Sinnarajah, A., Chochinov, H. M., & Sinclair, S. (2018). Healthcare providers' perspectives on perceived barriers and facilitators of compassion: Results from a grounded theory study. *Journal of Clinical Nursing, 27*(9–10), 2083–2097. doi: 10.1111/jocn.14357 Reprinted with permission from John Wiley and Sons.

impact the flow of compassion provides insight to address existing challenges to compassionate collaboration within the NICU (Figure 7.1; Singh et al., 2018).

Paternalistic values and a lack of shared decision-making and patient-centered care persist in healthcare organizations. Compassionate, collaborative interdisciplinary teamwork must address the power inequities that exist in hierarchical healthcare systems. The adoption of compassionate collaborative and empowering approaches will improve care delivery and outcomes for patients, families, and professionals in complex healthcare environments (Ocloo et al., 2020).

EVIDENCE-BASED STRATEGIES TO FACILITATE COMPASSIONATE FAMILY COLLABORATIVE CARE FOR THE CLINICIAN

Core competencies for interprofessional collaborative practice underpin CFCC (Table 7.4). *Interprofessional collaborative practice* is defined as the partnership among clinicians, patients,

Table 7.4 Core Competencies for Interprofessional Collaborative Practice

Competency 1	Work with individuals of other professions to maintain a climate of mutual respect and shared values.
Competency 2	Use the knowledge of one's own role and those of other professions to appropriately assess and address the healthcare needs of patients and to promote and advance the health of populations.
Competency 3	Communicate with patients, families, communities, and professionals in health and other fields in a responsive and responsible manner that supports a team approach to the promotion and maintenance of health and the prevention and treatment of disease.
Competency 4	Apply relationship-building values and the principles of team dynamics to perform effectively in different team roles to plan, deliver, and evaluate patient-/population-centered care and population health programs and policies that are safe, timely, efficient, effective, and equitable.

Source: Reprinted with permission from the Interprofessional Education Collaborative. (2016). *Core competencies for interprofessional collaborative practice: 2016 update.* https://hsc.unm.edu/ipe/resources/ipec-2016-core-competencies.pdf

and their families in shared decision-making, coordination, and cooperation (Morley & Cashell, 2017). Building confidence, competence, and process in interprofessional collaborative practice opens the way for CFCC.

Cultivating compassion, empathy, and emotional competence humanizes the healthcare experience, enabling nurses to align with their core values and achieve both professional satisfaction and compassion satisfaction. Humanizing the NICU experience is a process of communication and support for the family in crisis with the goal of transforming and transcending their lived experience of trauma (del Carmen Perez-Fuentes et al., 2020). Humanization-based interventions increase physical and emotional closeness while promoting partnerships through compassionate collaboration (del Carmen Perez-Fuentes et al., 2020). Examples of humanized care include mitigating and managing pain and stress, providing psychosocial support, respecting language needs, ensuring access to accurate information, and respectful communication, privacy and continuity of care (del Carmen Perez-Fuentes et al., 2020).

Strategies to counter unconscious bias (gender, ethnic, and other) is not only relevant for clinicians but families as well. Mitigating this pervasive phenomenon requires an intentional, multidimensional approach (Marcelin et al., 2019). Personal- and organizational-level strategies are presented in Figures 7.2 and 7.3 to address and mitigate unconscious bias in the practice setting.

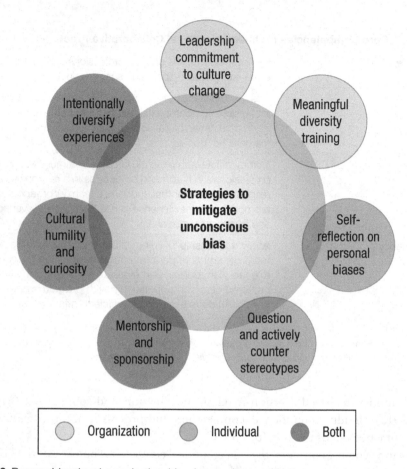

Figure 7.2 Personal-level and organizational-level strategies to mitigate unconscious bias.

Source: Marcelin, J. R., Siraj, D. S., Victor, R., Kotadia, S., & Maldonado, Y. A. (2019). The impact of unconscious bias in healthcare: How to recognize and mitigate it. *Journal of Infectious Disease, 220* (Suppl. 2), s62–s73. doi: 10.1093/infdis/jiz214 Reprinted with permission from Oxford University Press.

As advocates for patients and families in crisis, it is imperative that nurses have the self-efficacy to communicate effectively. Speaking up assertively when patient safety is at risk is a moral and ethical obligation. Assertiveness communication training builds skills and builds intention in a hierarchical healthcare context (Omura et al., 2017, 2019a, 2019b). Preceptorship programs and role modeling byseasoned nursing staff foster these skills in clinical practice (Mansour & Mattukoyya, 2019).

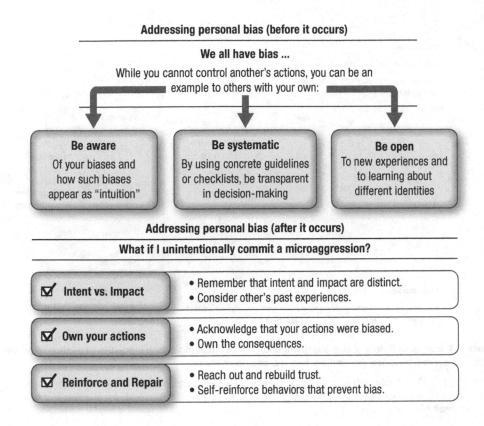

Addressing personal bias (before it occurs)

We all have bias ...

While you cannot control another's actions, you can be an example to others with your own:

Be aware
Of your biases and how such biases appear as "intuition"

Be systematic
By using concrete guidelines or checklists, be transparent in decision-making

Be open
To new experiences and to learning about different identities

Addressing personal bias (after it occurs)

What if I unintentionally commit a microaggression?

☑ **Intent vs. Impact**
- Remember that intent and impact are distinct.
- Consider other's past experiences.

☑ **Own your actions**
- Acknowledge that your actions were biased.
- Own the consequences.

☑ **Reinforce and Repair**
- Reach out and rebuild trust.
- Self-reinforce behaviors that prevent bias.

Figure 7.3 Strategies to address personal bias before and after it occurs.

Source: Marcelin, J. R., Siraj, D. S., Victor, R., Kotadia, S., & Maldonado, Y. A. (2019). The impact of unconscious bias in healthcare: How to recognize and mitigate it. *Journal of Infectious Disease, 220* (Suppl. 2), s62–s73. doi: 10.1093/infdis/jiz214 Reprinted with permission from Oxford University Press.

COMPASSIONATE FAMILY COLLABORATIVE CARE AND THE FAMILY

The capacity for mothers and families of critically ill infants to partner with clinicians in the care of their infant is influenced by a myriad of factors. Physical and emotional health, economic and social resources, culture, medical establishments, social policy, and structural injustice impact parenting behaviors in the NICU and more broadly the individual's health trajectory over the life span (Figure 7.4; Krieger, 2020; Pineda et al., 2018). Understanding these factors and how they play out in the life of the family in crisis is critical to cocreate compassionate, collaborative, and supportive relationships in the NICU (see Chapter 6).

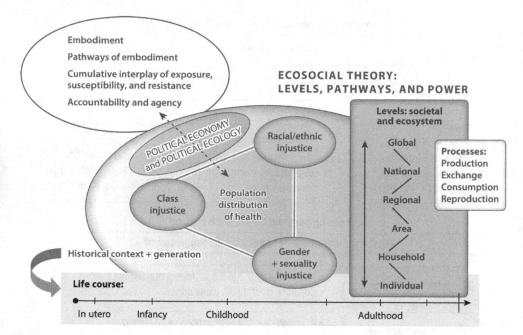

Figure 7.4 Ecosocial theory of disease distribution conceptualizing health inequities in relation to power levels, life course, historical generation, biology, and ecosystems.

Source: Krieger, N. (2020). Measures of racism, sexism, heterosexism, and gender binarism for health equity research: From structural injustice to embodied harm—An ecosocial analysis. *Annual Review of Public Health, 41,* 37–62. doi: 10.1146/annurev-publhealth-040119-094017

The hierarchical structure of healthcare often silences the voice of the patient and family who are perceived as ranking lower in the hierarchy (Griscti et al., 2017). Social discrimination further compounds this hierarchical structure. Social discrimination is differentiating the treatment of an individual based on their actual or perceived characteristics and adds to the burden of socially disadvantaged groups (D'Anna et al., 2018).

Social discrimination occurs across gender, ethnicity, and even includes weight bias and obesity discrimination (refer to Chapter 6; Jones & Jomeen, 2017; Mulherin et al., 2013; Phelan et al., 2015; Spahlholz et al., 2015). Social discrimination threatens the health and well-being of individuals, the family, and society. Nurses' primary commitments are to the patient, promoting, advocating, and protecting the rights, health, and safety of those in their charge with compassion and respect for the inherent dignity, worth, and unique attributes of every person (American Nurses Association, 2015).

Racial, ethnic, and sociodemographic disparities in satisfaction with healthcare are well documented, where Black and Hispanic parents are twice as likely to report dissatisfaction with their child's care as their White counterparts (Lilo et al., 2016). Black parents report dissatisfaction with a lack of support, compassion, and respectful communication with NICU nurses (Martin et al., 2016). White parents express dissatisfaction with inconsistent nursing care, a lack of informative exchanges, and a desire for education about their

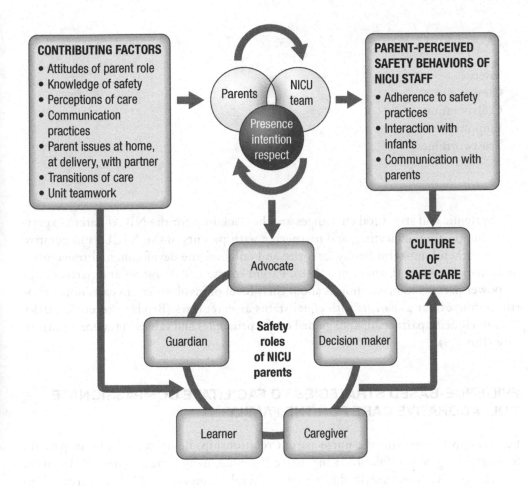

Figure 7.5 Conceptual model of parents as partners in NICU patient safety.

Source: Ottosen, M. J., Engebretson, J., Etchegaray, J., Arnold, C., & Thomas, E. J. (2019). An ethnography of parents' perceptions of patient safety in the neonatal intensive care unit. *Advances in Neonatal Care, 19*(6), 500–508. doi: 10.1097/ANC.0000000000000657 Reprinted with permission from Wolters Kluwer Health, Inc.

infant's short- and long-term needs (Martin et al., 2016). This reality creates a safety risk for all infants and their families.

Parent presence and infant care by the parent reduces the length of hospital stay, decreases hospital readmission rates, and improves infant outcomes to include breastfeeding rates and weight gain (Lee & O'Brien, 2014). Family-based interventions reduce the experience of toxic stress and are linked to improved parental mental well-being, sensitive parenting behaviors, and the infant's cognitive and socioemotional development (Lean et al., 2018; Weber & Harrison, 2019). Parent partnerships with clinicians improve safety through validation of parental role identity and promoting the delivery of safe care for the infant (Figure 7.5; Ottesen et al., 2019).

BOX 7.4 PRINCIPLES AND VALUES OF TRAUMA-INFORMED CARE

Safety
Choice
Collaboration
Empowerment
Trustworthiness

Systemic and structural challenges are the backdrop for the NICU parent experience. Supporting, educating, and partnering with parents in the NICU is imperative to strengthen long-term family integrity and enhance the developmental trajectories of high-risk infants (Lean et al., 2018). Parent–nurse collaboration and partnerships empower parents to make choices about their level of involvement in care, not as substitute nurses but as *parents* with equal status as caregivers (Brodsgaard et al., 2019). Parent–clinician partnerships are guided by the principles and values of trauma-informed care (Box 7.4).

EVIDENCE-BASED STRATEGIES TO FACILITATE COMPASSIONATE COLLABORATIVE CARE FOR THE FAMILY

Partnership begins with the nurse–parent relationship. Being considerate of parent's feelings, being respectful, practicing active listening, demonstrating trust and sharing knowledge have been described by parents as fundamental to establishing partnerships with clinicians (Brodsgaard et al., 2019). Ottosen et al. (2019) provide definitions and exemplars of parent roles in the NICU to guide nurses in fostering parent–clinician partnerships (Table 7.5).

A. Bry and Wigert (2019) explored the psychosocial needs of NICU parents and how staff can support these needs during the NICU stay. Four themes emerged to guide how NICU nurses can build congruent relationships with parents that support CFCC (Table 7.6). Hall et al. (2016) published 10 recommendations to create comprehensive family support in the NICU that also enhances CFCC (Box 7.5). For additional family support resources, visit the resource section of this chapter.

Table 7.5 Definitions and Exemplars of Parent Roles to Promote Safe Care

Role	Definition	Exemplar
Advocate	Speak up for my infant's needs to the healthcare team in the NICU.	"It definitely is frustrating when a nurse is trying to tell you something different. And I'm trying to educate you about my baby so I can leave and be comfortable."
Caregiver	Recognize and provide the activities of care that my infant needs.	"Once they get into the crib, there are certain milestones that they have to hit before we take them upstairs. And then we'll get a chance to interact with the babies a little bit more, get used to being around them and identifying what their needs are. So, when we get them home it'll be, you know, easier."
Decision-maker	Help make decisions about my infant's care.	"(Mom was told) We're gonna go through the weekend and if it's still bad by Monday, we'll give her the medicine." And my thing was why? Why are we waiting until Monday? It's not like it's going to change. This is something you already know, so let's just be proactive. So I don't want to wait until Monday."
Guardian	Protect my infant from uncertain harms and ensure my baby is in a safe environment.	"You (as the mom) want to know who's coming in the room, who's going to touch my baby, or if somebody's looking at him, like who are you? Who you with?"
Learner	Learn how to provide individualized care for my infant's needs.	"My responsibilities while I'm in here, basically just to try my best to know my baby's needs. So when I go home, her needs—her concern—what to look for—what not to look for ... I tell nurses all the time, what you tell me (about my baby) is gold."

Source: Ottosen, M. J., Engebretson, J., Etchegaray, J., Arnold, C., & Thomas, E. J. (2019). An ethnography of parents' perceptions of patient safety in the neonatal intensive care unit. *Advances in Neonatal Care, 19*(6), 500–508. doi: 10.1097/ANC.0000000000000657
Reprinted with permission from Wolters Kluwer Health, Inc.

Table 7.6. Themes, Subthemes, and Strategies to Support Psychosocial Needs of Parents in the NICU

Theme	Subthemes	Strategies
1. Emotional support	• Empathic treatment by staff • Other parents as a unique source of support • Unclear roles of the various professions	• Establish personal practices to cultivate loving-kindness (refer to Chapter 5 and the ten caritas processes). • Review/address unconscious biases (seeFigure 7.3). • Organize a peer-to-peer parent support group (Box 7.5). • Develop resource materials for families that clarify roles and responsibilities of the various disciplines in the NICU (an example is Quantum Caring for Parents, see Reader Resources section of this chapter).
2. Feeling able to trust the healthcare provider	• Quality of information • Timeliness of information • Familiarity/relationship with staff • Trustworthiness of staff	• Require communication skills training for all NICU staff (K. Bry et al., 2016; Hall et al., 2015; investigate the "Orsini Way" of communication training—link is available in the Reader Resources section of this chapter). • Develop trusting interpersonal caring relationships (refer to Chapter 5).
3. Support in balancing time spent with the infant and other responsibilities	• Understanding the complexity of the family's situation • Incongruent expectations	• Engage in transpersonal teaching–learning experiences (refer to Chapter 5). • Provide staff education on the psychosocial needs of NICU parents (Hall et al., 2015). • Find link to staff course of psychosocial support endorsed by the National Perinatal Association.
4. Privacy	• Private rooms did not guarantee privacy • Lack of quiet spaces to withdraw for moments of reflection • Involuntary exposure to other family's problems	• Implement best practices to afford family privacy in the NICU (private rooms, speaking in soft tones, knocking before entering a room, etc.). • Identify quiet spaces that may be dedicated toparents. • Discusswith families the suitability of the space with families; explore options; engage family. • Ensure confidentiality and privacy for conversations (between staff, family, etc.).

Source: Adapted from Bry, A., & Wigert, H. (2019). Psychosocial support for parents of extremely preterm infants in neonatal intensive care: A qualitative interview study. *BMC Psychology, 7,* 76. https://doi.org/10.1186/s40359-019-0354-4

BOX 7.5 TOP 10 RECOMMENDATIONS TO CREATE COMPREHENSIVE FAMILY SUPPORT IN NICUS

1. Policies are in place to guide how NICU staff routinely mentor parents in the developmental care of their babies.
2. Parent participation in medical rounds and nursing shift-change reports is welcomed and encouraged. Parents are involved as 24/7 members of the care team.
3. The NICU has, or is affiliated with, a parent-to-parent peer-support program, which is offered to all parents. Best practice includes a paid position for a parent support coordinator.
4. NICUs with more than 20 beds have a dedicated master's-level social worker *and* a full- or part-time PhD psychologist on staff or available by consultation to provide verbal therapeutic support to parents according to a layered levels of support model as well as to support staff as needed. Larger NICUs should have proportionally more NICU mental health professionals (NMHPs) on staff.
5. NMHPs should strive to meet with all parents/primary caregivers within 1 to 3 days of admission to establish a working relationship, normalize emotional distress, and evaluate risk factors for all forms of emotional distress. Screening of both mothers and fathers should be done within the first week and repeated when practical, especially before discharge and when concerns arise.
6. The NICU has policies for palliative and bereavement care, and staff have been educated in how to deliver this care.
7. A NICU point person is responsible for coordinating predischarge needs of families, including specific educational needs, scheduling of appointments, ordering home supplies and equipment, and communicating with follow-up providers. Planning for transition to outpatient care should begin at admission to ensure that appropriate care continues beyond discharge.
8. At NICU discharge, every family is connected with some type of follow-up support, whether provided through a phone contact or in-person visit by a community-based public health home visiting program, a NICU nurse, therapist, or developmental specialist or a continued relationship with a peer mentor. Postdischarge support should include screening for emotional distress and paraprofessional therapeutic support.
9. NICU staff regularly (once a year or more frequently) receive education on the psychosocial needs of parents and how to meet these needs, as well as education on self-care to minimize burnout.
10. A pastoral care staff person is embedded in the NICU staff team, to provide both parents and staff with support.

Source: Hall, S. L., Phillips, R., & Hynan, M. T. (2016). Transforming NICU care to provide comprehensive family support. *Newborn and Infant Nursing Reviews*, 16(2), 69–73. https://doi.org/10.1053/j.nainr.2016.03.008 Reprinted with permission from Elsevier.

COMPASSIONATE FAMILY COLLABORATIVE CARE AND THE INFANT

Hospitalized infants are at risk for socio-emotional deficits, disturbed executive function, cognitive and language delays and psychiatric disorders (Beebe et al., 2018; Porges et al., 2019). The paucity of mother–infant face-to-face communication in the NICU contributes to these deficits (Margolis et al., 2019). Alterations in bonding-related early-life experiences within the context of the NICU impairs hormonal, epigenetic, and neuronal development in preterm infants (Kommers et al., 2015).

Social relationships early in life are mediated by the neuropeptide hormone oxytocin. Oxytocin plays a critical role in early-life nurturing, social bonding, and attachment (Box 7.6; Filippa et al., 2019; Scatliffe et al., 2019). Skin-to-skin care increases oxytocin levels in both mothers and fathers and is an effective neuroprotective strategy for the immature brain of the critically ill hospitalized infant (Filippa et al., 2019; Zinni et al., 2018).

When parents take on the role of primary caregiver for their infant in the NICU, they experience significantly lower stress, anxiety, and depression (O'Brien et al., 2018; M. G. Welch, Halperin, et al., 2015). Infants cared for under a family integrated care model demonstrate a statistically significant increase in average daily weight gain when compared to controls with a higher frequency of exclusive breast-milk feedings at discharge (O'Brien et al., 2018). Maternal engagement in the NICU is linked to

---

BOX 7.6 ACTIONS OF OXYTOCIN

- Regulates autonomic nervous system.
- Increases social sensitivity.
- Modulates reactivity to stressors.
- Enhances social competence.
- Modulates pain expression.
- Modulates vocal learning circuits.

Sources: Adapted from Filippa, M., Poisbeau, P., Mairesse, J., Grazia Monaci, M., Baud, O., Huppi, P., Grandjean, D., & Kuhn, P. (2019). Pain, parental involvement, and oxytocin in the neonatal intensive care unit. *Frontiers in Psychology, 10,* 715. https://doi.org/10.3389/fpsyg.2019.00715; Scatliffe, N., Casavant, S., Vittner, D., & Cong, X. (2019). Oxytocin and early parent–infant interactions: A systematic review. *International Journal of Nursing Sciences, 6*(4), 445–453. https://doi.org/10.1016/j.ijnss.2019.09.009; Theofanopoulou, C., Boeckx, C., & Jarvis, E. D. (2017). A hypothesis on a role of oxytocin in the social mechanism of speech and vocal learning. *Proceedings in Biological Sciences, 284*(1861), 20170988. https://doi.org/10.1098/rspb.2017.0988

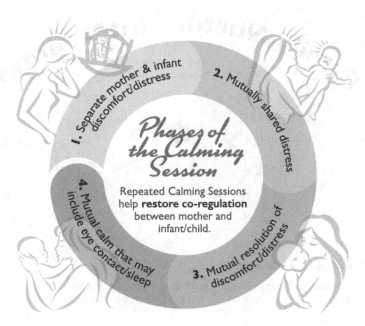

Figure 7.6 Phases of the calming-cycle session.

Source: Welch, M. G. (2016). Calming cycle theory: The role of visceral/autonomic learning in early mother and infant/child behavior and development. *Acta Paediatrica, 105*(11), 1266–1274. doi: 10.1111/apa.13547 Reprinted with permission from John Wiley and Sons.

improved infant outcomes, maternal health behavior, maternal mental health, caregiving behaviors, bonding, and breastfeeding outcomes (Beebe et al., 2018; Hane et al., 2015; Klawetter et al., 2019; M. G. Welch, Firestein, et al., 2015; M. G. Welch, Halperin, et al., 2015). Skin-to-skin care is the most studied maternal engagement activity responsible for these positive results.

The Family Nurture Intervention (FNI) has been shown to promote cerebral cortical development and accelerate brain maturation in preterm infants (Isler et al., 2018; C. D. Welch et al., 2017). The primary goal of the FNI is to establish co-regulation between infant and mother through mutual emotional expressions (M. G. Welch, 2016). In a randomized controlled study, infants who received sensory mediated mother–infant nurturing experiences demonstrated enhanced development of autonomic regulation and vagal efficiency reflecting neurophysiological maturation (Porges et al., 2019). Examples of nurturing experiences are represented through the calming cycle in Figures 7.6 and 7.7.

Social isolation for the developing human results in pervasive and lifelong perturbations to physical, psychological, and emotional development. Creating meaningful, role-validating experiences for NICU parents invariably benefits the infant and can mitigate short-term and long-term morbidity. Reducing the long-term morbidity in preterm infants is beyond the scope of technologically driven interventions and requires a return to the heart and soul of nursing care—unitary caring science (refer to Chapter 5).

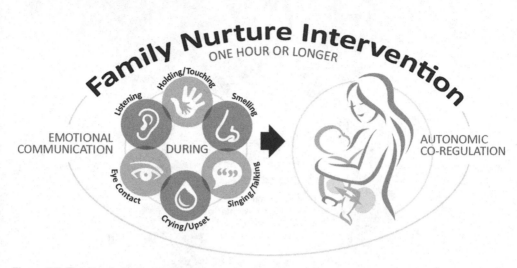

Figure 7.7 The Family Nurture Intervention.

Source: Welch, M. G. (2016). Calming cycle theory: The role of visceral/autonomic learning in early mother and infant/child behavior and development. *Acta Paediatrica, 105*(11), 1266–1274. doi: 10.1111/apa.13547 Reprinted with permission from John Wiley and Sons.

EVIDENCE-BASED STRATEGIES TO FACILITATE COMPASSIONATE FAMILY COLLABORATIVE CARE FOR THE INFANT

Reducing toxic stress for the critically ill hospitalized infant improves outcomes and is achieved through the compassionate and intentional actions of the neonatal nurse. Nurse-guided interventions that support parent–infant synchrony and co-regulation increase plasma oxytocin levels in the infant exposing the infant and family to the benefits of oxytocin described in Box 7.6. A sample of nurse guided interventions include:

- Promoting and facilitating early, frequent, and sustained experiences of skin-to-skin contact (Weber et al., 2018).
- Empowering parents to actively care for and parent their hospitalized infant (Hane et al., 2015; O'Brien et al., 2018).
- Providing comforting touch during caregiving encounters to include containment (aka "hand hugs") and swaddled holding (Weber et al., 2018).
- Minimizing stressors—*chronic stress dampens oxytocin secretion* (Weber et al., 2018).
- Speaking to the infant with a prosodic voice—"motherese" or infant-directed speech (Filippa et al., 2019).
- Promoting breastfeeding and/or breast-milk feeding (Weber et al., 2018).

Activating the calming cycle (Figures 7.6 and 7.7) facilitates emotional connection between the infant and parent and releases oxytocin (M. G. Welch & Ludwig, 2017). Interventions that facilitate parent–infant emotional connection include the exchange of

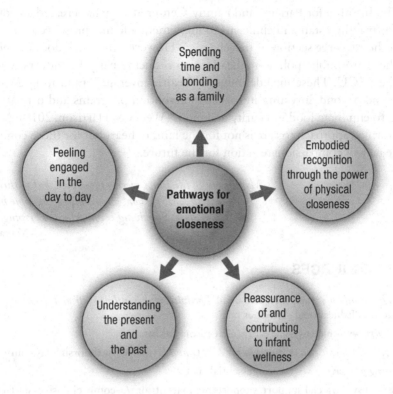

Figure 7.8 Pathways for emotional closeness.

Source: Flacking, R., Thomson, G., & Axelin, A. (2016). Pathways to emotional closeness in neonatal units—A cross-national qualitative study. *BMC Pregnancy Childbirth, 16,* 170. https://doi.org/10.1186/s12884-016-0955-3

a scented cloth (from infant and parent), skin-to-skin care and holding, comfort touch, eye contact, vocal soothing, listening, and deep emotional expression from the parent (M. G. Welch & Ludwig, 2017). These sensory engagements facilitate a coregulated release of oxytocin—the calming and connection hormone and the antithesis of cortisol.

Using a salutogenic approach (refer to Chapter 6), Flacking et al. (2016) pursued a qualitative study to understand pathways to emotional closeness for parents in the NICU. Five themes emerged to guide NICU nurses in supporting and facilitating emotional closeness (Figure 7.8). Nursing skill to facilitate closeness evolves over time and with experience (Skelton et al., 2019). Developing a robust, competency-based education and mentorship program for new nurses and new hires to build the requisite knowledge, skills, and attitudes that facilitate physical and emotional closeness is a best practice. Standardizing practice to promote parental proximity physically and emotionally ensures that all infants and parents experience the benefits of closeness in the NICU and beyond.

The evidence is overwhelming. Supporting and facilitating parent–infant closeness, engagement, and self-efficacy improves outcomes for the infant, the family, and society at large. The Institute for Patient- and Family-Centered Care has created an educational resource for frontline staff and clinicians to implement a family presence policy (refer to the link in the resource section of this chapter). However, the work does not end in the NICU. There are public policy implications to reducing early-life adversity and toxic stress in the NICU. These include universal health coverage, eradicating disparities in healthcare and beyond, investing in earlier intervention programs and primary preventive efforts to eliminate food insecurity and more (Weber & Harrison, 2019). Adopting a trauma-informed approach to care is not for the faint of heart but for those committed to leaving a legacy of compassionate action for the future.

> *My mission in life is not merely to survive, but to thrive; and to*
> *do so with some passion, some compassion, some humor, and*
> *some style. Surviving is important. Thriving is elegant.*
> —Maya Angelou

READER RESOURCES

Implementing a family presence policy: Educational activities for frontline staff and clinicians: ipfcc.org/bestpractices/Educational-Activities.pdf

NICU Awareness: www.nicuawareness.org/nicu-resources.html

The Orsini way—Difficult conversations in the NICU and beyond: www.theorsiniway.com

Quantum caring for parents: www.caringessentials.net

Staff course for psychosocial support: support4nicuparents.org/a-comprehensive-staff-education-course-on-psychosocial-support

Support 4 NICU Parents: support4nicuparents.org

REFERENCES

American Nurses Association. (2015). *Code of ethics for nurses with interpretive statements.* Nursesbooks.org. https://www.nursingworld.org/practice-policy/nursing-excellence/ethics/code-of-ethics-for-nurses/coe-view-only

Amoo, N., Malby, R., & Mervyn, K. (2016). Innovation and sustainability in a large-scale healthcare improvement collaborative–seven propositions for achieving system-wide innovation and sustainability. *International Journal of Sustainable Strategic Management, 5*(2), 149–179. https://doi.org/10.1504/IJSSM.2016.080465

Beebe, B., Myers, M. M., Lee, S. H., Lange, A., Ewing, J., Rubinchik, N., Andrews, H., Austin, J., Hane, A., Margolis, A. E., Hofer, M., Ludwig, R. J., & Welch, M. G. (2018). Family Nurture Interception for preterm infants facilitates positive mother-infant face-to-face engagement at four months. *Developmental Psychology, 54*(11), 2016–2031. https://doi.org/10.1037/dev0000557

Brodsgaard, A., Pedersen, J. T., Larsen, P., & Weis, J. (2019). Parents' and nurses' experiences of partnership in neonatal intensive care units: A qualitative review and meta-synthesis. *Journal of Clinical Nursing, 28*(17–18), 3117–3139. https://doi.org/10.1111/jocn.14920

Brown, S. S., Lindell, D. F., Dolansky, M. A., & Garber, J. S. (2014). Nurses' professional values and attitudes toward collaboration with physicians. *Nursing Ethics, 22*(2), 205–216. https://doi.org/10.1177/0969733014533233

Bry, A., & Wigert, H. (2019). Psychosocial support for parents of extremely preterm infants in neonatal intensive care: A qualitative interview study. *BMC Psychology, 7*, 76. https://doi.org/10.1186/s40359-019-0354-4

Bry, K., Bry, M., Hentz, E., Karlsson, H. L., Kyllonen, H., Lundkvist, M., & Wigert, H. (2016). Communication skills training enhances nurses' ability to respond with empathy to parents' emotions in a neonatal intensive care unit. *Acta Paediatrica, 105*(4), 397–406. https://doi.org/10.1111/apa.13295

Callister, L. C., & Edwards, J. E. (2017). Sustainable development goals and the ongoing process of reducing maternal mortality. *Journal of Obstetric, Gynecologic & Neonatal Nursing, 46*(3), e56–e64. https://doi.org/10.1016/j.jogn.2016.10.009

D'Anna, L., Hansen, M., Mull, B., Canjura, C., Lee, E., & Sumstine, S. (2018). Social discrimination and healthcare: A multidimensional framework of experiences among a low-income multiethnic sample. *Social Work & Public Health, 33*(3), 187–201. https://doi.org/10.1080/19371918.2018.1434584

del Carmen Perez-Fuentes, M., Herrera-Peco, I., del Mar Molero-Jurado, M., Oropesa Ruiz, N. F., Ayuso-Murillo, D., & Gazquez Linares, J. J. (2020). A cross-sectional study of empathy and emotion management: Key to a work environment for humanized care in nursing. *Frontiers in Psychology, 11*, 706. https://doi.org/10.3389/fpsyg.2020.00706

Edwards, P. B., Rea, J. B., Oermann, M. H., Hegarty, E. J., Prewitt, J. R., Rudd, M., Silva, S., Nagler, A., Turner, D. A., & DeMeo, S. D. (2017). Effect of peer-to-peer nurse-physician collaboration on attitudes toward the nurse-physician relationship. *Journal for Nurses in Professional Development, 33*(1), 13–18. https://doi.org/10.1097/NND.0000000000000310

Feeney, B. C., & Collins, N. L. (2015a). New look at social support: A theoretical perspective on thriving through relationships. *Personality and Social Psychology Review, 19*(2), 113–147. https://doi.org/10.1177/1088868314544222

Feeney, B. C., & Collins, N. L. (2015b). Thriving through relationships. *Current Opinions in Psychology, 1*, 22–28. https://doi.org/10.1016/j.copsyc.2014.11.001

Filippa, M., Poisbeau, P., Mairesse, J., Grazia Monaci, M., Baud, O., Huppi, P., Grandjean, D., & Kuhn, P. (2019). Pain, parental involvement, and oxytocin in the neonatal intensive care unit. *Frontiers in Psychology, 10*, 715. https://doi.org/10.3389/fpsyg.2019.00715

Flacking, R., Thomson, G., & Axelin, A. (2016). Pathways to emotional closeness in neonatal units—A cross-national qualitative study. *BMC Pregnancy Childbirth, 16*, 170. https://doi.org/10.1186/s12884-016-0955-3

GBD 2016 SDG Collaborators. (2017). Measuring progress and projecting attainment on the basis of past trends of the health-related Sustainable Development Goals in 188 countries: An analysis from the Global Burden of Disease Study 2016. *Lancet, 390*(10100), 1423–1459. https://doi.org/10.1016/S0140-6736(17)32336-X

Georgiou, E., Papathanassoglou, E. D. E., & Pavlakis, A. (2017). Nurse-physician collaboration and associations with perceived autonomy in Cypriot critical care nurses. *Nursing Critical Care, 22*(1), 29–39. https://doi.org/10.1111/nicc.12126

Goodridge, D., Henry, C., Watson, E., McDonald, M., New, L., Harrison, E. L., Scharf, M., Penz, E., Campbell, S., & Rotter, T. (2018). Structured approaches to promote patient and family engagement in treatment in acute care hospital settings: Protocol for a systematic scoping review. *Systematic Reviews, 7*, 35. https://doi.org/10.1186/s13643-018-0694-9

Griscti, O., Aston, M., Warner, G., Martin-Misener, R., & McLeod, D. (2017). Power and resistance within the hospital's hierarchical system: The experiences of chronically ill patients. *Journal of Clinical Nursing, 26*(1–2), 238–247. https://doi.org/10.1111/jocn.13382

Hall, S. L., Cross, J., Selix, N. W., Patterson, C., Segre, L., Chuffo-Siewert, R., Geller, P. A., & Martin, M. L. (2015). Recommendations for enhancing psychosocial support of NICU parents through staff education and support. *Journal of Perinatology*, *35*, s29–s36. https://doi.org/10.1038/jp.2015.147

Hall, S. L., Phillips, R., & Hynan, M. T. (2016). Transforming NICU care to provide comprehensive family support. *Newborn and Infant Nursing Reviews*, *16*(2), 69–73. https://doi.org/10.1053/j.nainr.2016.03.008

Hane, A. A., Myers, M. M., Hofer, M. A., Ludwig, R. J., Halperin, M. S., Austin, J., Glickstein, S. B., & Welch, M. G. (2015). Family Nurture Intervention improves the quality of maternal caregiving in the neonatal intensive care unit: Evidence from a randomized controlled trial. *Journal of Developmental & Behavioral Pediatrics*, *36*, 188–196. https://doi.org/10.1097/DBP.0000000000000148

House, S., & Havens, D. (2017). Nurses' and physicias'' perceptions of nurse-physician collaboration: A systematic review. *Journal of Nursing Administration*, *47*(3), 165–171. https://doi.org/10.1097/NNA.0000000000000460

Isler, J. R., Stark, R. I., Grieve, P. G., Welch, M. G., & Myers, M. M. (2018). Integrated information in the EEG of preterm infants increases with family nurture intervention, age and conscious state. *PLoS One*, *13*(10), e0206237. https://doi.org/10.1371/journal.pone.0206237

Jones, C., & Jomeen, J. (2017). Women with a BMI ≥ 30 kg/m² and their experience of maternity care: A meta ethnographic synthesis. *Midwifery*, *53*, 87–95. https://doi.org/10.1016/j.midw.2017.07.011

Karanikola, M. N. K., Albarran, J. W., Drigo, E., Giannakopoulou, M., Kalafati, M., Mpouzika, M., Tsiaousis, G. Z., & Papathanassoglou, E. D. E. (2014). Moral distress, autonomy and nurse-physician collaboration among intensive care unit nurses in Italy. *Journal of Nursing Management*, *22*(4), 472–484. https://doi.org/10.1111/jonm.12046

Khayatzadeh-Mahani, A., Labonte, R., Ruckert, A., & de Leeuw, E. (2019). Using sustainability as a collaborations magnet to encourage multi-sector collaborations for health. *Global Health Promotion*, *26*(1), 100–104. https://doi.org/10.1177/1757975916683387

Klawetter, S., Greenfield, J. C., Speer, S. R., Brown, K., & Hwang, S. S. (2019). An integrative review: Maternal engagement in the neonatal intensive care unit and health outcomes for U.S.-born preterm infants and their parents. *AIMS Public Health*, *6*(2), 160–183. https://doi.org/10.3934/publichealth.2019.2.160

Kommers, D., Oei, G., Chen, W., Feijs, L., & Oetomo, S. B. (2015). Suboptimal bonding impairs hormonal, epigenetic and neuronal development in preterm infants, but these impairments can be reversed. *Acta Paediatrica*, *105*(7), 738–751. https://doi.org/10.1111/apa.13254

Krieger, N. (2020). Measures of racism, sexism, heterosexism, and gender binarism for health equity research: From structural injustice to embodied harm—An ecosocial analysis. *Annual Review of Public Health*, *41*, 37–62. https://doi.org/10.1146/annurev-publhealth-040119-094017

Kruk, M. E., Gage, A. D., Arsenault, C., Jordan, K., Leslie, H. H., Roder-DeWan, S., Adeyi, O., Barker, P., Daelmans, B., Doubova, S. V., English, M., Garcia Elorrio, E., Guanais, F., Gureje, O., Hirschhorn, L. R., Jiang, L., Kelley, E., Lemango, E. T., Liljestrand, J., … Pate, M. (2018). High-quality health systems in the sustainable development goals era: Time for a revolution. *Lancet Global Health*, *6*(11), e1196–e1252. https://doi.org/10.1016/S2214-109X(18)30386-3

Lean, R. E., Rogers, C. E., Paul, R. A., & Gerstein, E. D. (2018). NICU hospitalization: Long-term implications on parenting and child behaviors. *Current Treatment Options in Pediatrics*, *4*(1), 49–69. https://doi.org/10.1007/s40746-018-0112-5

Lee, S. K., & O'Brien, K. (2014). Parents as primary caregivers in the neonatal intensive care unit. *Canadian Medical Association Journal*, *186*(11), 845–847. https://doi.org/10.1503/cmaj.130818

Lilo, E. A., Shaw, R. J., Corcoran, J., Storfer-Isser, A., & Horwitz, S. M. (2016) Does she think she's supported? Maternal perceptions of their experiences in the neonatal intensive care unit. *Patient Experience Journal*, *3*(1), 4. https://pxjournal.org/journal/vol3/iss1/4

Lown, B. A., McIntosh, S., Gaines, M. E., McGuinn, K., & Hatem, D. (2016). Integrating compassionate collaborative care (the "Triple C") into health professional education to advance the triple aim of health care. *Academic Medicine*, *91*(3), 310–316. https://doi.org/10.1097/ACM.0000000000001077

Maghsoudi, T., Cascon-Pereira, R., & Hernandez Lara, A. B. (2020). The role of collaborative healthcare in improving social sustainability: A conceptual framework. *Sustainability*, *12*, 3195. https://doi.org/10.3390/su12083195

Mansour, M., & Mattukoyya, R. (2019). Development of assertive communication skills in nursing preceptorship programmes: A qualitative insight from newly qualified nurses. *Nursing Management*, *26*(4), 29–35. https://doi.org/10.7748/nm.2019.e1857

Marcelin, J. R., Siraj, D. S., Victor, R., Kotadia, S., & Maldonado, Y. A. (2019). The impact of unconscious bias in healthcare: How to recognize and mitigate it. *Journal of Infectious Disease*, *220*(Suppl. 2), s62–s73. https://doi.org/10.1093/infdis/jiz214

Margolis, A. E., Lee, S. H., Peterson, B. S., & Beebe, B. (2019). Profiles of infant communicative behavior. *Developmental Psychology*, *55*(8), 1594–1604. https://doi.org/10.1037/dev0000745

Martin, A. E., D'Agostino, J. A., Passarella, M., & Lorch, S. A. (2016). Radial differences in parental satisfaction with neonatal intensive care unit nursing care. *Journal of Perinatology*, *36*(11), 1001–1007. https://doi.org/10.1038/jp.2016.142

Migotto, S., Garlatti Costa, G., Ambrosi, E., Pittino, D., Bortoluzzi, G., & Palese, A. (2019). Gender issues in physician-nurse collaboration in healthcare teams: Finding from a cross-sectional study. *Journal of Nursing Management*, *27*(8), 1773–1783. https://doi.org/10.1111/jonm.12872

Morley, L., & Cashell, A. (2017). Collaboration in health care. *Journal of Medical Imaging and Radiation Sciences*, *48*, 207–216. https://doi.org/10.1016/j.jmir.2017.02.071

Mulherin, K., Miller, Y. D., Barlow, F. K., Diedrichs, P. C., & Thompson, R. (2013). Weight stigma in maternity care: Women's experiences and care providers' attitudes. *BMC Pregnancy and Childbirth*, *13*, 19. https://doi.org/10.1186/1471-2393-13-19

O'Brien, K., Robson, K., Bracht, M., Cruz, M., Lui, K., Alvaro, R., da Silva, O., Monterrosa, L., Narvey, M., Ng, E., Soraisham, A., Ye, X. Y., Mirea, L., Tarnow-Mordi, W., Lee, S. K.; FICare Study Group and FICare Parent Advisory Board. (2018). Effectiveness of family integrated care in neonatal intensive care units on infant and parent outcomes: A multicenter, multinational, cluster-randomized controlled trial. *Lancet Child & Adolescent Health*, *2*(4), 245–254. https://doi.org/10.1016/S2352-4642(18)30039-7

Ocloo, J., Goodrich, J., Tanaka, H., Birchall-Searle, J., Dawson, D., & Farr, M. (2020). The importance of power, context and agency in improving patient experience through a patient and family centered care approach. *Health Research, Policy and Systems*, *18*, 10. https://doi.org/10.1186/s12961-019-0487-1

Omura, M., Levett-Jones, T., & Stone, T. E. (2019a). Evaluating the impact of an assertiveness communication training programme for Japanese nursing students: A quasi-experimental study. *Nursing Open*, *6*(2), 463–472. https://doi.org/10.1002/nop2.228

Omura, M., Levett-Jones, T., & Stone, T. E. (2019b). Design and evaluation of an assertiveness communication training programme for nursing students. *Journal of Clinical Nursing*, *28*(9–10), 1990–1998. https://doi.org/10.1111/jocn.14813

Omura, M., Maguire, J., Levett-Jones, T., & Stone, T. E. (2017). The effectiveness of assertiveness communication training programs for healthcare professionals and students: A systematic review. *International Journal of Nursing Studies, 76*, 120–128. https://doi.org/10.1016/j.ijnurstu.2017.09.001

Omura, M., Stone, T. E., & Levett-Jones, T. (2018a). Cultural factors influencing Japanese nurses' assertive communication. Part 1: Collectivism. *Nursing & Health Sciences, 20*(3), 283–288. https://doi.org/10.1111/nhs.12411

Omura, M., Stone, T. E., & Levett-Jones, T. (2018b). Cultural factors influencing Japanese nurses' assertive communication: Part 2—Hierarchy and power. *Nursing & Health Sciences, 20*(3), 289–295. https://doi.org/10.1111/nhs.12418

Ottosen, M. J., Engebretson, J., Etchegaray, J., Arnold, C., & Thomas, E. J. (2019). An ethnography of parents' perceptions of patient safety in the neonatal intensive care unit. *Advances in Neonatal Care, 19*(6), 500–508. https://doi.org/10.1097/ANC.0000000000000657

Oude Maatman, S. M., Bohlin, K., Lillieskold, S., Garberg, H. T., Uitewaal-Poslawsky, I., Kars, M. C., & van den Hoogen, A. (2020). Factors influencing implementation of family-centered care in a neonatal intensive care unit. *Frontiers in Pediatrics, 8*, 222. https://doi.org/10.3389/fped.2020.00222

Pfaff, K., & Markaki, A. (2017). Compassionate collaborative care: An integrative review of quality indicators in end-of-life care. *BMC Palliative Care, 16*, 65. https://doi.org/10.1186/s12904-017-0246-4

Phelan, S. M., Burgess, D. J., Yeazel, M. W., Hellerstedt, W. L., Griffin, J. M., & van Ryn, M. (2015). Impact of weight bias and stigma on quality of care and outcomes for patients with obesity. *Obesity Reviews, 16*(4), 319–326. https://doi.org/10.1111/obr.12266

Pineda, R., Bender, J., Hall, B., Shabosky, L., Annecca, A., & Smith, J. (2018). Parent participation in the neonatal intensive care unit: Predictors and relationships to neurobehavior and developmental outcomes. *Early Human Development, 117*, 32–38. https://doi.org/10.1016/j.earlhumdev.2017.12.008

Porges, S. W., Davila, M. I., Lewis, G. F., Kolacz, J., Okonmah-Obazee, S., Hane, A. A., Kwon, K. Y., Ludwig, R. J., Myers, M. M., & Welch, M. G. (2019). Autonomic regulation of preterm infants is enhanced by family nurture intervention. *Developmental Psychobiology, 61*(1), 1–11. https://doi.org/10.1002/dev.21841

Profit, J., Sharek, P. J., Kan, P., Rigdon, J., Desai, M., Nisbet, C. C., Tawfik, D. S., Thomas, E. J., Lee, H. C., & Sexton, J. B. (2017). Teamwork in the NICU setting and its association with healthcare-associated infections in very low birth weight infants. *American Journal of Perinatology, 34*(10), 1032–1040. https://doi.org/10.1055/s-0037-1601563

Scatliffe, N., Casavant, S., Vittner, D., & Cong, X. (2019). Oxytocin and early parent–infant interactions: A systematic review. *International Journal of Nursing Sciences, 6*(4), 445–453. https://doi.org/10.1016/j.ijnss.2019.09.009

Singh, P., Raffin-Bouchal, S., McClement, S., Hack, T. F., Stajduhar, K., Hagen, N. A., Sinnarajah, A., Chochinov, H. M., & Sinclair, S. (2018). Healthcare providers' perspectives on perceived barriers and facilitators of compassion: Results from a grounded theory study. *Journal of Clinical Nursing, 27*(9–10), 2083–2097. https://doi.org/10.1111/jocn.14357

Skelton, H., Dahlen, H. G., Psaila, K., & Schmied, V. (2019). Facilitating closeness between babies with congenital abnormalities and their parents in the NICU: A qualitative study of neonatal nurses' experiences. *Journal of Clinical Nursing, 28*(15–16), 2979–2989. https://doi.org/10.1111/jocn.14894

Soltys, F., Philpott-Streiff, S. E., Fuzzell, L., & Politi, M. C. (2020). The importance of shared-decision-making in the neonatal intensive care unit. *Journal of Perinatology, 40*, 504–509. https://doi.org/10.1038/s41372-019-0507-6

Spahlholz, J., Baer, N., Honig, H.-H., Riedel-Heller, S. G., & Luck-Silkorski, C. (2015). Obesity and discrimination—A systematic review and meta-analysis of observational studies. *Obesity Reviews, 17*(1), 43–55. https://doi.org/10.1111/obr.12343

Tawfik, D. S., Sexton, J. B., Adair, K. C., Kaplan, H. C., & Profit, J. (2017). Context in quality of care: Improving teamwork and resilience. *Clinica in Perinatology, 44*(3), 541–552. https://doi.org/10.1016/j.clp.2017.04.004

Umberger, E., Canvasser, J., & Hall, S. L. (2018). Enhancing NICU parent engagement and empowerment. *Seminars in Pediatric Surgery, 27*(1), 19–24. https://doi.org/10.1053/j.sempedsurg.2017.11.004

United Nations. Department of Economic and Social Affairs: Sustainable Development. (n.d.). *The 127 goals*. sdgs.un.org/goals

Weber, A., & Harrison, T. M. (2019). Reducing toxic stress in the NICU to improve infant outcomes. *Nursing Outlook, 67*(2), 169–189. https://doi.org/10.1016/j.outlook.2018.11.002

Weber, A., Harrison, T. M., Sinnott, L., Shoben, A., & Steward, D. (2018). Associations between nurse-guided variables and plasma oxytocin trajectories in premature infants during initial hospitalization. *Advances in Neonatal Care, 18*(1), e12–e23. https://doi.org/10.1097/ANC.0000000000000452

Welch, C. D., Check, J., & O'Shea, T. M. (2017). Improving care collaboration for NICU patients to decrease length of stay and readmission rate. *BMJ Open Quality, 6*(2), e000130. https://doi.org/10.1136/bmjoq-2017-000130

Welch, M. G. (2016). Calming cycle theory: The role of visceral/autonomic learning in early mother and infant/child behavior and development. *Acta Paediatrica, 105*(11), 1266–1274. https://doi.org/10.1111/apa.13547

Welch, M. G., Firestein, M. R., Austin, J., Hane, A. A., Stark, R. I., Hofer, M. A., Garland, M., Glickstein, S. B., Brunelli, S. A., Ludwig, R. J., & Myers, M. M. (2015). Family Nurture Intervention in the neonatal intensive care unit improves social-relatedness, attention, and neurodevelopment of preterm infants at 18 months in a randomized controlled trial. *Journal of Child Psychology and Psychiatry, 56*(11), 1202–1211. https://doi.org/10.1111/jcpp.12405

Welch, M. G., Halperin, M. S., Austin, J., Stark, R. I., Hofer, M. A., Hane, A. A., & Myers, M. M. (2015). Depression and anxiety symptoms of mothers of preterm infants are decreased at 4 months corrected age with Family Nurture Intervention in the NICU. *Archives of Womens Mental Health, 19*, 51–61. https://doi.org/10.1007/s00737-015-0502-7

Welch, M. G., & Ludwig, R. J. (2017). Calming cycle theory and the coregulation of oxytocin. *Psychodynamic Psychiatry, 45*(4), 519–541. https://doi.org/10.1521/pdps.2017.45.4.519

Welch, M. G., Stark, R. I., Grieve, P. G., Ludwig, R. J., Isler, J. R., Barone, J. L., & Myers, M. M. (2017). Family nurture intervention in preterm infants increases early development of cortical activity and indepe3ndence of regional power trajectories. *Acta Paediatrica, 106*(12), 1952–1960. https://doi.org/10.1111/apa.14050

Zinni, M., Colella, M., Novais, A. R. B., Baud, O., & Mairesse, J. (2018). Modulating the oxytocin system during the perinatal period: A new strategy for neuroprotection of the immature brain? *Frontiers in Neurology, 9*, 229. https://doi.org/10.3389/fneur.2018.00229

8

Protected Sleep

Protecting sleep is critical for health and safety. This chapter presents the latest research regarding the importance of sleep for the hospitalized infant, the family, and the healthcare professional.

WHAT IS SLEEP?

The National Institute of Mental Health (NIMH) defines *sleep* and *wakefulness* as "endogenous, recurring, behavioral states that reflect coordinated changes in the dynamic functional organization of the brain and that optimize physiology, behavior and health" (NIMH, 2013). Sleep health is influenced by genetics, disease, and lifestyle; in turn, these factors impact the quality of one's sleep (Figure 8.1; Buysse, 2014). Specific dimensions of sleep have been linked to disturbances in health outcomes.

The five most relevant dimensions of sleep quality impacting overall health and well-being include: (a) duration, (b) efficiency and continuity, (c) timing, (d) alertness, and (e) satisfaction (Figure 8.1).

Duration

Sleep duration is the total amount of time spent asleep in a 24-hour period. Total sleep needs vary across the life span, with very premature infants requiring up to 21 hours of sleep per day. The National Sleep Foundation updated their sleep-duration recommendations for newborns through older adults in 2015 after performing a rigorous systematic review of the global scientific literature linking sleep duration to health, performance, and safety outcomes (Table 8.1; National Sleep Foundations, 2015).

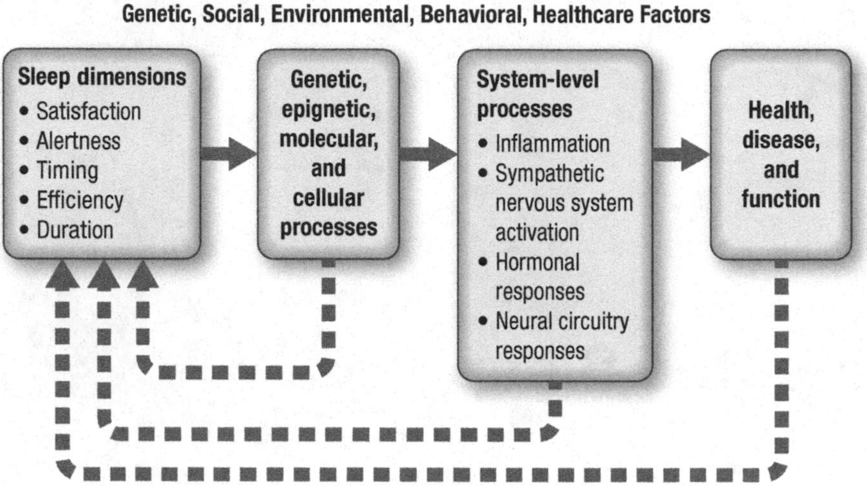

Genetic, Social, Environmental, Behavioral, Healthcare Factors

Figure 8.1 Conceptual model of sleep health.

Source: Reprinted with permission from Buysse, D. J. (2014). Sleep health: Can we define it? Does it matter? *Sleep,* 37(1), 9–17. doi: 10.5665/sleep.3298

Table 8.1 National Sleep Foundation's Sleep-Duration Recommendations, 2015

Age Group	Recommended	May Be Appropriate	Not Recommended
Newborns (0–3 months)	14–17 hours/day	11–13 hours 18–19 hours	Less than 11 hours More than 19 hours
Infants (4–11 months)	12–15 hours/day	10–11 hours 16–18 hours	Less than 10 hours More than 18 hours
Toddlers (1–2 years)	11–14 hours/day	9–10 hours 15–16 hours	Less than 9 hours More than 16 hours
Preschoolers (3–5 years)	10–13 hours/day	8–9 hours 14 hours	Less than 8 hours More than 14 hours
School-aged children (6–13 years)	9–11 hours/day	7–8 hours 12 hours	Less than 7 hours More than 12 hours
Teenagers (14–17 years)	8–10 hours/day	7 hours 11 hours	Less than 7 hours More than 11 hours
Younger adults (18–25 years)	7–9 hours/day	6 hours 10–11 hours	Less than 6 hours More than 11 hours
Adults (25–64 years)	7–9 hours/day	6 hours 10 hours	Less than 6 hours More than 10 hours
Older adults (65+)	7–8 hours/day	5–6 hours 9 hours	Less than 5 hours More than 9 hours

Efficiency and Continuity

Sleep efficiency and *continuity* refer to the ease with which one can fall asleep and stay asleep. In general, it should take about 10–20 minutes to fall asleep, this period is called *sleep latency*. If it takes longer than an hour to fall asleep, this may indicate insomnia or a disturbance in the circadian rhythm (such as jet lag). If one falls asleep as soon as their head hits the pillow, this may be an indicator of sleep deprivation and an accruing sleep debt warranting immediate attention.

Timing

Timing refers to when sleep is placed within the 24-hour day. We are biologically wired to sleep at night and be awake during the day; we follow a diurnal, circadian rhythm. Every cell in the body has its own circadian rhythm. The master circadian pacemaker is the suprachiasmatic nucleus, located in the hypothalamus, which controls the timing of sleep–wake cycles (Moore, 2007).

Alertness

Alertness or lack of alertness (aka sleepiness) speaks to how one can maintain an attentive state while awake. Although this dimension of sleep quality is influenced by the duration and timing of sleep, it can also be impacted by diet and disease as well as environment, lifestyle, and occupational factors (Dahlgren et al., 2016; St-Onge et al., 2016).

Satisfaction

One's sleep satisfaction, which is purely subjective, answers the question: Was the sleep "good" or "poor?" The Epworth Sleepiness Scale (Johns, 1991) is the most popular sleep assessment tool. However, it is limited to assessing sleepiness and does not address the other dimensions of sleep health and sleep quality. The Satisfaction Alertness Timing Efficiency and Duration (SATED) scale (Exhibit 8.1), developed by a team at the University of Pittsburgh, is a user-friendly, self-report sleep health assessment scale (Buysse, 2014). This scale assesses the five dimensions of sleep quality, including specific quantitative aspects of sleep, that have been identified as physiologically relevant in the literature (Buysse, 2014).

Summary

Sleep is regulated by an overlap of the circadian system, which endogenously synchronizes biologic rhythms, and sleep–wake homeostasis, which drives the body toward sleep or waking (Bathory & Tomopoulos, 2017). Disruptions or perturbations to sleep quality in adults are linked to cardiovascular disease, obesity, dementia, and even cancer. For developing individuals, such as preterm infants, newborns, and young children, poor sleep health compromises brain growth and development and is linked to cognitive, behavioral, and neurodevelopmental impairments (Table 8.2; Gogou et al., 2019; Williamson et al., 2019).

EXHIBIT 8.1 SATED SCALE

		Rarely/ Never (0)	Sometimes (1)	Usually/ Always (2)
<u>S</u>atisfaction	Are you satisfied with your sleep?			
<u>A</u>lertness	Do you stay awake all day without dozing?			
<u>T</u>iming	Are you asleep (or trying to sleep) between 2 a.m. and 4 a.m.?			
<u>E</u>fficiency	Do you spend less than 30 minutes awake at night? (This includes the time it takes to fall asleep and awakenings from sleep.)			
<u>D</u>uration	Do you sleep between 6 and 8 hours per day?			

Total for all for items ranges from 0 to 10

0 = Poor Sleep Health   Good Sleep Health = 10

Source: Reprinted with permission from Buysse, D. J. (2014). Sleep health: Can we define it? Does it matter? *Sleep*, *37*(1), 9–17. doi: 10.5665/sleep.3298

SLEEP AND THE CLINICIAN

The biological relevance of sleep for overall health, wellness, and survival is significantly downplayed in modern day-to-day life, especially among healthcare professionals. We all know we need sleep; we know it's important, but for the most part, we pay little attention to those activities, habits, and choices that undermine healthy sleep. Table 8.2 outlines the attributes and examples of the protected sleep core measure.

When we are sleepy on the job, we pose a safety hazard to our patients, their families, our colleagues, and ourselves. Shift work additionally challenges our efforts to protect and promote sleep health. In addition to shift work, job stress and workload

Table 8.2 Protected Sleep Core Measure Attributes and Examples

Attributes	Examples
Sleep integrity and circadian rhythmicity are protected for infants, families, and clinicians.	*Infant:* Scheduled, nonemergent care is provided during wakeful states. *Family:* Sleep education is provided to all families; single-family rooms are equipped with sleep protection resources (cycled lighting, recommended sound levels, comfortable sleeping surfaces, etc.). *Staff:* Shift-workers are provided with sleep education for self-health and safety.
Strategies that support sleep for infants, families, and clinicians are an integral component of care and self-care.	*Infant:* Skin-to-skin care is an integral component in the daily care of eligible infants. *Family:* Education on the importance of sleep hygiene routines for infants and families is provided. *Staff:* Supportive sleep routines are endorsed and encouraged by staff and the organization.
Safe sleep practices for infants, families, and clinicians are adopted, role-modeled, and incorporated into daily routine.	*Infant:* Infants are transitioned to safe sleep practices in the hospital with consistency and reliability. *Family:* Parents demonstrate competency in safe sleep practices for their infant and themselves to discharge to home. *Staff:* Strategies to ensure staff safety regarding the sleep displacement/disruption associated with shift work are supported by staff peers and the organization at large.

Source: Reprinted with permission from Caring Essentials Collaborative, LLC.

also impact sleep. Job demands have been negatively linked to sleep quality, emotional exhaustion, presenteeism (showing up to work ill), and lower levels of relaxation (Gillet et al., 2020).

Short intervals between shifts, defined as less than 11 hours between the end of one shift and the beginning of the next, is associated with shorter sleep durations and reduced sleep quality (Dahlgren et al., 2016). This misalignment with circadian rhythms increases the risk of workplace accidents and injuries by inducing sleep deficiency, sympathovagal and hormonal imbalances, inflammation, impaired glucose metabolism, and dysregulated cell cycles (James et al., 2017).

James et al. (2017) highlight four domains of health adversely impacted by shift work (Figure 8.2). Beyond circadian misalignment, shift work determines when a person will eat, exercise, socialize, and engage in sexual activity, all of which have ramifications on physical and mental health (James et al., 2017). A recent systematic review of shift work and nurses'

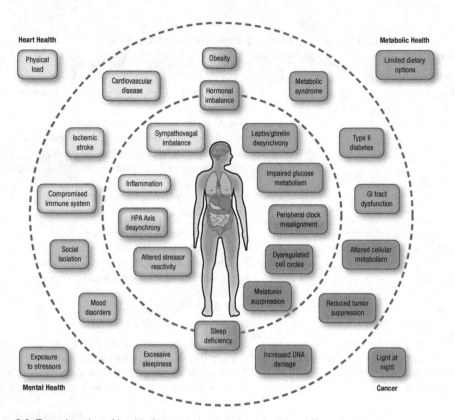

Figure 8.2 Four domains of health that are adversely impacted by shift work.

GI, gastrointestinal; HPA, hypothalamic–pituitary–adrenal.
Source: Reprinted with permission from James, S. M., Honn, K. A., Gaddameedhi, S., & Van Dongen, H. P. A. (2017). Shift work: Disrupted circadian rhythms and sleep—Implications for health and well-being. *Current Sleep Medicine Reports, 3*(2), 104–112. doi: 10.1007/s40675-017-0071-6

health (Rosa et al., 2019) revealed that, in addition to the lifestyle disturbances, shift work is a risk factor for stress, sleep disorders, metabolic syndromes, diabetes, cardiovascular disease, and breast cancer.

The International Commission on Occupational Health launched a series of consensus papers developed by the Working Time Society to provide guidance on managing fatigue associated with shift work (Wong et al., 2019). They developed a fatigue risk trajectory, which outlines a sequence of events that may lead to fatigue-related errors and incidents (Wong et al., 2019). Elements of the trajectory included opportunities for sleep, actual sleep obtained, behavioral symptoms of fatigue, fatigue-related errors, and, fatigue-related incidents (Wong et al., 2019). Although this trajectory has implications and accountability at the individual level, there is also a responsibility to mitigate fatigue-related errors and incidents at the organizational level.

Stressful psychosocial characteristics of the nurse's professional practice environment include decreased nurse manager support, nurse–physician collaboration, and distressing patient events that negatively affect the behaviors, attitudes, and psychological well-being of healthcare professionals with implications for sleep quality (Gillet et al., 2020; Knupp et al., 2019). Psychological detachment from work when off shift allows the individual to disengage from work-related activities, feelings, and thoughts (Hulsheger et al., 2018). The level of disengagement influences the quality of sleep, crucial for the day-to-day recovery of the clinician as optimal sleep quality restores, refreshes, and replenishes the body, mind, and spirit (Hulsheger et al., 2018).

Opportunities to mitigate fatigue-related errors and incidents in the NICU include scheduling patterns, shift length and shift rotation, rest breaks, general staff education and training regarding sleep health, promoting self-care routines for staff, as well as leadership support (Barger et al., 2018; Hulsheger et al., 2018; Knupp et al., 2019; Wong et al., 2017). In a scoping review of the literature, Dall'Ora et al. (2016) reveal the complexity of shift work and identify shift characteristics that impact job performance and professional well-being. In general, 12-hour shifts are associated with decreased quality of care, patient safety, increased errors, and reduced participation in continuing-education programs (Dall'Ora et al., 2016, 2020). Regardless of shift length, shift work, workload, emotional dissonance, and compromised personal wholeness pose a hazard to the patient, the individual, and the organization both on shift and off (Gillet et al., 2020; Knupp et al., 2019; Rosa et al., 2019; Wickwire et al., 2017).

EVIDENCE-BASED STRATEGIES TO PROTECT CLINICIAN SLEEP

Assessing quality of sleep is a first step in protecting sleep. The SATED questionnaire (see Exhibit 8.1) is a reliable and valid measure used to assess sleep health in the general population (Benitez et al., 2020). In addition to assessing sleep quality, chronicling sleep-hygiene routines with a sleep diary can help uncover aspects of one's daily routine that may be hindering sleep quality and sleep health.

The American Nurses Association (ANA) issued a position statement in 2014 calling for collaboration between employers and nurses to reduce the risk of nurse fatigue and the sleepiness associated with shift work and long work hours. In its statement, the ANA urges the implementation of evidence-based strategies to proactively address nurse fatigue and sleepiness (ANA, 2014). Evidence-based strategies that reduce fatigue and sleepiness on duty include exposure to bright light, physical exercise, and naps (Richter et al., 2016; Slanger et al., 2016; Wickwire et al., 2017). Scheduled naps in the workplace for healthcare professionals is recommended by The Joint Commission (2018) to reduce sleepiness and fatigue.

Benefits of night-shift napping include:

- Reduced sleepiness,
- Enhanced well-being,
- Improved psychomotor vigilance,

- Improved job performance,
- Reduced drowsy driving post shift (Geiger Brown et al., 2016; Li et al., 2019; Ruggiero et al., 2014).

Barriers to night-shift napping adoption include:

- Lack of appropriate dedicated space to support restful napping,
- No clear supportive policies,
- Lack of peer support,
- Paucity of shared responsibility among nursing administrators to develop evidence-based programs to counteract the effects of nurse fatigue (Dalky et al., 2018; Edwards et al., 2014; Knupp et al., 2018).

Light "showers" or exposure to bright light during night-shift work has been shown to reset the human central circadian clock (Cuesta et al., 2017). This poses a problem in the patient care area, where bright light may adversely impact the sleep quality of the patients. Portable light-therapy glasses have been shown to significantly reduce sleepiness, enhance vigilance and cognition, while improving mood (Comtet et al., 2019). This resource may have value in settings where the professional is unable to leave the work area but is experiencing sleepiness in the workplace. However, the use of phototherapy (aka light therapy) to reduce sleepiness isn't a "one size fits all" solution; the phase resetting that does occur is based on individual light-exposure patterns relative to an individual's baseline circadian phase (Stone et al., 2018).

Bursts of physical activity or exercise during night-shift work boosts alertness and has been shown to be more effective than acute exposure to blue-enriched lighting (Barba et al., 2018; Slanger et al., 2016). Like exposure to light, exercise has been shown to elicit significant circadian phase-shifting effects and has an additive effect when combined with bright light (Youngstedt et al., 2016, 2019). In the hospital setting, this might mean climbing stairs in a brightly lit stairwell, going for a brisk walk around the facility or, if your organization has a gym, planning for a gym break to boost your alertness. Exercise not only boosts alertness on night shift but has also shown to enhance sleep quality off duty as well (Barba et al., 2018).

Strategies aimed at reducing stress have been shown to improve sleep quality and sleep health for healthcare professionals and are recommended as an integral component to a healthy sleep hygiene routine. Mind-body interventions include a variety of treatments that have a direct impact on health and wellness. Regular yoga practice can reduce work stress while improving sleep quality in staff nurses (Fang & Li, 2015). In a retrospective analysis of outcome data comparing the health benefits of two hospital-provided mind–body interventions (yoga and meditation), the results revealed a significant decrease in depression, anxiety and stress levels while improving sleep quality (Mohapatra & Marshall, 2019).

Sleep is the best meditation.
—Dalai Lama

SLEEP AND THE NICU FAMILY

At baseline, the sleep costs of having children are significant and the incurred sleep debt never resolves. The most pronounced effects of sleep loss are experienced by first-time parents versus repeat parents, mothers more so than fathers, and in breastfeeding compared with bottle-feeding families (Richter et al., 2019). The sleep disturbances experienced by parents in the NICU are complicated by the life-threatening nature of NICU hospitalization and the subsequent disruption to the family's sense of safety and security as the trauma unfolds (Baumgartel & Facco, 2018; Coughlin, 2016).

Poor sleep quality in pregnancy has been associated with perinatal mood disturbances (Gonzalez-Mesa et al., 2019). In a scoping review of the literature, maternal total maternal sleep time was reported to be less than 7 hours/day disrupted by frequent nighttime awakenings with an increase in daytime sleeping (Haddad et al., 2019; Marthinsen et al., 2018). Positive correlations among sleep quality and maternal fatigue, anxiety, stress, and depression have also been reported (Marthinsen et al., 2018). Although mothers seem to experience more stress, anxiety, and depression related to their NICU experience than fathers, both parents experience similar disturbances to their sleep quality (Al Maghaireh et al., 2017). The long-term implications of an accruing sleep debt may jeopardize marital relationships, family dynamics, and the parent–infant relationship (Al Maghaireh et al., 2017; Haddad et al., 2019).

Daily exposure to high stress is directly linked to poor sleep quality (Edell-Gustafsson et al., 2015; Haddad et al., 2019). The types of stressors that negatively impact both mothers and fathers in the NICU include alterations in their parenting role, the infant's appearance and behavior, the sights and sounds of the NICU environment, seeing their infant in pain, being unable to comfort or help their infant, separation, and breathing problems (Al Maghaireh et al., 2017; Matricardi et al., 2013; Prouhet et al., 2018).

Beyond NICU specific stressors, the background of the parents will also influence the degree of psychological distress they experience and can contribute to sleep disturbances (Lange et al., 2019; Muzik et al., 2013; Narayan et al., 2018). Applying a socio-ecological model to the NICU parent experience, Loewenstein (2018) describes variables across intrapersonal, interpersonal, institutional, community, and public policy variables that can affect parent mental health and consequently influence sleep quality.

Mothers of hospitalized newborns experience both nocturnal sleep problems and disturbed circadian rhythms (S.-H. Lee et al., 2010). Poor sleep quality in mothers of premature infants is associated with depression independent of other risk factors to include depression during pregnancy, poor partner relationship, previous experience with depression and stressful life events over the past year (Schaffer et al., 2013). The prevalence rate of postpartum posttraumatic stress disorder (PP-PTSD) is approximately 9% and is caused by a real or perceived intrapartum/postpartum trauma. PP-PTSD in mothers of preterm infants has been reported to be as high as 41% (Shaw et al., 2013).

Causes of PP-PTSD:

- Prolapsed cord,
- Unplanned cesarean section,

- The use of a vacuum extractor or forceps,
- The infant requires NICU care,
- Feelings of powerlessness, poor communication, and/or lack of support and reassurance during the delivery,
- A history of previous trauma in the setting of pregnancy related complications (Postpartum Support International, 2020).

The link between emotional well-being and sleep is irrefutable. Emerging research suggests a link between maternal sleep duration and fetal outcomes, such as low birthweight and preterm birth in mothers who sleep less than 7 hours per day (Warland et al., 2018). Trauma-informed interventions that can improve sleep quality for NICU parents have lifelong implications for the infant, the family, and society at large.

EVIDENCE-BASED STRATEGIES TO PROTECT SLEEP FOR THE NICU FAMILY

Evidence-based strategies that protect sleep for clinicians can also be effective for parents. Parent education regarding the importance of sleep and its association with health and wellness for the entire family can be very empowering and is a preventive strategy that protects sleep health.

Proactive interventions to improve sleep for NICU parents include:

- Skin-to-skin care,
- Bright-light therapy,
- Guided imagery,
- Muscle relaxation techniques,
- Consistent sleep-hygiene practices,
- Aromatherapy (Baumgartel & Facco, 2018; Keshavarz Afshar et al., 2015; Lillehei et al., 2015).

Skin-to-skin care improves bonding and is an effective stress-reducing strategy that improves relaxation and sleep for NICU parents (Edell-Gustafsson et al., 2014). Promoting and facilitating skin-to-skin encounters in the NICU, however, can be fraught with challenges around consistency, a paucity of fall-prevention strategies and resources, nursing beliefs regarding the importance of skin-to-skin care, and rigid routines and rituals that may disempower parents from advocating for this evidence-based intervention. Skin-to-skin care is an evidence-based best practice in the provision of trauma-informed, age-appropriate care for the family in crisis (Eliades, 2018; Sanders & Hall, 2018).

Bright-light therapy used to promote sleep in mothers of low-birth-weight infants resets circadian rhythmicity, which can become desynchronized from stress and dim lighting in the NICU environment (S. Y. Lee et al., 2013). When combined with sleep education, bright-light therapy improves total sleep time, reduces feelings of anxiety and depression, and enhances maternal perception of health-related quality of life (S. Y. Lee et al., 2013). The American Academy of Sleep Medicine recommends light therapy for individuals who experience disruptions to circadian rhythmicity that undermine sleep quality (Auger et al., 2015).

Guided imagery and muscle relaxation have also been found to improve sleep quality (Baumgartel & Facco, 2018). Schaffer et al. (2013) examined the relationship between an 8-week relaxation guided-imagery intervention, sleep quality, and depressive symptoms in a cohort of preterm mothers. The use of relaxation guided imagery was well accepted by the study cohort and improved sleep quality in those mothers who engaged in the intervention. As the average amount of time spent listening to the relaxation guided imagery increased, the Pittsburgh Sleep Quality Index (PSQI) scores decreased, indicating improved sleep quality (Schaffer et al., 2013).

Karbandi et al. (2015) examined the effect of progressive muscle relaxation on the sleep quality of mothers of preterm infants with similar results. In their randomized controlled trial, mothers were taught the relaxation techniques and were then provided with an audio disc and a self-report checklist to record the frequency in which they engaged in the relaxation technique (Karbandi et al., 2015). At the end of 4 and 8 weeks, the intervention group demonstrated statistically significant improvements in their PSQI scores when compared to a control group (Karbandi et al., 2015).

The use of lavender essentials oils in a cohort of postpartum mothers resulted in a statistically significant improvement in sleep quality scores ($p <.05$; Keshavarz Afshar et al., 2015). Lavender aromatherapy during the early postpartum period has been shown to reduce maternal pain and fatigue while boosting maternal mood (Vaziri et al., 2017). Combining the use of lavender aromatherapy with optimal sleep-hygiene practices has demonstrated a lasting positive effect on sleep quality in the general population (Lillehei et al., 2015).

Optimizing sleep quality for NICU parents in the hospital setting can improve parent partnership and participation in the care of their critically ill infant; reduce parental stress, anxiety, and depression; and increase the potential for improved long-term health for the infant and family (Schaffer et al., 2013).

SLEEP AND THE HOSPITALIZED INFANT

Sleep development begins during early fetal life once central and peripheral neural networks are laid out and functional neural circuitry emerges through synaptogenesis, at around 16 weeks of gestation (Bennet et al., 2018). As sleep unfolds during the second trimester, distinct sleep states appear; this evolution in sleep behavior reflects brain maturation and development. As depicted in Figure 8.3, a variety of events can derail healthy development of sleep architecture in the preterm infant with implications for neurogenesis and, ultimately, impaired neurodevelopmental outcomes (Bennet et al., 2018).

The fetus and preterm infant spend most of their 24-hour day asleep. Insufficient sleep in newborns and young infants is linked with increased adiposity, poor emotional regulation, poor overall well-being, and decreased academic performance (Barbeau & Weiss, 2017).

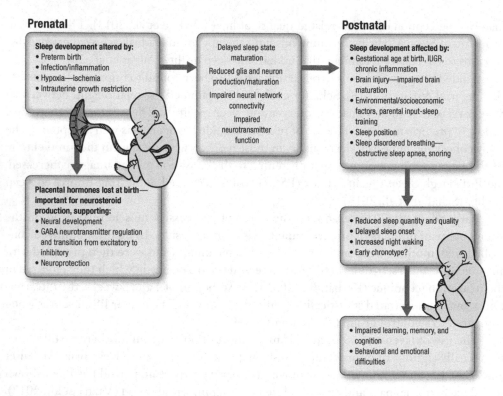

Figure 8.3 Illustration of how adverse experiences before and during preterm birth can alter brain maturation and sleep development.

GABA, gamma-aminobutyric acid; IUGR, intrauterine growth restriction.
Source: Bennet, L., Walker, D. W., & Horne, R. S. C. (2018). Waking up too early—The consequences of preterm birth on sleep develop-ment. *Journal of Physiology*, *23*, 5687–5708. doi: 10.1113/JP274950 Reprinted with permission from John Wiley & Sons.

Sleep states after birth include active sleep (a precursor to rapid eye movement [REM] sleep), quiet sleep (a precursor to no-REM sleep), indeterminate or transitional sleep, and wakefulness (Barbeau & Weiss, 2017; Bennet et al., 2018). As gestation progresses, the total amount of sleep time decreases, from a high of 90% of the 24-hour day in very preterm infants to 70% at term gestation (Barbeau & Weiss, 2017). When compared to full-term infants, premature infants have significant differences in their sleep structure, which impacts total sleep time and arousal threshold (Gogou et al., 2019).

In addition to total sleep time, the configuration of sleep state shifts as the infant matures. In the youngest preterm infant, 80% of sleep time is spent in active sleep (Figure 8.4). During active sleep, the brain is in a rapid state of growth and maturation as neural networks associated with sensory system development, organization, and other critical brain functions are evolving in their complexity (Bennet et al., 2018; Del Rio-Bermudez & Blumberg, 2018).

Quiet sleep is also crucial for brain development. As the infant ages, the proportion of quiet sleep to total sleep time increases (Bennet et al., 2018). Quiet sleep promotes synaptic remodeling through the replaying and processing of experiential input received

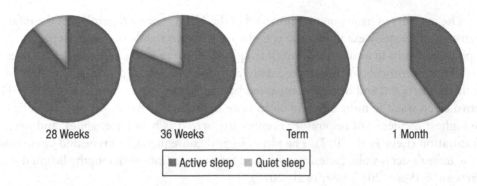

Figure 8.4 Progression of active sleep and quiet sleep.

Source: Barbeau, D. Y., & Weiss, M. D. (2017). Sleep disturbances in newborns. *Children, 4*(10), 90. https://doi.org/10.3390/children4100090

during wakefulness—this is how the infant learns about the world and adapts (Bennet et al., 2018). Neurons that fire together, wire together (Hebb, 1949). Consequently, any disruption to sleep, both active and quiet, compromises the development of neural networks that regulate sleep architecture and brain maturation (Bennet et al., 2018).

In a prospective study, Lan et al. (2019) examined the sleep–wake patterns in a cohort of premature infants over 3 days. Sleep efficiency, total sleep time, average duration and frequency of sleep–wake bouts were collected. The researchers uncovered a link among sleep quality, gender, severity of illness, age (both chronological and corrected), and body weight. Overall, preterm infants demonstrated inadequate sleep efficiency exacerbated by severity of illness, female gender, advanced chronological and corrected age, and birthweight (Lan et al., 2019). The physical, emotional and practice domains associated with the NICU environment further undermines the fragmented sleep intrinsic to hospitalized preterm infants.

Attributes of the physical environment have been associated with sleep disturbances in preterm infants (Casavant et al., 2017; Gogou et al., 2019; Orsi et al., 2017). Preterm infants exhibit a lower arousal threshold that makes them particularly vulnerable to environmental stimuli in the NICU (Gogou et al., 2019). Small increases in light levels increase sleep disruptions in very preterm infants, even when lighting levels are within the recommended range from the American Academy of Pediatrics (AAP; Zores et al., 2018). Kuhn et al. (2013) reported a significant increase in awakenings associated with sound peaks ranging from 5 to 15 decibels above background noise levels. Despite sound level recommendations by the AAP, NICU noise levels consistently exceed 45 decibels (Casavant et al., 2017).

Hospitalized infants are exposed to repeated painful and stressful procedures during their hospital stay (Cong et al., 2017). Pain and sleep are interdependent; pain interferes with the quantity and quality of sleep and insufficient sleep increases an infant's pain sensitivity and somatic symptomatology (Bonan et al., 2014). Pain, stress, and sleep deprivation induce an oxidative stress response that compromises brain growth and development and increases adenosine triphosphate utilization which further reduces the infant's already limited energy stores (Slater et al., 2012; Tan et al., 2018). Please refer to Chapter 4 for more information regarding the energy costs of prematurity.

The majority of hands-on care provided in the NICU occurs regardless of the infant's sleep state. In a study examining the correlation between hands-on care, sleep state, and respiratory events in a cohort of convalescing NICU patients, the researchers discovered that despite protocols for developmentally appropriate clustered care, infant sleep was routinely disrupted and often accompanied by respiratory instability (Levy et al., 2017). Active sleep was the most frequent sleep state disturbed by hands-on care and elicited the highest incidence of respiratory events categorized as hypopnea, apnea, and oxygen desaturation (Levy et al., 2017). The physiological consequences of repeated disruptions of the infant's sleep-wake cycle are magnified for those infant's with lengthy hospital stays (Barbeau & Weiss, 2017; Levy et al., 2017).

Feeding and sleeping patterns of preterm infants are inextricably linked to the NICU routine. However, studies reveal NICU feeding schedules mask infants' natural, endogenous biologic rhythms, inducing an ultradian rhythm (Bueno & Menna-Barreto, 2016). Park et al. (2019) demonstrated an association between sleep–wake cycle maturation and oral feeding skill progression. The maturation of sleep–wake cycles fosters neurobehavioral competence, enabling infants to develop their capacity to interact with the environment physically and emotionally (Park et al., 2019). Sleep–wake states are an indicator of central nervous system maturation as well as a neurobehavioral indicator of the infant's readiness for an oral feeding encounter (Park et al., 2019). Maturation cannot be trained and must unfold on its own trajectory. Expectations for feeding skills not aligned with the infant's physiologic capacity are extremely distressing and potentially damaging to the infant's developmental trajectory (Lubbe, 2018). Supporting and protecting sleep consistently over the hospital experience promotes maturation of sleep–wake cycles and, in turn, supports the maturation of emerging feeding skills that are requisite for optimal feeding outcomes (Lubbe, 2018; Park et al., 2019).

EVIDENCE-BASED STRATEGIES TO PROTECT SLEEP FOR THE INFANT

The gold standard for assessing infant sleep state is polysomnography (Bennet et al., 2016). However, in the immediate clinical setting, attuning to several behavioral indicators provides the trauma-informed clinician with sufficient information to distinguish active sleep from quiet sleep from wakefulness. In active sleep, the infant's eyes will be closed, and eye movements will be evident behind the closed lids. In addition, the infant can exhibit an irregular respiratory pattern, negative facial expressions, and/or sucking movements and random startle-like movements of their extremities in active sleep (Coughlin, 2016). Quiet sleep behaviors include closed eyes without eye movement behind closed lids, regular rhythmic respirations, quiet facies, and an absence of extraneous movement (Coughlin, 2016). The Neonatal Sleep Wake Assessment Tool, developed by Caring Essentials Collaborative, LLC, is an effective teaching tool to build clinicians confidence and competence assessing infant sleep state (Exhibit 8.2).

EXHIBIT 8.2 NEONATAL SLEEP WAKE ASSESSMENT TOOL

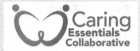

Indicator	0	1	2	Total Score
Eyes	Lids closed with intermittent REM	Lids closed; no REM observed	Lids open	
Respirations	Uneven respirations	Relatively regular and abdominal	Regular respirations, may be crying	
Facial expressions	Negative facial expressions (crying face or a frown)	Quiet facies, occasional sigh/startle	Interactive facies	
Motor activity	Sporadic motor movements, muscle tone low between movements	Tonic level of motor tone is maintained and motor activity is limited to startles or sighs	Motor activity varies but is usually high	
				Cumulative score

Score <3: Neonate is in clear sleep state, do not disturb unless there is a medical emergency.

Score 3–6: If care is indicated, infant should be aroused gently with soft vocalizations and firm but gentle tactile input to a nonvulnerable area (i.e., placing caregiver's hand on the infant's back); increase verbal and tactile input as the infant's arousal level rises.

Score >6: Infant is waking/awake and ready for care.

Neo SWAT, Neonatal Sleep Wake Assessment Tool; REM, rapid eye movement.

Source: Reprinted with permission from Caring Essentials Collaborative, LLC.

Evidence-based environmental strategies to protect sleep in the NICU include (Coughlin, 2016):

- Promote parental proximity and partnership in sleep-hygiene routines.
- Facilitate skin-to-skin care encounters.
- Establish cycled lighting and a quiet acoustic environment.
- Adopt a cue-based approach to care guided by the infant's sleep–wake state.
- Mitigate stress and distress for the baby.
- Support optimal posture for safe, restorative sleep (Coughlin, 2016).

A systematic review of nonpharmacological interventions to promote sleep for preterm infants in the NICU revealed a significant increase in total sleep time and improved active sleep efficiency with the use of remolding mattresses and cycled lighting strategies (Liao et al., 2018). The adoption of "quiet time" practices has been reported to increase total sleep time and decrease sound levels inside the infant's incubator during the quiet-time period (Pugliesi et al., 2018). Quite-time initiatives have decreased ambient noise levels in the NICU, improved infant sleep patterns, and changed nursing staff attitudes about noise-reduction strategies (Casavant et al., 2017). Exposure to cycled lighting in the NICU for infants as young as 28 weeks of gestational age and younger has shown to improve weight gain, reduce length of hospital stay, decrease fussiness and crying behaviors, and promote maturation of sleep architecture (Brandon et al., 2017; Guyer et al., 2012, 2015).

Promoting parent presence and proximity through skin-to-skin care improves infant sleep development while validating parent role identity (Feeley et al., 2016; Ludington-Hoe et al., 2006; Makela et al., 2018; Shorey et al., 2016). Skin-to-skin contact (aka kangaroo care) results in maturation of sleep architecture and brain development. The benefits of skin-to-skin care touch on all five core measures of trauma-informed care.

Benefits of skin-to-skin care include:

- Consistently increases time spent in deep sleep,
- Enhances the infant's ability to sustain quiet, awake and alert states,
- Promotes self-regulatory behaviors (Bastani et al., 2017; Feldman et al., 2002).

Barriers to the adoption of skin-to-skin care for mothers include:

- Issues with limited resources and the facility environment,
- Staff attitudes,
- Safety concerns,
- Lack of support facilitating skin-to-skin care,
- Limited awareness of the benefits of skin-to-skin care (Seidman et al., 2015).

Barriers to the adoption of skin-to-skin care for nurses include:

- Increased workload,
- Concerns about the medical status of the infant,

- Lack of clear guidelines and training,
- Lack of buy-in,
- The belief that skin-to-skin care causes additional work (Seidman et al., 2015).

Education is not enough to change practice; successful change requires engagement, empowerment, and process. Adopting a systematic approach to practice improvement specific to skin-to-skin care can result in a statistically significant increase in the adoption, documentation, and sustainability of skin-to-skin care practices (Coughlin, 2015).

Managing pain consistently and reliably can improve sleep in the hospitalized infant (Bonan et al., 2014). Lan et al. (2018) studied the effectiveness of a supportive-care bundle for procedural pain on infant sleep variables. The supportive-care bundle was provided during each intrusive procedure during the study period. Bundle elements included adjusting light and sound levels, gently waking infant for the procedure with warm hands and a quiet voice, providing the infant with nonnutritive sucking, oral sucrose, and facilitated tucking throughout the intervention (Lan et al., 2018). Preterm infants who received the supportive-care bundle demonstrated a significant increase in sleep efficiency and total sleep time with a decrease in sleep latency and awakenings (Lan et al., 2018). Mitigating infant pain and distress during intrusive procedures provides a dual benefit of pain relief and sleep protection and is the perfect exemplar of a trauma-informed approach to the care of the hospitalized infant.

Infant position during sleep has implications for cardiovascular and cerebrovascular function. Prone sleeping position in both term and preterm infants has been associated with increased heart rate, decreased blood pressure, heart rate variability and baroreflex sensitivity (Shepherd et al., 2018). In healthy term infants past the first 6 months of life, prone sleeping position resulted in decreased cerebral oxygenation despite oxygen saturations remaining stable; these adverse effects are amplified in the premature infant (Shepherd et al., 2018). Sleep position ensures a safe sleep environment for the hospitalized infant prior to and following discharge to home and requires all stakeholders to not only receive education but role modeling and demonstration of safe sleep practices in the hospital and home settings (Dowling et al., 2018; Shepherd et al., 2018).

Nurses caring for infants in the hospital setting are inconsistent in their adoption and implementation of safe sleep practices (Table 8.3; Barsman et al., 2015; Gelfer et al., 2013; Newberry, 2019; Patton et al., 2015). Barriers include lack of knowledge, unsubstantiated beliefs about safety and the supine position, absent or outdated safe sleep policies, and a lack of process and accountability related to the transition of the infant to safe sleep practices (Naugler & DiCarlo, 2018). Addressing these barriers in partnership with parents and clinicians through educational interventions and quality improvement initiatives can ensure safe sleep environments for vulnerable infants in the hospital and at home (Gelfer et al., 2013; Leong et al., 2019; Naugler & DiCarlo, 2018).

Your future depends on your dreams, so go to sleep.
—Mesut Barazany

Table 8.3 American Academy of Pediatrics Safe Sleep Recommendations 2011 and 2016

Topic	2011 AAP Guidelines	2016 AAP Guidelines
Sleep surface	Firm mattress	Firm mattress; no type of sitting device
Crib setup	No bumpers, blankets, or pillows	Fitted sheet, no soft materials or objects; supine
Sleeping position	Supine is recommended, side sleeping is not safe and not advised	Supine
Room sharing	Room sharing without bed sharing is recommended	Separate sleep surface in the parent's room for at least 6 months, preferably for a year
Bed sharing	Not recommended	Not recommended, but mothers may breastfeed in the bed if they think they will fall asleep during feeding if all blankets and pillows are removed in advance
Breastfeeding	Recommended and protective against SIDS	Recommended and protective against SIDS
Pacifier use	Nap and bedtime	Nap and bedtime
Infant monitors	Do not use	Do not use
Vaccinations	Should be immunized	Encourage all infant vaccines recommended by APP and CDC
Tummy time	When awake and supervised to prevent plagiocephaly	When awake and supervised for development
Swaddling	Not mentioned	Snug at chest but provide ample room at hips and knees; stop swaddling when infant can roll
Preterm infants	Should be placed supine as soon as clinically stable and by 32 weeks' postmenstrual age	Should be placed supine as soon as possible, at least from 32 weeks' postmenstrual age onward

AAP, American Academy of Pediatrics; CDC, Centers for Disease Control and Prevention; SIDS, sudden infant death syndrome.
Source: Newberry, J. A. (2019). Creating a safe sleep environment for the infant: What the pediatric nurse needs to know. *Journal of Pediatric Nursing, 44,* 119–122. doi: 10.1016/j.pedn.2018.12.001 Reprinted with permission from Elsevier.

READER RESOURCES

Arianna Huffington's sleep resources: https://www.ariannahuffington.com/sleep-resources

National Sleep Foundation sleep diary: www.sleepfoundation.org/sites/default/files/inline-files/SleepDiaryv6.pdf

7-Minute bedtime yoga–Yoga with Adriene: www.youtube.com/watch?v=LI9upn4t9n8&list=PLui6Eyny-UzwiUzvhM2BjxThodiRWZ2JR&index=2

What happens to your body and brain if you don't get sleep | The human body: www.youtube.com/watch?v=Y-8b99rGpkM

REFERENCES

Al Maghaireh, D. F., Abdullah, K. L., Chong, M. C., Chua, Y. P., & Al Kawafha, M. M. (2017). Stress, anxiety, depression and sleep disturbances among Jordanian mothers and fathers of infants admitted to neonatal intensive care unit: A preliminary study. *Journal of Pediatric Nursing, 36,* 132–140. https://doi.org/10.1016/j.pedn.2017.06.007

American Nurses Association. (2014). *Position statement. Addressing nurse fatigue to promote safety and health: Joint responsibilities of registered nurses and employers to reduce risks.* https://www.patientsafetysolutions.com/docs/December_2_2014_ANA_Position_Statement_on_Nurse_Fatigue.htm

Auger, R. R., Burgess, H. J., Emens, J. S., Deriy, L. V., Thomas, S. M., & Sharkey, K. M. (2015). Clinical practice guideline for the treatment of intrinsic circadian rhythm sleep-wake disorders: Advanced sleep-wake phase disorder (ASWPD), delayed sleep-wake phase disorder (DSWPD), non-24-hour sleep-wake rhythm disorder (N24SWD), and irregular sleep-wake rhythm disorder (ISWRD). An update for 2015. *Journal of Clinical Sleep Medicine, 11*(10), 1199–1236. https://doi.org/10.5664/jcsm.5100

Barba, A., Padilla, F., Luque-Casado, A., Sanabria, D., &. Correa, A. (2018). The role of exercise-induced arousal and exposure to blue-enriched lighting on vigilance. *Frontiers in Human Neuroscience, 12,* 499. https://doi.org/10.3389/fnhum.2018.00499

Barbeau, D. Y., &. Weiss, M. D. (2017). Sleep disturbances in newborns. *Children, 4*(10), 90. https://doi.org/10.3390/children4100090

Barger, L. K., Runyon, M. S., Renn, M. L., Moore, C. G., Weiss, P. M., & Condle, J. P. (2018). Effect of fatigue training on safety, fatigue, and sleep in emergency medical services personnel and other workers: A systematic review and meta-analysis. *Prehospital Emergency Care, 22*(Suppl. 1), 58–68. https://doi.org/10.1080/10903127.2017.1362087

Barsman, S. G., Dowling, D. A., Damato, E. G., & Czeck, P. (2015). Neonatal nurses' beliefs, knowledge, and practices in relation to sudden infant death syndrome risk-reduction recommendations. *Advances in Neonatal Care, 15*(3), 209–219. https://doi.org/10.1097/ANC.0000000000000160

Bastani, F., Rajai, N., Farsi, Z., & Als, H. (2017). The effects of kangaroo care on the sleep and wake states of preterm infants. *Journal of Nursing Research, 25*(3), 231–239. https://doi.org/10.1097/JNR.0000000000000194

Bathory, E., & Tomopoulos, S. (2017). Sleep regulation, physiology and development, sleep duration and patterns, and sleep hygiene in infants, toddlers, and preschool-age children. *Current Problems in Pediatric and Adolescent Health Care, 47*(2), 29–42. https://doi.org/10.1016/j.cppeds.2016.12.001

Baumgartel, K. L., & Facco, F. (2018). An integrative review of the sleep experiences of mothers of hospitalized preterm infants. *Nursing for Women's Health*, *22*(4), 310–326. https://doi.org/10.1016/j.nwh.2018.05.003

Benitez, I., Roure, N., Pinilla, L., Sapina-Beltran, E., Buysse, D. J., Barbe, F., & de Batlle, J. (2020). Validation of the Satisfaction Alertness Timing Efficiency and Duration (SATED) questionnaire for sleep health measurement. *Annals of the American Thoracic Society*, *17*, 338–343. https://doi.org/10.1513/AnnalsATS.201908-628OC

Bennet, L., Fyfe, K. L., Yiallourou, S. R., Merk, H., Wong, F. Y., & Horne, R. S. C. (2016). Discrimination of sleep states using continuous cerebral bedside monitoring (amplitude-integrated electroencephalography) compared to polysomnography in infants. *Acta Paediatrica*, *105*(12), e582–e587. https://doi.org/10.1111/apa.13602

Bennet, L., Walker, D. W., & Horne, R. S. C. (2018). Waking up too early—The consequences of preterm birth on sleep development. *Journal of Physiology*, *23*, 5687–5708. https://doi.org/10.1113/JP274950

Bonan, K. C., Pimentel Filho, J. C., Tristao, R. M., Jesus, J. A., & Campos Junior, D. (2014). Sleep deprivation, pain and prematurity: A review study. *Arquivos de Neuro-Psiquiatria*, *73*(2), 147–154. https://doi.org/10.1590/0004-282X20140214

Brandon, D. H., Silva, S. G., Park, J., Malcolm, W., Kamhawy, H., & Holditch-Davis, D. (2017). Timing for the introduction of cycled light for extremely preterm infants: A randomized controlled trial. *Research in Nursing and Health*, *40*(4), 294–310. https://doi.org/10.1002/nur.21797

Bueno, C., & Menna-Barreto, L. (2016). Environmental factors influencing. Biologic rhythms in newborns: From neonatal intensive care units to home. *Sleep Science*, *9*, 295–300. https://doi.org/10.1016/j.slsci.2016.10.004

Buysse, D. J. (2014). Sleep health: Can we define it? Does it matter? *Sleep*, *37*(1), 9–17. https://doi.org/10.5665/sleep.3298

Casavant, S. G., Bernier, K., Andrews, S., & Bourgoin, A. (2017). Noise in the neonatal intensive care unit: What does the evidence tell us? *Advances in Neonatal Care*, *17*(4), 265–273. https://doi.org/10.1097/ANC.0000000000000402

Comtet, H., Geoffroy, P. A., Frisk, M. K., Hubbard, J., Robin-Choteau, L., Calvel, L., Hugueny, L., Viola, A. U., & Bourgin, P. (2019). Light therapy with boxes or glasses to counteract effects of acute sleep deprivation. *Scientific Reports*, *9*(18073), 1–9. https://doi.org/10.1038/s41598-019-54311-x.

Cong, X., Wu, J., Vittner, D., Xu, W., Hussain, N., Galvin, S., Fitzsimmons, M., McGrath, J. M., & Henderson, W. A. (2017). The impact of cumulative pain/stress on neurobehavioral development of preterm infants in the NICU. *Early Human Development*, *108*, 6–16. https://doi.org/10.1016/j.earlhumdev.2017.03.003

Coughlin, M. (2015). The sobreviver (survive) project. *Newborn and Infant Nursing Reviews*, *15*(4), 169–173. https://doi.org/10.1053/j.nainr.2015.09.010

Coughlin, M. (2016). *Trauma-informed care in the NICU: Evidence-based practice guidelines for neonatal clinicians*. Springer Publishing Company.

Cuesta, M., Boudreau, P., Cermakian, N., & Boivin, D. B (2017). Rapid resetting of human peripheral clocks by phototherapy during simulated night shift work. *Scientific Reports*, *7*(1), 16310. https://doi.org/10.1038/s41598-017-16429-8

Dahlgren, A., Tucker, P., Gustavsson, P., & Rudman, A. (2016). Quick returns and night work as predictors of sleep quality, fatigue, work–family balance and satisfaction with work hours. *Chronobiology International*, *33*(6), 759–767. https://doi.org/10.3109/07420528.2016.1167725

Dalky, H. F., Raeda, A. F., & Esraa, A. A. (2018). Nurse managers' perception of night-shift napping: A cross-sectional survey. *Nursing Forum*, *53*(2), 173–178. https://doi.org/10.1111/nuf.12239

Dall'Ora, C., Ball, J., Recio-Saucedo, A., & Griffiths, P. (2016). Characteristics of shift work and their impact on employee performance and wellbeing: A literature review. *International Journal of Nursing Studies*, *57*(1), 12–27. https://doi.org/10.1016/j.ijnurstu.2016.01.007

Dall'Ora, C., Griffiths, P., Emmanuel, T., Rafferty, A. M., Ewings, S.; RN4CAST Consortium. (2020). 12-hr shifts in nursing: Do they remove unproductive time and information loss, or do they reduce education and discussion opportunities for nurses? A cross-sectional study in 12 European countries. *Journal of Clinical Nursing*, *29*(1–2), 53–59. https://doi.org/10.1111/jocn.14977

Del Rio-Bermudez, C., &. Blumberg, M. S. (2018). Active sleep promotes functional connectivity in developing sensorimotor networks. *Bioassays*, *40*(4), e1700234. https://doi.org/10.1002/bies.201700234

Dowling, D. A., Barsman, S. G., Forsythe, P., & Damato, E. G. (2018). Caring about preemies' safe sleep (CaPSS): An educational program to improve adherence to safe sleep recommendations by mothers of preterm infants. *Journal of Perinatal and Neonatal Nursing*, *32*(4), 366–372. https://doi.org/10.1097/JPN.0000000000000345

Edell-Gustafsson, U., Angelhoff, C., Johnsson, E., Karlsson, J., & Morelius, E. (2015). Hindering and buffering factors for parental sleep in neonatal care: a phenomenographic study. *Journal of Clinical Nursing*, *24*(5–6), 717–727. https://doi.org/10.1111/jocn.12654

Edwards, M. P., McMillan, D. E., & Fallis, W. M. (2014). Napping during breaks on night shift: A critical care nurse managers' perceptions. *Dynamics*, *24*(4), 30–35.

Eliades, C. (2018). Mitigating infant medical trauma in the NICU: Skin-to-skin contact as a trauma-informed, age-appropriate best practice. *Neonatal Network*, *37*(6), 343–350. https://doi.org/10.1891/0730-0832.37.6.343

Fang, R. & Li, X. (2015). A regular yoga intervention for staff nurse sleep quality and work stress: A randomized controlled trial. *Journal of Clinical Nursing*, *24*, 3374–3379. https://doi.org/10.1111/jocn.12983

Feeley, N., Genest, C., Niela-Vilen, H., Charbonneau, L., & Axelin, A. (2016). Parents and nurses balancing parent–infant closeness and separation: A qualitative study of NICU nurses' perceptions. *BMC Pediatrics*, 16, 134. https://doi.org/10.1186/s12887-016-0663-1

Feldman, R., Weller, A., Sirota, L., & Eidelman, A. I. (2002). Skin-to-skin contact (kangaroo care) promotes self-regulation in premature infants: Sleep-wake cyclicity, arousal modulation, and sustained exploration. *Developmental Psychology*, *38*(2), 194–207. https://doi.org/10.1037//0012-1649.38.2.194

Geiger Brown, J., Sagherian, K., Zhu, S., Wieroniey, M., Blair, L., Warren, J., Hinds, P., & Szeles, R. (2016). Napping on the night shift: A two-hospital implementation project. *American Journal of Nursing*, *116*(5), 26–33. https://doi.org/10.1097/01.NAJ.0000482953.88608.80

Gelfer, P., Cameron, R., Masters, K., & Kennedy, K. A. (2013). Integrating "back to sleep" recommendations into neonatal ICU practice. *Pediatrics*, *131*(4), 1264–1270. https://doi.org/10.1542/peds.2012-1857

Gillet, N., Huyghebaert-Zouaghi, T., Reveillere, C., Colombat, P., & Fouquereau, E. (2020). The effects of job demands on nurses' burnout and presenteeism through sleep quality and relaxation. *Journal of Clinical Nursing*, *29*(3–4), 583–592. https://doi.org/10.1111/jocn.15116

Gogou, M., Haidopoulou, K., & Pavlou, E. (2019). Sleep and prematurity: Sleep outcomes in preterm children and influencing factors. *World Journal of Pediatrics*, *15*(3), 209–218. https://doi.org/10.1007/s12519-019-00240-8

Gonzalez-Mesa, E., Cuenca-Marin, C., Suarez-Arana, M., Tripiana-Serrano, B., Ibrahim-Diez, N., Gonzalez-Cazorla, A., & Blasco-Alono, M. (2019). Poor sleep quality is associated with perinatal depression. A systematic review of last decade scientific literature and meta-analysis. *Journal of Perinatal Medicine*, 47(7), 689–703. https://doi.org/10.1515/jpm-2019-0214

Guyer, C., Huber, R., Fontijn, J., Bucher, H. U., Nicolai, H., Werner, H., Molinari, L., Latal, B., & Jenni, O. G. (2012). Cycled light exposure reduces fussing and crying in very preterm infants. *Pediatrics*, 130(1), e145–e151. https://doi.org/10.1542/peds.2011-2671

Guyer, C., Huber, R., Fontijn, J., Bucher, H. U., Nicolai, H., Werner, H., Molinari, L., Latal, B., & Jenni, O. G. (2015). Very preterm infants show earlier emergence of 24-hour sleep-wake rhythms compared to term infants. *Early Human Development*, 91(1), 37–42. https://doi.org/10.1016/j.earlhumdev.2014.11.002

Haddad, S., Dennis, C. L., Shah, P. S., & Stremler, R. (2019). Sleep in parents of preterm infants: A systematic review. *Midwifery*, 73, 35–48. https://doi.org/10.1016/j.midw.2019.01.009

Hebb, D. O. (1949). *The organization of behavior*. John Wiley & Sons.

Hulsheger, U. R., Walkowiak, A., & Thommes, M. S. (2018). How can mindfulness be promoted? Workload and recovery experiences as antecedents of daily fluctuations in mindfulness. *Journal of Occupational and Organizational Psychology*, 91, 261–284. https://doi.org/10.1111/joop.12206

James, S. M., Honn, K. A., Gaddameedhi, S., & Van Dongen, H. P. A. (2017). Shift work: Disrupted circadian rhythms and sleep—Implications for health and well-being. *Current Sleep Medicine Reports*, 3(2), 104–112. https://doi.org/10.1007/s40675-017-0071-6

Johns, M. W. (1991). A new method for measuring daytime sleepiness: The Epworth sleepiness scale. *Sleep*, 14, 540–545. https://doi.org/10.1093/sleep/14.6.540

Karbandi, S., Hosseini, S. M., Masoudi, R., Hosseini, S. A., Sadeghi, F., & Moghaddam, M. H. (2015). Recognition of the efficacy of relaxation program on sleep quality of mothers with premature infants. *Journal of Education and Health Promotion*, 4, 97. https://doi.org/10.4103/2277-9531.171811

Keshavarz Afshar, M., Behboodi Moghadam, Z., Taghizadeh, Z., Bekhradi, R., Montazeri, A., & Mokhtari, P. (2015). Lavender fragrance essential oil and the quality of sleep in postpartum women. *Iranian Red Crescent Medical Journal*, 17(4), e25880. https://doi.org/10.5812/ircmj.17(4)2015.25880

Knupp, A. M., Patterson, E. S., Ford, J. L., Zurmehly, J., & Patrick, T. (2018). Associations among nurse fatigue, individual nurse factors, and aspects of the nursing practice environment. *Journal of Nursing Administration*, 48(12), 642–648. https://doi.org/10.1097/NNA.0000000000000693

Kuhn, P., Zores, C., Langlet, C., Escande, B., Astruc, D., & Dufour, A. (2013). Moderate acoustic changes can disrupt the sleep of very preterm infants in their incubator. *Acta Paediatrica*, 102(10), 949–954. https://doi.org/10.1111/apa.12330

Lan, H.-Y., Yang, L., Hsieh, K.-H., Yin, T., Chang, Y.-C., & Liaw, J.-J. (2018). Effects of a supportive care bundle on sleep variables of preterm infants during hospitalization. *Research in Nursing and Health*, 41(3), 281–291. https://doi.org/10.1002/nur.21865

Lan, H.-Y., Yin, T., Chen, J.-L., Chang, Y.-C., & Liaw, J.-J. (2019). Factors associated with preterm infants' circadian sleep/wake patterns at the hospital. *Clinical Nursing Research*, 28(4), 456–472. https://doi.org/10.1177/1054773817724960

Lange, B. C., Callinan, L. S., & Smith, M. V. (2019). Adverse childhood experiences and their relation to parenting stress and parenting practices. *Community Mental Health Journal*, 55(4), 651–662. https://doi.org/10.1007/s10597-018-0331-z

Lee, S.-H., Lee, K. A., Aycock, D., & Decker, M. (2010). Circadian activity rhythms for mothers with an infant in the ICU. *Frontiers in Neurology*, *1*, 155. https://doi.org/10.3389/fneur.2010.00155

Lee, S. Y., Aycock, D. M., & Moloney, M. F. (2013). Bright light therapy to promote sleep in mothers of low-birth-weight infants: A pilot study. *Biological Research for Nursing*, *15*(4), 398–406. https://doi.org/10.1177/1099800412445612

Leong, T., Billaud, M., Agarwal, M., Miller, T., McFadden, T., Johnson, J., & Lazarus, S. G. (2019). As easy as ABC: Evaluation of safe sleep initiative on safe sleep compliance in a freestanding pediatric hospital. *Injury Epidemiology*, *6*(Suppl. 1), 26. https://doi.org/10.1186/s40621-019-0205-z

Levy, J., Hassan, F., Plegue, M. A., Sokoloff, M. D., Kushwaha, J. S., Chervin, R. D., Barks, J. D. E., & Shellhaas, R. A. (2017). Impact of hands-on care on infant sleep in the neonatal intensive care unit. *Pediatric Pulmonology*, *52*(1), 84–90. https://doi.org/10.1002/ppul.23513

Li, H., Shao, Y., Xing, Z., Li, Y., Wang, S., Zhang, M., Ying, J., Shi, Y., & Sun, J. (2019). Napping on night-shifts among nursing staff: A mixed-methods systematic review. *Journal of Advanced Nursing*, *75*(2), 291–312. https://doi.org/10.1111/jan.13859

Liao, J.-H., Hu, R.-F., Su, L.-J., Wang, S., Xu, Q., Qian, X. F., & He, H.-G. (2018). Nonpharmacological interventions for sleep promotion on preterm infants in neonatal intensive care unit: A systematic review. *World Views on Evidence-Based Nursing*, *15*(5), 386–393. https://doi.org/10.1111/wvn.12315

Lillehei, A. S., Halcon, L. L., Savik, K., & Reis, R. (2015). Effect of inhaled lavender and sleep hygiene on self-reported sleep issues: A randomized controlled trial. *Journal of Alternative and Complimentary Medicine*, *21*(7), 430–438. https://doi.org/10.1089/acm.2014.0327

Loewenstein, K. (2018). Parent psychological distress in the neonatal intensive care unit within the context of the social ecological model: A scoping review. *Journal of the American Psychiatric Nursing Association*, *24*(6), 495–509. https://doi.org/10.1177/1078390318765205

Lubbe, W. (2018). Clinicians guide for cue-based transition to oral feeding in preterm infants: An easy-to-use clinical guide. *Journal of Evaluation in Clinical Practice*, *24*(1), 80–88. https://doi.org/10.1111/jep.12721

Ludington-Hoe, S. M., Johnson, M. W., Morgan, K., Lewis, T., Gutman, J., Wilson, P. D., & Scher, M. S. (2006). Neurophysiologic assessment of neonatal sleep organization: Preliminary results of a randomized, controlled trial of skin contact with preterm infants. *Pediatrics*, *117*(5), e909–e923. https://doi.org/10.1542/peds.2004-1422

Makela, H., Axelin, A., Feeley, N., & Niela-Vilen, H. (2018). Clinging to closeness: The parental view on developing a close bond with their infants in the NICU. *Midwifery*, *62*, 183–188. https://doi.org/10.1016/j.midw.2018.04.003

Marthinsen, G. N., Helseth, S., & Fegran, L. (2018). Sleep and its relationship to health in parents of preterm infants: A scoping review. *BMC Pediatrics*, *18*(1), 352. https://doi.org/10.1186/s12887-018-1320-7

Matricardi, S., Agostino, R., Fedeli, C., & Montirosso, R. (2013). Mothers are not fathers: Differences between parents in the reduction of stress levels after a parental intervention in a NICU. *Acta Paediatrica*, *102*(1), 8–14. https://doi.org/10.1111/apa.12058

Mohapatra, B., & Marshall, R. S. (2019). Psychosomatic and physical well-being factors after mind-body interventions in a hospital setting. *Advances in Mind Body Medicine*, *33*(3), 4–11.

Moore, R. Y. (2007). Suprachiasmatic nucleus in sleep-wake regulation. *Sleep Medicine*, *8*(Suppl. 3), 27–33. https://doi.org/10.1016/j.sleep.2007.10.003

Muzik, M., Ads, M., Bonham, C., Rosenblum, K., Broderick, A., & Kirk, R. (2013). Perspectives on trauma-informed care from mothers with a history of childhood maltreatment: A qualitative study. *Child Abuse & Neglect*, *37*(12), 1215–1224. https://doi.org/10.1016/j.chiabu.2013.07.014

Narayan, A. J., Rivera, L. M., Bernstein, R. E., Harris, W. W., & Lieberman, A. F. (2018). Positive childhood experiences predict less psychopathology and stress in pregnant women with childhood adversity: A pilot study of the benevolent childhood experiences (BCEs) scale. *Child Abuse & Neglect*, *78*, 19–30. https://doi.org/10.1016/j.chiabu.2017.09.022

National Institute of Mental Health. (2013). *Arousal and regulatory systems: Workshop proceedings.* https://www.nimh.nih.gov/research/research-funded-by-nimh/rdoc/arousal-and-regulatory-systems-workshop-proceedings.shtml

National Sleep Foundations. (2015, February 2). *National sleep foundation recommends new sleep times.* https://www.sleepfoundation.org/press-release/national-sleep-foundation-recommends-new-sleep-times

Naugler, M. R. & DiCarlo, K. (2018). Barriers to and interventions that increase nurses' and parents' compliance with safe sleep recommendations for preterm infants. *Nursing for Womens Health*, *22*(1), 24–39. https://doi.org/10.1016/j.nwh.2017.12.009

Newberry, J. A. (2019). Creating a safe sleep environment for the infant: What the pediatric nurse needs to know. *Journal of Pediatric Nursing*, *44*, 119–122. https://doi.org/10.1016/j.pedn.2018.12.001

Orsi, K. C., Avena, M. J., Lurdes de Cacia Pradella-Hallinan, M., da Luz Goncalves Pedreira, M., Tsunemi, M. H., Machado Avelar, A. F., & Pinheiro, E. M. (2017). Effects of handling and environment on preterm newborns sleeping in incubators. *Journal of Obstetric, Gynecologic, and Neonatal Nursing*, *46*(2), 238–247. https://doi.org/10.1016/j.jogn.2016.09.005

Park, J., Silva, S. G., Thoyre, S. M., & Brandon, D. H. (2019). Sleep–wake states and feeding progression in preterm infants. *Nursing Research*, *69*(1), 22–30. https://doi.org/10.1097/NNR.0000000000000395

Patton, C., Stiltner, D., Wright, K. B., & Kautz, D. D. (2015). Do nurses provide a safe sleep environment for infants in the hospital setting? An integrative review. *Advances in Neonatal Care*, *15*(1), 8–22. https://doi.org/10.1097/ANC.0000000000000145

Postpartum Support International. (2020). *Post-traumatic stress disorder.* https://www.postpartum.net/learn-more/postpartum-post-traumatic-stress-disorder/

Prouhet, P. M., Gregory, M. R., Russell, C. L., & Yaeger, L. H. (2018). Fathers' stress in the neonatal intensive care unit: A systematic review. *Advances in Neonatal Care*, *18*(2), 105–120. https://doi.org/10.1097/ANC.0000000000000472

Pugliesi, R. R., Campillos, M. S., Calado Orsi, K. C. S., Avena, M. J., Pradella-Hallinan, M. L. C., Tsunemi, M. H., Avelar, A. F. M., & Pinheiro, E. M. (2018). Correlation of premature infant sleep/wakefulness and noise levels in the presence or absence of "quiet time." *Advances in Neonatal Care*, *18*(5), 393–399. https://doi.org/10.1097/ANC.0000000000000549

Richter, D., Kramer, M. D., Tang, N. K. Y., Montgomery-Downs, H. E., & Lemola, S. (2019). Long-term effects of pregnancy and childbirth on sleep satisfaction and duration of first-time and experienced mothers and fathers. *Sleep*, *42*(4), 1–10. https://doi.org/10.1093/sleep/zsz015

Richter, K., Acker, J., Aam, S., & Niklewski, G. (2016). Prevention of fatigue and insomnia in shift workers—A review of non-pharmacological measures. *EPMA Journal*, *7*(1), 16. https://doi.org/10.1186/s13167-016-0064-4

Rosa, D., Terzoni, S., Dellafiore, F., & Destrebecq, A. (2019). Systematic review of shift work and nurses' health. *Occupational Medicine*, *69*(4), 237–243. https://doi.org/10.1093/occmed/kqz063

Ruggiero, J. S., & Redeker, N. S. (2014). Effects of napping on sleepiness and sleep-related performance deficits in night-shift workers: a systematic review. *Biologic Research in Nursing*, *16*(2), 134–142. https://doi.org/10.1177/1099800413476571

Sanders, M. R. & Hall, S. L. (2018). Trauma-informed care in the newborn intensive care unit: Promoting safety, security and connectedness. *Journal of Perinatology*, *38*, 3–10. https://doi.org/10.1038/jp.2017.124

Schaffer, L., Jallo, N., Howland, L., James, K., Glaser, D., & Arnell, K. (2013). Guided imagery: An innovative approach to improving maternal sleep quality. *Journal of Perinatal & Neonatal Nursing*, *27*(2), 151–159. https://doi.org/10.1097/JPN.0b013e3182870426

Seidman, G., Unnikrishnan, S., Kenny, E., Myslinski, S., Cairns-Smith, S., Mulligan, B., & Engmann, C. (2015). Barriers and enablers of kangaroo mother care practice: A systematic review. *PLoS One*, *10*(5), e0125643. https://doi.org/10.1371/journal.pone.0125643

Shaw, R. J., Bernard, R. S., Storfer-Isser, A., Rhine, W., & Horwitz, S. M. (2013). Parental coping in the neonatal intensive care unit. *Journal of Clinical Psychology in Medical Settings*, *20*(2), 135–142. https://doi.org/10.1007/s10880-012-9328-x

Shepherd, K. L., Yiallourou, S. R., Horne, R. S. C., & Wong, F. Y. (2018). Prone sleeping position in infancy: Implications for cardiovascular and cerebrovascular function. *Sleep Medicine Reviews*, *39*, 174–186. https://doi.org/10.1016/j.smrv.2017.10.001

Shorey, S., He, H.-G., & Morelius, E. (2016). Skin-to-skin contact by fathers and the impact on infant and paternal outcomes: An integrative review. *Midwifery*, *40*, 207–217. https://doi.org/10.1016/j.midw.2016.07.007

Slanger, T. E., Gross, J. V., Pinger, A., Morfeld, P., Bellinger, M., Duhme, A. L., Reichardt. Ortega, R. A., Costa, G., Driscoll, T. R., Foster, R. G., Fritschi, L., Sallinen, M., Liira, J., & Erren, T. C. (2016). Person-directed, non-pharmacological interventions for sleepiness at work and sleep disturbances caused by shift work. *Cochrane Database of Systematic Reviews*, *23*(8), CD010641. https://doi.org/10.1002/14651858.CD010641.pub2

Slater, L., Asmerom, Y., Boskovic, D. S., Bahjri, K., Plank, M. S., Angeles, K. R., Phillips, R., Deming, D., Ashwal, S., Hougland, K., Fayard, E., & Angeles, D. M. (2012). Procedural pain and oxidative stress in premature neonates. *Journal of Pain*, *13*(6), 590–597. https://doi.org/10.1016/j.jpain.2012.03.010

Stone, J. E., Sletten, T. L., Magee, M., Ganesan, S., Mulhall, M. D., Collins, A., Howard, M., Lockley, S. W., & Rajaratnam, S. M. W. (2018). Temporal dynamics of circadian phase shifting response to consecutive night shifts in healthcare workers: Role of light-dark exposure. *Journal of Physiology*, *12*, 2381–2395.

St-Onge, M.-P., Mikic, A., & Pietrolungo, C. E. (2016). Effects of diet on sleep quality. *Advances in Nutrition*, *7*(5), 938–949. https://doi.org/10.3945/an.116.012336

Tan, J. B. C., Boskovic, D. S., & Angeles, D. M. (2018). The energy costs of prematurity and the neonatal intensive care unit (NICU) experience. *Antioxidants*, *7*(3), 37. https://doi.org/10.3390/antiox7030037

The Joint Commission (2018). *Health care worker fatigue and patient safety*. https://www.jointcommission.org/-/media/tjc/documents/resources/patient-safety-topics/sentinel-event/sea_48_hcw_fatigue_final_w_2018_addendum.pdf

Vaziri, F., Shiravani, M., Najib, F. S., Pourahmad, S., Salehi, A., & Yazdanpanahi, Z. (2017). Effect of lavender oil aroma in the early hours of postpartum period on maternal pains, fatigue, and mood: A randomized clinical trial. *International Journal of Preventive Medicine, 8*(1), 29. https://doi.org/10.4103/ijpvm.IJPVM_137_16

Warland, J., Dorrian, J., Morrison, J. L., & O'Brien, L. M. (2018). Maternal sleep during pregnancy and poor fetal outcomes: A scoping review of the literature with meta-analysis. *Sleep Medicine Reviews, 41*, 197–219. https://doi.org/10.1016/j.smrv.2018.03.004

Wickwire, E. M., Geiger-Brown, J., Scharf, S. M., & Drake, C. L. (2017). Shift work and shift work sleep disorder: Clinical and organizational perspectives. *Chest, 151*(5), 1156–1172. https://doi.org/10.1016/j.chest.2016.12.007

Williamson, A., Mindell, J. A., Hiscock, H., & Quach, J. (2019). Sleep problem trajectories and cumulative socio-ecological risks: Birth to school-age. *Journal of Pediatrics, 215*, 229–237. https://doi.org/10.1016/j.jpeds.2019.07.055

Wong, I. S., Popkin, S., & Folkard, S. (2019). Working Time Society consensus statements: A multi-level approach to managing occupational sleep-related fatigue. *Industrial Health, 57*(2), 228–244. https://doi.org/10.2486/indhealth.SW-6

Youngstedt, S. D., Elliott, J. A., & Kripke, D. F. (2019). Human circadian phase-response for exercise. *Journal of Physiology, 597*(8), 2253–2268. https://doi.org/10.1113/JP276943

Youngstedt, S. D., Kline, C. E., Elliott, J. A., Zielinski, M. R., Devlin, M. S., & Moore, T. A. (2016). Circadian phase-shifting effects of bright light, exercise, and bright light + exercise. *Journal of Circadian Rhythms, 14*(1), 2. https://doi.org/10.5334/http://doi.org/10.5334/jcr.137

Zores, C., Dufour, A., Pebayle, T., Dahan, I., Astruc, D., & Kuhn, P. (2018). Observational study found that even small variations in light can wake up very preterm infants in a neonatal intensive care unit. *Acta Paediatrica, 107*(7), 1191–1197. https://doi.org/10.1111/apa.14261

9

Pain and Stress

Preventing, assessing, and managing pain and stress are not only important aspects of quality healthcare, but are moral and ethical imperatives. This chapter presents the latest research and evidence-based best practices related to pain and stress for the hospitalized infant, the family, and the healthcare professional.

WHAT ARE PAIN AND STRESS?

Pain

The first official definition of *pain*, issued in 1979 by the International Association for the Study of Pain (IASP), described pain as *an unpleasant sensory and emotional experience associated with actual or potential tissue damage or described in terms of such damage* (Aydede, 2019, p. 1). The definition survived four decades and withstood much criticism. In late 2019, the IASP's Definition of Pain Task Force proposed a new definition of pain; a definition that clearly recognizes that verbal descriptions of pain represent only one of several behaviors associated with pain expression (IASP, 2019). The proposed new definition of *pain* describes it as *an aversive sensory and emotional experience typically caused by, or resembling that caused by, actual or potential tissue injury* (IASP, 2019, p. 1). The IASP Task Force clarifies this definition further in their accompanying notes (Box 9.1).

The IASP's definition of *pain* captures the sensory (intensity) and affective (unpleasantness) dimensions of the pain experience (Talbot et al., 2019). However, this two-dimensional view fails to acknowledge a third component of the subjective pain experience. Pain-related suffering represents a cognitive-evaluative dimension of the pain experience distinct from intensity and unpleasantness (Bustan et al., 2015), with suffering defined as an unpleasant and even anguishing experience with psychophysiological and existential implications (Bueno-Gomez, 2017). Despite the unpleasantness of pain and pain-related suffering, the majority of medical interventions and treatments provided to patients have painful consequences and often lead to some form of suffering (Bueno-Gomez, 2017). Pain's intensity,

BOX 9.1 ACCOMPANYING NOTES TO SUPPORT THE PROPOSED IASP DEFINITION OF *PAIN*

- Pain is always a subjective experience that is influenced to varying degrees by biological, psychological, and social factors.
- Pain and nociception are different phenomena: The experience of pain cannot be reduced to activity in sensory pathways.
- Through their life experiences, individuals learn the concept of pain and its applications.
- A person's report of an experience as pain should be accepted as such and respected.
- Although pain usually serves an adaptive role, it may have adverse effects on function and social and psychological well-being.
- Verbal description is only one of several behaviors used to express pain; inability to communicate does not negate the possibility that a human or a nonhuman animal experiences pain.

Source: International Association for the Study of Pain. (2019, August 7). *Proposed new definition of pain released for comment.* https://www.iasp-pain.org/PublicationsNews/NewsDetail.aspx?ItemNumber=9218

unpleasantness, and degree of associated suffering affect the whole person—body, mind, and spirit— inviting clinicians and healthcare systems at large to reexamine the goals of medicine and adopt a holistic, whole person perspective.

Stress

All pain is stress, but not all stress is pain. *Stress* was introduced into the medical lexicon by the work of Hans Selye, a prolific researcher who connected the hypothalamic–pituitary–adrenal (HPA) axis with the body's capacity to cope with stress (Godoy et al., 2018; S. Y. Tan & Yip, 2018). *Stress* is basically defined as a biological response to any intrinsic or extrinsic stimulus or stressor (Godoy et al., 2018; Yaribeygi et al., 2017). All stress is not bad. In fact, positive stress helps us grow, adapt, and learn. The stress response is activated in the setting of real or potential threat and is composed of physiological and behavioral mechanisms that strive to restore homeostasis and promote adaptation (Figure 9.1; Godoy et al., 2018).

Stressful situations activate complex mechanisms that integrate brain and body systems for the individual to process and cope with a stressor. Once the stressor is identified, two major constituents of the stress system, the sympathetic–adreno–medullar (SAM) axis and the HPA axis release critical mediating chemicals. The SAM axis secretes noradrenaline and

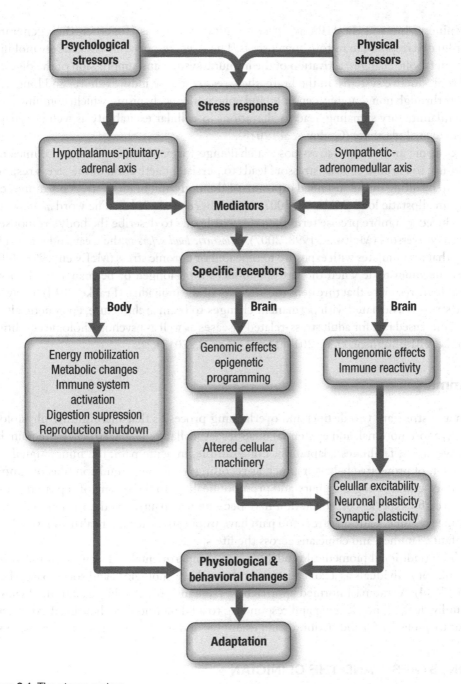

Figure 9.1 The stress system.

Source: Godoy, L. D., Rossignoli, M. T., Delfino-Pereira, P., Garcia-Cairasco, N., & de Lima Umeoka, E. H. (2018). A comprehensive overview on stress neurobiology: Basic concepts and clinical implications. *Frontiers in Behavioral Neuroscience, 12*, 127. doi: 10.3389/fnbeh.2018.00127

norepinephrine and the HPA axis secretes glucocorticoids. Together, they generate a coordinated response to restore homeostasis. The stress response initiates energy mobilization, metabolic changes, activation of the immune system and suppression of the digestive and reproductive systems. In the brain, the stress response induces short- and long-term effects through nongenomic, genomic, and epigenetic mechanisms, which, combined with pro-inflammatory signaling, lead to alterations in cellular excitability as well as synaptic and neuronal plasticity (Godoy et al., 2018).

Chronic and/or toxic stress poses a challenge for patients, families, and clinicians.o Exposure to chronic or toxic stressors leads to persistent activation of the stress response system, resulting in the sustained exposure of the body and brain to stress hormones creating an allostatic load (McEwen, 2007, 2012; Shern et al., 2016). The word *allostasis* was introduced as a more precise term than the word *stress* to describe the body's response to everyday stressors (McEwen, 1998, 2007). *Allostatic load refers to* the wear and tear on the body that accumulates with exposure to repeated or chronic stress (McEwen, 1998, 2007). Stress becomes toxic when the stressor induces a prolonged or permanently abnormal physiologic response that threatens the integrity of the individual (Franke, 2014). Early-life toxic stress is associated with permanent changes to brain architecture, epigenetic alterations, increased risk for adult stress-related diseases as well as psychopathologic conditions (Franke, 2014; Johnson et al., 2013; Shonkoff et al., 2012).

Summary

Pain and stress are two distinct and overlapping processes that share similar physiological, psycho-emotional, and existential qualities (Abdallah & Geha, 2017). Acute pain, like positive stress, facilitates adaptation. For example, in acute pain, the injury signals the initiation of protective behaviors, such as recoiling from the painful stimulus or limping to reduce exacerbating the injury and promote healing. In the setting of repeated painful and stressful experiences, adaptation may become maladaptive as the pain and/or stress becomes chronic. Chronic stress and pain have implications for the health and well-being of infants, families, and clinicians across the life span.

The traditional biomedical model offers a compartmentalized view of an individual. It thinks of individuals as a collection of biological, psychological, and social parts (Lima et al., 2014). A trauma-informed approach to pain and stress embraces a unified view of the individual, acknowledging and responding to all dimensions of their lived experience. Refer to Table 9.1 for the attributes and examples of the pain and stress core measure set.

PAIN, STRESS, AND THE CLINICIAN

Pain and stress are a pervasive part of life. The persistence of pain and stress over time is maladaptive, compromises health and well-being, and is now recognized as a global health problem characterized by high prevalence and significant physiological,

Table 9.1 Pain and Stress Core Measure Attributes and Examples

Attributes	Examples
1. Prevention of pain and stress is a daily expressed goal for infants, families, and clinicians	*Infant:* The prevention of pain and stress is an expressed goal of the healthcare team; each care encounter is guided by the infant's behavioral cues of readiness, stress, and pain *Family:* Families receive education and resources to effectively reduce their pain and distress during their NICU stay *Staff:* Staff adopt proactive effective strategies aimed at managing and mitigating the pain and stress they experience as part of their daily life and their work
2. Pain and/or stress is assessed, managed, and reassessed continuously for infants, families, ,and clinicians.	*Infant:* A validated, age-appropriate, and contextually accurate tool is used to assess pain and/or stress; pain and stress behaviors guide all interventions to include the use of pharmacologic and nonpharmacologic strategies to manage and mitigate pain and/or stress. *Family:* Families receive competency-based education on infant pain and stress cues and effective comfort measures for their baby; in addition, families are able to recognize and respond to their own pain and stress and adopt effective strategies to optimize their own health and wellness. Staff: Staff and team members support each other in managing and mitigating the pain and/or stress experienced on duty (i.e., code lavender).
3. Family and/or social networks are integral to the nonpharmacologic management and mitigation of pain and/or stress for infants, families, and clinicians.	*Infant:* Painful and/or stressful events and experiences are supported consistently through the presence of a dedicated person who comforts the infant. *Family:* Families, in partnership with the healthcare team, identify social and/or medical supports and resources that will assist them in managing and mitigating pain, stress, and distress over their hospital stay and beyond. *Staff:* Strategies to ensure a healthy work environment are supported and cultivated by staff and leadership.

Source: Reprinted with permission from Caring Essentials Collaborative, LLC.

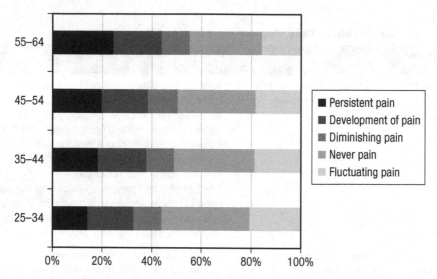

Figure 9.2 The prevalence of 15-year pain trajectories by 10-year age groups at baseline.

Source: Picavet, H. S. J., Monique Verschuren, W. M., Groot, L., Schaap, L., & van Oostrom, S. H. (2019). Pain over the adult life course: 15-year pain trajectories—The Doetinchem Cohort Study. *European Journal of Pain, 23*(9), 1723–1732. doi: 10.1002/ejp.1450 Reprinted with permission from John Wiley & Sons.

psychological, and economic associated costs physiologically, psychologically, and economically (Abdallah & Geha, 2017; Yang & Chang, 2019).

Using data from a longitudinal prospective cohort study of adults, Picavet et al. (2019) examined pain trajectories in adults to understand the prevalence and impact of pain in the general population. The researchers followed the cohort over 15 years. The prevalence of reported pain over the 15 years was 67.8% in the study population (Figure 9.2; Picavet et al., 2019). Experiences of pain were associated with gender differences (female greater than male), smoking, short-sleep duration, obesity, chronic disease, and poor perceived health status (Picavet et al., 2019).

Nursing is stressful by nature: physiologically, emotionally, and existentially, and is associated with a high level of burnout (Fernandez-Castro et al., 2017; Larson et al., 2017). Work-related stress is superimposed on a backdrop of the individual's life history of stress and pain and compounded by the inherent day-to-day life stressors we all experience. The totality of the nurse's life experiences is brought to bear on the nurse's professional practice. Nurse health, to include the physical, psychoemotional, and spiritual dimensions, impacts quality of care and patient safety (Chiang et al., 2016; June & Cho, 2011; Letvak et al., 2012).

Presenteeism, which is the opposite of absenteeism, occurs when an employee shows up for work with a reduced performance capacity due to illness, pain, or some other reason. Compared with other occupations, nurses are 4 times more likely to exhibit presenteeism (Lui & Johnston, 2019). Studies examining presenteeism in nurses report anywhere from

Table 9.2 **Estimated Annual Costs of Presenteeism in the United States**

Basis for Cost Estimates	Cost/RN	Total U.S. Cost ($ Millions)
Decreased productivity	$15,541	$22,667
Decreased quality of care	$2,791	$4,070
Increased patient falls and medication errors		
Baseline	$1,346	$1,964
Upper boundary	$9,067	$13,244

Source: Letvak, S. A., Ruhm, C. J., & Gupta, S. N. (2012). Nurses' presenteeism and its effects on self-reported quality of care and costs. *American Journal of Nursing, 112*(2), 30–38. doi: 10.1097/01.NAJ.0000411176.15696.f9 Reprinted with permission from Wolter Kluwer Health Inc.

17% to 89% of nurses work with some form of musculoskeletal disorder, pain, or both (Letvak et al., 2012). In the Letvak et al. (2012) cohort, presenteeism was associated with an increase in patient falls, a higher number of medication errors, lower quality-of-care scores, and significant financial costs (Table 9.2).

Stressors for neonatal nurses include confrontations with life-and-death situations, moral and ethical dilemmas, challenges associated with complex conditions, the inherent complexities in working with families in crisis, as well as their work environment (Buckley et al., 2020; Doede et al., 2018; Larson et al., 2017; Lavoie-Tremblay et al., 2016). Work-related stress and professional burnout in NICU nurses is associated with a multitude of health complaints (Figure 9.3; Skorobogatova et al., 2017). Nurses' personal experiences with pain and stress shape how they perceive these phenomena in others. In the NICU, clinician perceptions influence engagement with the patient and their family as well as how they interpret physiologic and behavioral expressions of pain and stress (D'Agata et al., 2018). These perceptions, combined with knowledge gaps specific to the short-term and long-term implications of underrecognized and undermanaged pain and stress in the hospitalized infant, threatens the safety of this extremely vulnerable population (Polkki et al., 2018).

Understanding how pain and stress play out in our daily lives is critical to managing, mitigating, and reducing the negative consequences of pain and stress for ourselves and others. Understanding of the pain experience calls for self-reflection and introspection. In general, nurses are less healthy than the average person. They are more likely to be overweight, have higher levels of stress, and get less sleep which can exacerbate existing medical conditions (Stanulewicz et al., 2020). We cannot give what we do not have; we cannot support health in others if we do not support health for ourselves.

And what nursing has to do… is to put the [body] in the best condition for nature to act upon.
—Florence Nightingale (1969)

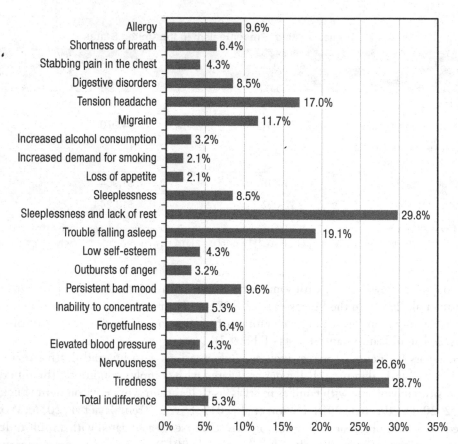

Figure 9.3 Prevalence of frequent health complaints in nurses.

Source: Skorobogatova, N., Zemaitiene, N., Smigelskas, K., & Tameliene, R. (2017). Professional burnout and concurrent health complaints in neonatal nursing. *Open Medicine, 12*, 328–334. doi: 10.1515/med-2017-0047 Reprinted with permission from the author.

EVIDENCE-BASED STRATEGIES TO REDUCE PAIN AND STRESS FOR CLINICIANS

The healthy nurse actively focuses on creating and maintaining balance and synergy with the physical, intellectual, emotional, spiritual, personal, and professional domains of well-being (Exhibit 9.1). Nurses must take an active role in ensuring their own health and wellness to ensure that safe, compassionate, quality care is provided to patients and families in crisis. Interventions aimed at improving nurse health, well-being, and job-related stress have shown positive outcomes with regard to nutrition, body composition, physical activity, and stress (Stanulewicz et al., 2020).

Simple strategies aimed at reducing stress and chronic pain include the practice of loving-kindness, meditation, and forgiveness. Yoga and mindfulness-based interventions have been shown to reduce stress, anxiety, and acute and chronic pain in healthcare workers

EXHIBIT 9.1 DOMAINS OF HEALTH AND WELL-BEING

Physical– exercise, walking, yoga, swimming, dance, play, etc.	Intellectual– reading, writing, reflection, journaling etc.	Emotional– connecting with others and nature, self-expression etc.	Spiritual– meditation, religious practices, retreats, etc.	Personal– self-care, manicure, pedicure, hygiene routines, etc.	Professional– membership in professional organization, participate in quality-improvement work, etc.

(Bernier Carney et al., 2020; Bischoff et al., 2019; Cocchiara et al., 2019; La Torre et al., 2020; McClintock et al., 2019). Kundalini yoga, a practice that focuses on creating vitality in the body, balance in the mind, and openness to the spirit, was shown over a 3-month period to statistically significantly reduce salivary cortisol levels and stress scores in program participants when compared with the control group (Garcia-Sesnich et al., 2017). In addition, regular yoga practice has been shown to improve sleep quality while decreasing stress in staff nurses (Fang & Li, 2015).

The Cleveland Clinic introduced the idea of a "code lavender" back in 2008 to meet the emotional and spiritual needs of patients and clinicians during a painful or stressful situation. Davidson et al. (2017) evaluated the feasibility and impact of the code lavender program across four target units to include a 49-bed NICU at a large urban university teaching hospital. The intervention included a care package that contained a vial of lavender essential oil, a piece of chocolate, a small card with encouraging quotes, and a referral card for free access to psychological counseling at the recipient's discretion. Although the intervention did not impact staff members' Professional Quality of Life scores, the intervention was overwhelmingly embraced and used, with 100% of staff reporting it was helpful in reducing their stress (Davidson et al., 2017). As a follow-up intervention, the same research team expanded the concept of code lavender to include the use of peer supporters. Peer supporters received 8-hours of training by a qualified psychologist and then reached out to staff who were experiencing workplace stress to provide emotional support. One suicide was prevented, the emotion of feeling cared for improved, and 100% of staff found the support helpful and would recommend it to others (Graham et al., 2019).

In addition to frontline clinicians, nursing leaders are exposed to a unique set of stressors that may hinder their ability to function optimally, both personally and professionally. These stressors include ensuring high-quality care against a backdrop of resource restrictions, financial constraints, high nurse turnover, and nurse shortages with inconsistent support from their chain of command (Haggman-Laitila & Romppanen, 2017). Interventions described as most effective to reduce stress in nurse leaders included mindfulness meditation, healing touch training, and spirituality training (Haggman-Laitila & Romppanen, 2017).

BOX 9.2 DAILY ACTIVITIES LIMITED BY POSTPARTUM (PUERPERAL) PAIN

- Self-care
- Newborn care
- Mobility
- Rest

PAIN, STRESS, AND THE NICU FAMILY

Admission to the NICU is an unexpected traumatic event that undermines the stability, health, and wellness of the family. Beyond the admission, additional factors can overwhelm the family, including surgical interventions, the highly technological environment of the NICU, the infant's appearance, anxiety over infant survival and outcomes, as well as disruptions and alterations in the family's role identity (Joseph et al., 2019). This stress is compounded by the family's history of pain, stress, and trauma. The findings from the Picavet et al. (2019) study regarding the pervasiveness of pain in adults invite clinicians to see the family's experience of pain and stress beyond the scope of the NICU.

Pain is a subjective biopsychosocial phenomenon that always has a physical correlate (Beneitez & Nieto, 2017). Postpartum pain compromises a woman's ability to perform necessary daily activities (Box 9.2), which can result in physical, psychological, and emotional issues (Pereira et al., 2017). These limitations in functional activity can hinder maternal participation and presence at the bedside of the critically ill infant, which creates additional stress and distress for the mother and possibly the mother's partner.

Chronic postpartum pain is often reported following cesarean section (Kainu et al., 2016; Lavand'Homme, 2019). Cesarean section is one of the most common surgical procedures performed around the world (Lavand'Homme, 2019). Two percent to 10% of women who deliver vaginally report chronic postpartum pain of higher intensity than their cesarean section counterparts, affecting quality of life and mood (Lavand'Homme, 2019). Both acute and chronic postpartum pain, and the associated psychological burden of pain experienced by mothers whose babies are admitted to the NICU, warrant attention and the adoption of evidence-based best practices to manage and mitigate this source of pain, stress, and trauma.

Prouhet et al. (2018) completed a systematic review examining psychological stress and types of stressors experienced by fathers with infants in the NICU (Box 9.3). The authors concluded fathers indeed experience stress, which increases with decreasing gestational age of their baby. Similar to mothers of preterm infants, fathersexperienced stress related to the infant's appearance, the NICU environment, and alterations in the parental role.

> **BOX 9.3** STRESSORS IMPACTING THE FATHER'S PSYCHOLOGICAL STATE
>
> - Father's employment status
> - Inability to comfort the infant
> - Separation from the infant
> - A lack of support and communication
> - Feelings of exclusion and isolation
>
> *Sources:* Adapted from Prouhet, P. M., Gregory, M. R., Russell, C. L., & Yaeger, L. H. (2018). Fathers' stress in the neonatal intensive care unit: A systematic review. *Advances in Neonatal Care, 18*(2), 105–120. doi: 10.1097/ANC.0000000000000472; Sisson, H., Jones, C., Williams, R., & Lachanudis, L. (2015). Meta-ethnographic synthesis of fathers' experiences of the neonatal intensive care unit environment during hospitalization of their premature infants. *Journal of Obstetric, Gynecologic, and Neonatal Nursing, 44*(4), 471–480. https://doi.org/10.1111/1552-6909.12662

Families of color report similar stressors during the perinatal period. Chronic worries about racial discrimination have been associated with preterm birth rates in Black women with higher incomes (Braverman et al., 2017). Refer to Chapter 7 for more information about social determinants of health and the maternal health crisis.

Fathers of color who have premature infants have described their feelings of stress as similar to a "roller coaster" ride, in which they experienced unmet information needs, a lack of support services, and communication challenges (Edwards et al., 2020). Edwards et al. (2020) uncovered four major themes associated with the father experience in men of color (Figure 9.4).

Understanding and recognizing that many of these fathers have experienced discrimination and mistrust in their encounters with healthcare professionals invites clinicians and organizations to adopt the "5 Rs of cultural humility" (Table 9.3; Masters et al., 2019).

EVIDENCE-BASED STRATEGIES TO REDUCE PAIN AND STRESS FOR FAMILIES

Similar to the benefits of mindfulness-based interventions for nurses, these same interventions have positive benefits for NICU parents. Mindfulness-based stress reduction (MBSR) increases an individual's awareness and acceptance of a given situation in the present moment. In the NICU setting, MBSR has been linked to decreased stress and increased milk production (Joseph et al., 2019). Additionally, MBSR enhances emotional well-being; manages symptoms of anxiety, depression, pain, and sleep problems; and improves family mental health-related quality of life (Joseph et al., 2019; refer to Chapter 5 for suggested strategies). See the end of this chapter for a Reader Resource.

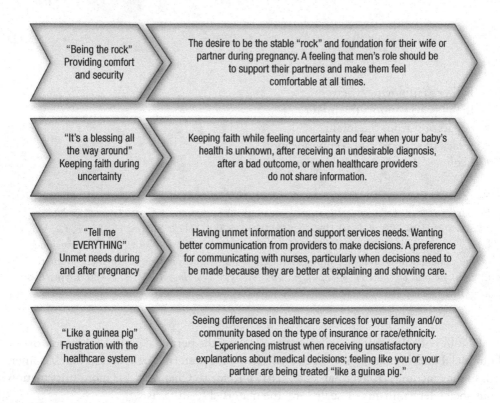

"Being the rock" Providing comfort and security	The desire to be the stable "rock" and foundation for their wife or partner during pregnancy. A feeling that men's role should be to support their partners and make them feel comfortable at all times.
"It's a blessing all the way around" Keeping faith during uncertainty	Keeping faith while feeling uncertainty and fear when your baby's health is unknown, after receiving an undesirable diagnosis, after a bad outcome, or when healthcare providers do not share information.
"Tell me EVERYTHING" Unmet needs during and after pregnancy	Having unmet information and support services needs. Wanting better communication from providers to make decisions. A preference for communicating with nurses, particularly when decisions need to be made because they are better at explaining and showing care.
"Like a guinea pig" Frustration with the healthcare system	Seeing differences in healthcare services for your family and/or community based on the type of insurance or race/ethnicity. Experiencing mistrust when receiving unsatisfactory explanations about medical decisions; feeling like you or your partner are being treated "like a guinea pig."

Figure 9.4 Four major themes of experiences of men of color during pregnancy and birth.

Source: Edwards, B. N., McLemore, M. R., Baltzell, K., Hodgkin, A., Nunez, O., & Franck, L. S. (2020). What about the men? Perinatal experiences of men of color whose partners were at risk for preterm birth, a qualitative study. *BMC Pregnancy and Childbirth, 20*(1), 91. https://doi.org/10.1186/s12884-020-2785-6

Despite the benefits of mindfulness-based interventions, racial and ethnic minorities may be underrepresented in these effective interventions. Watson-Singleton et al. (2019) propose a culturally responsive approach to mindfulness-based interventions for African Americans (Figure 9.5). Including Black facilitators, incorporating salient cultural values, using culturally familiar terminology, and ensuring the availability of culturally tailored resources, optimizes the benefits of mindfulness-based interventions in a culturally diverse population (Watson-Singleton et al., 2019).

Petteys and Adoumie (2018) examined the impact of parent education and participation on stress in mindfulness-based neurodevelopmental care in NICU parents. The intervention group received one-on-one education on mindfulness techniques and structured neurodevelopmental care training over a 10-day period following enrollment (Petteys & Adoumie, 2018). Parents in the intervention group demonstrated a statistically significant decrease in their overall stress scores from enrollment to discharge when compared to the control group (Petteys & Adoumie, 2018). In addition,

Table 9.3 The 5 Rs of Cultural Humility

Reflection	Approach each encounter with humility and understanding. There is always something to learn from everyone.
Respect	Treat every person with the utmost respect and preserve dignity at all times.
Regard	Hold every person in the highest regard. Do not allow unconscious biases to interfere in any interactions.
Relevance	Expect cultural humility to be relevant and apply this practice to every encounter.
Resiliency	Embody the practice of cultural humility to enhance personal resiliency and global compassion.

Source: Adapted from Masters, C., Robinson, D., Faulkner, S., Patterson, E., McIlraith, T., & Ansari, A. (2019). Addressing biases in patient care with the 5Rs of cultural humility, a clinician tool. *Journal of General Internal Medicine, 34,* 627–630. doi: 10.1007/s11606-018-4814-y

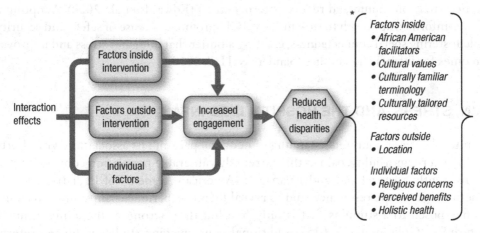

Figure 9.5 Proposed culturally responsive mindfulness-based intervention model.

Note: *Represents specific factors that emerged in the qualitative thematic analyses.
Source: Watson-Singleton, N. N., Black, A. R., & Spivey, B. N. (2019). Recommendations for a culturally responsive mindfulness-based intervention for African Americans. *Complementary Therapies in Clinical Practice, 34,* 132–138. doi: 10.1016/j.ctcp.2018.11.013 Reprinted with permission from Elsevier.

the infants in the intervention group were discharged 8 to 10 days earlier (Petteys & Adoumie, 2018).

Parental proximity and participation in care has also been associated with decreased stress in parents of infants hospitalized in the NICU. The Family Integrated Care model promotes and empowers parents to partner with NICU clinicians in the care of their infant and has demonstrated statistical significance in reducing maternal stress and anxiety in the NICU (C. Chen et al., 2019). Validating parental role identity through the consistent facilitation of skin-to-skin care encounters is a potent mediator of stress in the NICU for mothers and their partners (Eliades, 2018). Skin-to-skin care increases oxytocin levels in parents (and infants), which invokes a sense of calm and connectedness, reduces stress, supports social engagement, and promotes bonding (Cho et al., 2016; Pados, 2019; Vittner et al., 2018).

Affectionate touch is associated with psychological and physical well-being and is an effective stress-reduction intervention (Jakubiak & Feeney, 2017). Promoting affectionate and supportive touch among family members in crisis activates the release of oxytocin and endogenous opioids, leading to reduced stress and stress reactivity (Jakubiak & Feeney, 2017). Opportunities for parents to parent their hospitalized infant together in the NICU validates parental role identity, preserves the integrity of the couple, and reduces parental stress (Craig et al., 2015; De Bernardo et al., 2017; Ionia et al., 2016).

In addition to interpersonal support among family members, peer-to-peer support has also been shown to reduce parental stress in the NICU. The different types of support provided by veteran NICU parents include in-person or telephone support, parent support groups, and internet support groups (Hall et al., 2015). Interventions aimed at improving father-centered communication help build trust across the perinatal and neonatal continuum and reduce paternal stress (Edwards et al., 2020). Adopting a trauma-informed approach to care in the NICU promotes a sense of safety and security while fostering social connectedness, creating a buffer that mitigates stress and improves outcomes for infants and families (Sanders & Hall, 2018).

PAIN, STRESS, AND THE HOSPITALIZED INFANT

Despite advances in our understanding of neonatal pain and its association with short- and long-term morbidity, pain in this extremely vulnerable population continues to be inconsistently assessed and undermanaged (American Academy of Pediatrics, 2016). Functional magnetic resonance studies reveal infants experience pain similar to adults when exposed to a stimulus that is only one fourth as strong as the adult stimulus (Figure 9.6; Goksan et al., 2015). Additional neuroimaging studies indicate preterm infants have a 30% to 50% lower pain threshold than adults and a lower pain tolerance than older children (Perry et al., 2019).

All stress may not be pain, but all pain is stressful. Stressful and painful experiences are an inherent part of the NICU stay. Although premature infants make up the largest percentage of NICU patients (72.3%), a significant amount of NICU admissions are term born (27.7%; Williams & Lascelles, 2020). In the United States, approximately 460,000 newborns are admitted to the NICU each year and experience largely under- or unmanaged procedural, medical, and/or surgical pain, prolonging human suffering and compromising short-term and long-term physical, behavioral, and cognitive health (Anand et al., 2017; Williams & Lascelles, 2020).

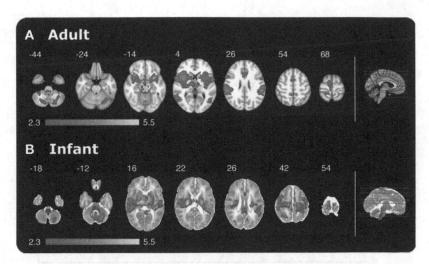

Figure 9.6 Noxious-evoked brain activity in response to the maximum presented stimulus in adults.

Source: Goksan, S., Hartley, C., Emery, F., Cockrill, N., Poorun, R., Moultrie, F., Rogers, R., Campbell, J., Sanders, M., Adams, E., Clare, S., Jenkinson, M., Tracey, I., & Slater, R. (2015). fMRI reveals neural activity overlap between adult and infant pain. *Elife*, 4. https://doi.org/10.7554/eLife.06356

Cong et al. (2017) evaluated the cumulative exposure of pain and stress on preterm infants using the Neonatal Infant Stressor Scale. During the first 28-days of NICU hospitalization,infants experienced on average 23 procedures per day and endured approximately 43 hours of chronic stress events (Figure 9.7; Cong et al., 2017). Due to the scoring metrics, infants may experience several chronic stressors simultaneously, so the score may exceed 24 hours. The most common daily stressors are shown in Figure 9.8.

Bellieni et al. (2017) completed a cross-sectional survey of physicians and nurses working in five Italian NICUs to assess the frequency of the self-reported use of nonpharmacologic therapies for skin-breaking procedures. Sixty-four percent of respondents reported using nonpharmacologic analgesia during a heel stick, 60% employed a nonpharmacologic strategy for venipuncture, and more than half of the respondents reported no form of analgesia for intramuscular injections (Bellieni et al., 2017). Venipuncture is the second most frequent skin-breaking procedure in the NICU. In the Epidemiology of Procedural PAin In Neonates (EPIPPAIN) 2 study, 76% of venipunctures were performed with pre-procedural analgesia and only 61.7% of venipunctures were successful on the first attempt, making this procedure high risk for repeated and recurrent pain (Courtois et al., 2016). Despite the availability of a myriad of pharmacologic and nonpharmacologic interventions, consistent pain management remains suboptimal for hospitalized newborns and infants (Balice-Bourgois et al., 2020)

Although procedural pain frequently occurs in the NICU, infants also experience chronic pain as a consequence of repeated undertreated pain mediated by inflammation and hypersensitization of nociceptive pathways (Anand et al., 2017; DiLorenzo et al., 2016; Williams & Lascelles, 2020). These types of pain are confounded by the infant's underlying

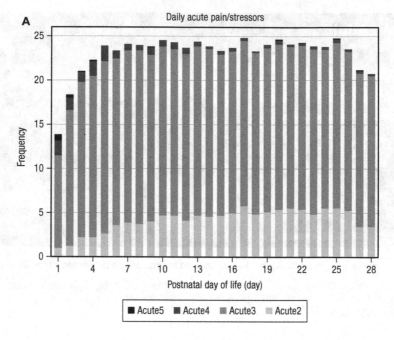

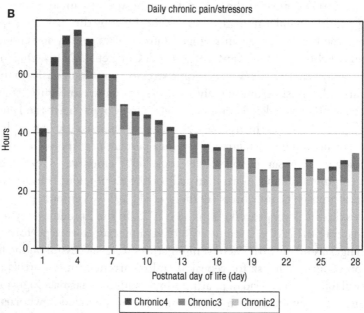

Figure 9.7 Daily mean stressors during the first 28 days in the NICU. Pain/stress severity labels: Acute2/Chronic2 = low, Acute3/Chronic3 = moderate, Acute4/Chronic4 = high, and Acute5/Chronic5 = extremely painful/stressful.

Source: Cong, X., Wu, J., Vittner, D., Xu, W., Hussain, N., Galvin, S., Fitzsimons, M., McGrath, J. M., & Henderson, W. A. (2017). The impact of cumulative pain/stress on neurobehavioral development of preterm infants in the NICU. *Early Human Development, 108,* 9–16. doi: 10.1016/j.earlhumdev.2017.03.003 Reprinted with permission from Elsevier.

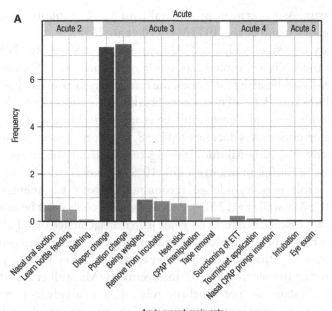

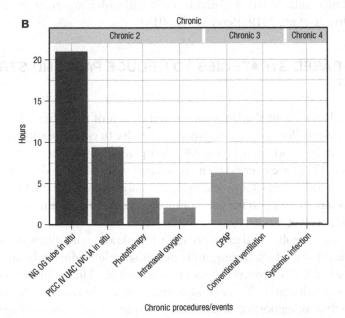

Figure 9.8 Common daily pain/stressors experienced during the first 28 postnatal days in the NICU. (**A**) Acute procedures (frequency); (**B**) daily chronic events (hours). Pain/stress severity levels: Acute2/Chronic 2 = low, Acute3/Chronic3 = moderate, Acute4/Chronic4 =high, and Acute5 = extremely painful/stressful.

CPAP, continuous positive airway pressure; ETT, endotracheal tube; NG, nasogastric; OG, orogastric; PICC, peripherally inserted central catheter. *Source:* Cong, X., Wu, J., Vittner, D., Xu, W., Hussain, N., Galvin, S., Fitzsimons, M., McGrath, J. M., & Henderson, W. A. (2017). The impact of cumulative pain/stress on neurobehavioral development of preterm infants in the NICU. *Early Human Development, 108,* 9–16. doi: 10.1016/j.earlhumdev.2017.03.003 Reprinted with permission from Elsevier.

disease-related pain. Assessment of procedural pain and continuous pain in the NICU remains suboptimal (Anand et al., 2017; Maxwell et al., 2019).

In a secondary analysis of study data, 242 newborns underwent a total of 10,469 painful procedures over their NICU hospitalization (Orovec et al., 2019). Separated into tissue-breaking and non-tissue-breaking categories, the researchers discovered that 56.6% of tissue breaking procedures and 12.2% of non-tissue-breaking procedures had a documented pain score associated with the painful event (Orovec et al., 2019). The use of nonpharmacologic pain-relieving interventions was documented in 58.5% of procedures (Orovec et al., 2019).

In a prospective, observational study investigating neonatal pain assessment practices in 243 NICUs across 18 European countries, only 10% of infants received daily assessments of continuous pain in spite of pain guidelines recommending pain assessments every 4–6 hours (Anand et al., 2017; Maxwell et al., 2019). Pain assessment tools must be valid, contextually accurate, and age appropriate to effectively guide pain management (Anand, 2017; Perry et al., 2018). Given this recommendation for assessment, however, there is no general consensus for a pain score threshold that would warrant treatment, and even in postoperative studies, pain scores rarely link to specific analgesic interventions (Maxwell et al., 2019).

Newborns and infants are preverbal and rely on their caregivers to accurately assess and manage their pain to avoid human suffering and the adverse sequalae related to unmanaged pain and pain-related stress (Anand, 2017; Clifford-Faugere et al., 2019; Maxwell et al., 2019; Orovec et al., 2019; Perry et al., 2018).

EVIDENCE-BASED STRATEGIES TO REDUCE PAIN AND STRESS FOR INFANTS

Given what we know about the frequency and duration of early-life pain experiences in the NICU, we must collectively and consistently resolve to eradicate the burden of pain on hospitalized newborns and infants (Box 9.4). Best practices in managing infant pain begin with assessment. There are over 40 pain assessment tools developed specifically to assess pain in newborns and infants. Choose a limited number of tools that address the needs of your unique patient population for age, context ,and type of pain and use it correctly and consistently (Maxwell et al., 2019).

A randomized controlled trial examined the effect of various nonpharmacologic strategies on preterm infant pain before, during, and after orogastric feeding-tube insertion (Figure 9.9). Cirik and Efe (2020) discovered the combination of swaddling plus the use of expressed breast milk provided the most effective nonpharmacologic pain relief for this invasive painful procedure. In addition, supporting nonnutritive sucking will facilitate feeding tube advancement, for both orogastric and nasogastric feeding tube insertion; as the infant swallows, the tube advances gently and organically with reduced distress and anatomic accuracy.

Gomes Neto et al. (2020) performed a systematic review and meta-analysis of the effectiveness of facilitated tucking as a nonpharmacologic pain intervention. The facilitated tucking position was shown to significantly reduce pain scores during endotracheal

BOX 9.4 EVIDENCE-BASED STRATEGIES TO MANAGE PROCEDURAL PAIN AND PAIN-RELATED STRESS

- Parental presence
- Breastfeeding/breast milk
- Skin-to-skin holding
- Facilitated tucking
- Swaddling
- Sucrose
- Nonnutritive sucking
- Music
- Massage
- Acupuncture

Sources: Adapted from Johnston, C., Campbell-Yeo, M., Disher, T., Benoit, B., Fernandes, A., Streiner, D., Inglis, D., & Zee, R. (2017). Skin-to-skin care for procedural pain in neonates. *Cochrane Database of Systematic Reviews*, 2, CD006275. https://doi.org/10.1002/14651858 .CD006275.pub3; Mangat, A. K., Oei, J.-L., Quah-Smith, I., & Schmolzer, G. M. (2018). A review of non-pharmacological treatments for pain management in newborn infants. *Children*, 5(10), 130. https://doi.org/10.3390/children5100130; Perry, M., Tan, Z., Chen, J., Weidig, T., Xu, W., & Cong, X. S. (2019). Neonatal pain: Perceptions and current practice. *Critical Care Nursing Clinics of North America*, 30(4), 549–561. https://doi.org/10.1016/j .cnc.2018.07.013; Pillai Riddell, R. R., Racine, N. M., Gennis, H. G., Turcotte, K., Uman, L. S., Horton, R. E., Ahola Kohut, S., Hillgrove Stuart, J., Stevens, B., & Lisi, D. M. (2015). Non-pharmacological management of infant and young child procedural pain. *Cochrane Database of Systematic Reviews*, 12, CD006275. https://doi.org/10.1002/14651858 .CD006275.pub3

intubation and heel stick procedures when compared to routine care (Gomes Neto et al., 2020). Contrasted to oral sucrose or opioid administration, facilitated tucking did not impact pain scores; however, it is an effective adjunctive therapy. Facilitated tucking as well as gentle human touch has shown to reduce pain scores during endotracheal suctioning in hospitalized infants (Fatollahzade et al., 2020). Adding facilitated tucking to nonnutritive sucking and breast milk during the heel stick procedure not only reduced pain scores during the procedure but also supported the infants' return to baseline in the postprocedure period (Peng et al., 2018; Perroteau et al., 2018).

Pain management during retinopathy of prematurity (ROP) eye examinations remains a challenge. The use of sucrose solution or breast milk decreased pain scores during the examination when compared to controls (Sener Taplak & Erdem, 2017; Sun et al., 2010).

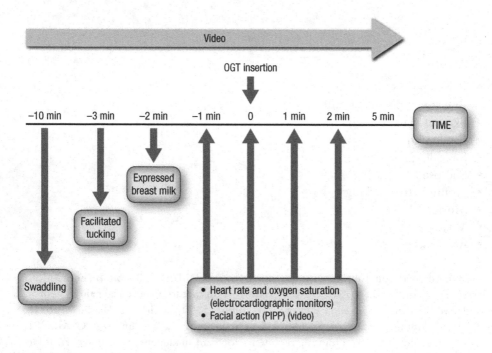

Figure 9.9 Study protocol for Cirik and Efe (2020).

OGT, orogastric tube; PIPP, Premature Infant Pain Profile.
Source: Cirik, V. A., & Efe, E. (2020). The effect of expressed breast milk, swaddling and facilitated tucking methods in reducing the pain caused by orogastric tube insertion in preterm infants: A randomized controlled trial. *International Journal of Nursing Studies, 104,* 103532. doi: 10.1016/j.ijnurstu.2020.103532 Reprinted with permission from Elsevier.

However, despite the benefit of the sweet solution, pain scores during the examination remain distressing and warrant further investigation to effectively treat infant pain during ROP exam and mitigate the infant's extreme adverse physiologic response to the exam (J. B. C. Tan et al., 2019).

Alternative and complementary therapies to reduce pain and stress for the hospitalized infant are becoming mainstream. In a randomized controlled trial, the use of mechanical vibration as an adjunct to sucrose and swaddling during heel stick was evaluated and demonstrated statistical significance in reducing infant pain scores (McGinnis et al., 2016). Auricular noninvasive magnetic acupuncture reduced pain scores during heel stick in preterm infants in a randomized controlled pilot study (K. L. Chen et al., 2017). Acupuncture and ear acupuncture have been studied for use in newborns with neonatal abstinence syndrome (NAS) and as a nonpharmacologic pain management therapy with positive results (Jackson et al., 2019b; Raith, 2018).

Managing the pain, stress, and distress of the infant experiencing NAS is a clinical challenge. The current standard of care focuses on a substitution weaning protocol supported by nonpharmacologic interventions. The use of acupuncture and acupressure has been studied in this unique population with favorable results. Both have proven safe for

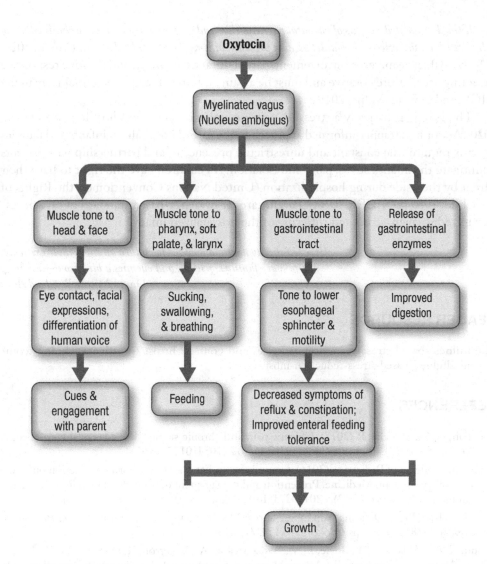

Figure 9.10 Effects of oxytocin and infant outcomes.

Source: Pados, B. F. (2019). Physiology of stress and use of skin-to-skin care as a stress-reducing intervention in the NICU. *Nursing for Women's Health, 23*(1), 59–70. doi: 10.1016/j.nwh.2018.11.002 Reprinted with permission from Elsevier.

use in infants and could reduce opioid withdrawal symptoms, decrease length of hospital stay, and reduce healthcare costs (Jackson et al., 2019a, 2019b).

Studies examining the benefits of skin-to-skin care in mitigating pain and stress in the hospitalized infant are prolific (Johnston et al., 2017; Pados & Hess, 2019). Skin-to-skin contact is the safest, most effective pain and stress management strategy for hospitalized infants (Moen, 2020). Skin-to-skin care promotes the release of oxytocin, a neuropeptide that plays a key role in fostering attachment bonds while also relieving stress and anxiety through systemic effects (Figure 9.10; Pados, 2019; Vittner et al., 2018).

If the documented benefits of parental participation and stress reduction could be obtained using a drug with no side effects, it would, based on present evidence, be a standard of care (Moen, 2020, p. 1709). Affective maternal involvement, parent-infant synchrony, and positive responsive parenting are neurorestorative and must be a pain and stress management mainstay in the NICU and beyond (Volpe, 2019).

The NICU is basically a stressful, pain-provoking, lonely, and hostile place (Moen, 2020). Adopting a trauma-informed approach to the care of hospitalized infants and families in crisis requires the constant and unrestricted presence of and partnership with parents to mitigate the infant's stress, pain, and isolation. All children have the right to have their parent by their side during hospitalization (United Nations Convention on the Rights of the Child, 1989 [UNICEF, 2020]). Parents are *the* evidence-based standard of care necessary to reduce pain, stress and suffering of the hospitalized infant.

> *[It's] selfish…to demand another to endure an intolerable existence,*
> *just to spare families, friends, and enemies a bit of soul-searching.*
> —David Mitchell, *Cloud Atlas*

READER RESOURCE

Mindfulness-based stress reduction exercises and courses: https://positivepsychology.com/mindfulness-based-stress-reduction-mbsr

REFERENCES

Abdallah, C. G., & Geha, P. (2017). Chronic pain and chronic stress: Two sides of the same coin? *Chronic Stress, 1*, 1–10. https://doi.org/10.1177/2470547017704763

American Academy of Pediatrics. (2016). Committee on Fetus and Newborn and Section on Anesthesiology and Pain Medicine. Prevention and management of procedural pain in the neonate: An update. *Pediatrics, 137*(2), e20154271. https://doi.org/10.1542/peds.2015-4271

Anand, K. J. S. (2017). Defining pain in newborns: Need for a uniform taxonomy? *Acta Paediatrica, 106*(9), 1438–1444. https://doi.org/10.1111/apa.13936

Anand, K. J. S., Eriksson, M., Boyle, E. M., Avila-Alvarez, A., Anderson, R. D., Sarafidis, K., Polkki, T., Matos, C., Papadouri, T., Attard-Montalto, S., Ilmoja, M. L., Simons, S., Tameliene, R., van Overmeire, B., Berger, A., Dobrzanska, A., Schroth, M., Bergqvist, L., Courtois, E., … EUROPAIN Survey Working Group of the NeoOpioid Consortium. (2017). Assessment of continuous pain in newborns admitted to NICUs in 18 European countries. *Acta Paediatrica, 106*(8), 1248–1259. https://doi.org/10.1111/apa.13810

Aydede, M. (2019). Does the IASP definition of pain need updating? *Pain Reports, 4*(5), e777. https://doi.org/10.1097/PR9.0000000000000777

Balice-Bourgois, C., Zumstein-Shaha, M., Vanoni, F., Jaques, C., Newman, C. J., & Simonetti, G. D. (2020). A systematic review of clinical practice guidelines for acute procedural pain on neonates. *Clinical Journal of Pain, 36*(5), 390–398. https://doi.org/10.1097/AJP.0000000000000808

Bellieni, C. V., Tei, M., Cornacchione, S., Di Lucia, S., Nardi, V., Verrotti, A., & Buonocore, G. (2017). Pain perception in NICU: A pilot questionnaire. *Journal of Maternal–Fetal & Neonatal Medicine, 31*(14), 1921–1923. https://doi.org/10.1080/14767058.2017.1332038

Beneitez, I., & Nieto, R. (2017). Do we understand pain from a biopsychosocial perspective? A review and discussion of the usefulness of some terms. *Pain Management*, 7(1), 41–48. https://doi.org/10.2217/pmt-2016-0024

Bernier Carney, K. M., Young, E. E., Guite, J. W., & Starkweather, A. R. (2020). A systematic review of biological mechanisms and chronic pain outcomes during stress reduction interventions. *Biological Research for Nursing*, 22(2), 205–216. https://doi.org/10.1177/1099800420907964

Bischoff, L. L., Otto, A. K., Hold, C., & Wollesen, B. (2019). The effect of physical activity interventions on occupational stress for health personnel: A systematic review. *International Journal of Nursing Studies*, 97, 94–104. https://doi.org/10.1016/j.ijnurstu.2019.06.002

Braverman, P., Heck, K., Egerter, S., Dominquez, T. P., Rinki, C., Marchi, K. S., & Curtis, M. (2017). Worry about racial discrimination: A missing piece of the puzzle of Black-White disparities in preterm birth? *PLoS One*, 12(10), e0186151. https://doi.org/10.1371/journal.pone.0186151

Buckley, L., Berta, W., Cleverley, K., Medeiros, C., & Widger, K. (2020). What is known about pediatric nurse burnout: A scoping review. *Human Resources for Health*, 18(9), https://doi.org/10.1186/s12960-020-0451-8

Bueno-Gomez, N. (2017). Conceptualizing suffering and pain. *Philosophy, Ethics, and Humanities in Medicine*, 12, 7. https://doi.org/10.1186/s13010-017-0049-5

Bustan, S., Gonzalez-Roldan, A. M., Kamping, S., Brunner, M., Loffler, M., Flor, H., & Anton, F. (2015). Suffering as an independent component of the experience of pain. *European Journal of Pain*, 19, 1035–1048. https://doi.org/10.1002/ejp.709

Chen, C., Franck, L. S., Ye, X. Y., Hutchinson, S. A., Lee, S. K., & O'Brien, K. (2019). Evaluating the effect of Family Integrated Care on maternal stress and anxiety in neonatal intensive care units. *Journal of Reproductive and Infant Psychology*, 1–14. https://doi.org/10.1080/02646838.2019.1659940

Chen, K. L., Lindrea, K. B., Quah-Smith, I., Schmolzer, G. M., Daly, M., Schindler, T., & Oei, J. L. (2017). Magnetic noninvasive acupuncture for infant comfort (MAGNIFIC)—A single-blinded randomized controlled pilot trial. *Acta Paediatrica*, 106(11), 1780–1786. https://doi.org/10.1111/apa.14002

Chiang, Y. C., Lee, H. C., Chu, T. L., Han, C. Y., & Hsiao, Y. C. (2016). The impact of nurses' spiritual health on their attitudes toward spiritual care, professional commitment, and caring. *Nursing Outlook*, 64(3), 215–224. https://doi.org/10.1016/j.outlook.2015.11.012

Cho, E.-S., Kim, S.-J., Kwon, M. S., Cho, H., Kim, E. H., Jun, E. M., & Lee, S. (2016). The effects of kangaroo care in the neonatal intensive care unit of physiological functions of preterm infants, maternal-infant attachment, and maternal stress. *Journal of Pediatric Nursing*, 31, 430–438. https://doi.org/10.1016/j.pedn.2016.02.007

Cirik, V. A., & Efe, E. (2020). The effect of expressed breast milk, swaddling and facilitated tucking methods in reducing the pain caused by orogastric tube insertion in preterm infants: A randomized controlled trial. *International Journal of Nursing Studies*, 104, 103532. https://doi.org/10.1016/j.ijnurstu.2020.103532

Clifford-Faugere, G., Aita, M., & Le May, S. (2019). Nurses' practices regarding procedural pain management of preterm infants. *Applied Nursing Research*, 45, 52–54. https://doi.org/10.1016/j.apnr.2018.11.007

Cocchiara, R. A., Peruzzo, M., Mannocci, A., Ottolenghi, L., Villari, P., Polimeni, A., Guerra, F., & La Torre, G. (2019). The use of yoga to manage stress and burnout in healthcare workers: A systematic review. *Journal of Clinical Medicine*, 8(3), 284. https://doi.org/10.3390/jcm8030284

Cong, X., Wu, J., Vittner, D., Xu, W., Hussain, N., Galvin, S., Fitzsimons, M., McGrath, J. M., & Henderson, W. A. (2017). The impact of cumulative pain/stress on neurobehavioral development of preterm infants in the NICU. *Early Human Development*, *108*, 9–16. https://doi.org/10.1016/j.earlhumdev.2017.03.003

Courtois, E., Cimerman, P., Dubuche, V., Goiset, M. F., Orfevre, C., Lagarde, A., Sgaggero, B., Guiot, C., Goussot, M., Huraux, E., Nanquette, M. C., Butel, C., Ferreira, A. M., Lacoste, S., Sejourne, S., Jolly, V., Lajoie, G., Maillard, V., Guedj, R., … Carbajal, R. (2016). The burden of venipuncture pain in neonatal intensive care units: EPIPPAIN 2, a prospective observational study. *International Journal of Nursing Studies*, *57*, 48–59. https://doi.org/10.1016/j.ijnurstu.2016.01.014

Craig, J. W., Glick, C., Phillips, R., Hall, S. L., Smith, J., & Browne, J. (2015). Recommendations for involving the family in developmental care of the NICU baby. *Journal of Perinatology*, *35*(Suppl. 1), s5–s8. https://doi.org/10.1038/jp.2015.142

D'Agata, A. L., Coughlin, M., & Sanders, M. R. (2018). Clinician perceptions of the NICU infant experience: Is the NICU hospitalization traumatic? *American Journal of Perinatology*, *35*(12), 1159–1167. https://doi.org/10.1055/s-0038-1641747

Davidson, J. E., Graham, P., Montross-Thomas, L., Norcross, W., & Zerbi, G. (2017). Code lavender: Cultivating intentional acts of kindness in response to stressful work situations. *Explore*, *13*(3), 181–185. https://doi.org/10.1016/j.explore.2017.02.005

De Bernardo, G., Svelto, M., Giordano, M., Sordino, D., & Riccitelli, M. (2017). Supporting parents in taking care of their infants admitted to a neonatal intensive care unit: A prospective cohort pilot study. *Italian Journal of Pediatrics*, *43*, 36. https://doi.org/10.1186/s13052-017-0352-1

DiLorenzo, M., Pillai Riddell, R., & Holsti, L. (2016). Beyond acute pain: Understanding chronic pain in infancy. *Children*, *3*(4), 26. https://doi.org/10.3390/children3040026

Doede, M., Trinkoff, A. M., & Gurses, A. P. (2018). Neonatal intensive care unit layout and nurses' work. *Health Environments Research & Design Journal*, *11*(1), 101–118. https://doi.org/10.1177/1937586717713734

Edwards, B. N., McLemore, M. R., Baltzell, K., Hodgkin, A., Nunez, O., & Franck, L. S. (2020). What about the men? Perinatal experiences of men of color whose partners were at risk for preterm birth, a qualitative study. *BMC Pregnancy and Childbirth*, *20*(1), 91. https://doi.org/10.1186/s12884-020-2785-6

Eliades, C. (2018). Mitigating infant medical trauma in the NICU: Skin-to-skin contact as a trauma-informed, age-appropriate best practice. *Neonatal Network*, *37*(6), 343–350. https://doi.org/10.1891/0730-0832.37.6.343

Fang, R., & Li, X. (2015). A regular yoga intervention for staff nurse sleep quality and work stress: A randomized controlled trial. *Journal of Clinical Nursing*, *24*(23–24), 3374–3379. https://doi.org/10.1111/jocn.12983

Fatollahzade, M., Parvizi, S., Kashaki, M., Haghani, H., & Alinejad-Naeini, M. (2020). The effect of gentle human touch during endotracheal suctioning on procedural pain response in preterm infant admitted to neonatal intensive care unit: A randomized controlled crossover study. *Journal of Maternal-Fetal & Neonatal Medicine*, 1–7. https://doi.org/10.1080/14767058.2020.1755649

Fernandez-Castro, J., Martinez-Zaragoza, F., Rovira, T., Edo, S., Solanes-Puchol, A., Martin-del-Rio, B., Garcia-Sierra, R., Benavides-Gil, G., & Doval, E. (2017). How does emotional exhaustion influence work stress? Relationships between stressor appraisals, hedonic tone, and fatigue in nurses' daily tasks: a longitudinal cohort study. *International Journal of Nursing Studies*, *75*, 43–50. https://doi.org/10.1016/j.ijnurstu.2017.07.002

Franke, H. A. (2014). Toxic stress: Effects, prevention and treatment. *Children*, *1*(3), 390–402. https://doi.org/10.3390/children1030390

Garcia-Sesnich, J. N., Garrido Flores, M., Hernandez Rios, M., & Gamonal Aravena, J. (2017). Longitudinal and immediate effect of kundalini yoga on salivary levels of cortisol and activity of alpha-amylase and its effect on perceived stress. *International Journal of Yoga*, *10*(2), 73–80. https://doi.org/10.4103/ijoy.IJOY_45_16

Godoy, L. D., Rossignoli, M. T., Delfino-Pereira, P., Garcia-Cairasco, N., & de Lima Umeoka, E. H. (2018). A comprehensive overview on stress neurobiology: Basic concepts and clinical implications. *Frontiers in Behavioral Neuroscience*, *12*, 127. https://doi.org/10.3389/fnbeh.2018.00127

Goksan, S., Hartley, C., Emery, F., Cockrill, N., Poorun, R., Moultrie, F., Rogers, R., Campbell, J., Sanders, M., Adams, E., Clare, S., Jenkinson, M., Tracey, I., & Slater, R. (2015). fMRI reveals neural activity overlap between adult and infant pain. *Elife*, *4*. https://doi.org/10.7554/eLife.06356

Gomes Neto, G., da Silva Lopes, I. A., Araujo, A. C. C. L. M., Oliveira, L. S., & Saquetto, M. B. (2020). The effect of facilitated tucking position during painful procedure in pain management of preterm infants in neonatal intensive care unit: A systematic review and meta-analysis. *European Journal of Pediatrics*, *179*(5), 699–709. https://doi.org/10.1007/s00431-020-03640-5

Graham, P., Zerbi, G., Norcross, W., Montross-Thomas, L., Lobbestael, L., & Davidson, J. (2019). Testing of a caregiver support team. *Explore*, *15*(1), 19–26. https://doi.org/10.1016/j.explore.2018.07.004

Haggman-Laitila, A., & Romppanen, J. (2017). Outcomes of interventions for nurse leaders' wellbeing at work: A quantitative systematic review. *Journal of Advanced Nursing*, *74*(1), 34–44. https://doi.org/10.1111/jan.13406

Hall, S. L., Ryan, D. J., Beatty, J., & Grubbs, L. (2015). Recommendations for peer-to-peer support for NICU parents. *Journal of Perinatology*, *35*, s9– s13. https://doi.org/10.1038/jp.2015.143

International Association for the Study of Pain. (2019, August 7). *Proposed new definition of pain released for comment*. https://www.iasp-pain.org/PublicationsNews/NewsDetail.aspx?ItemNumber=9218

Ionio, C., Colombo, C., Brazzoduro, V., Mascheroni, E., Confalonieri, E., Castoldi, F., & Lista, G. (2016). Mothers and fathers in NICU: The impact of preterm birth on parental distress. *Europe's Journal of Psychology*, *12*(4), 604–621. https://doi.org/10.5964/ejop.v12i4.1093

Jackson, H. J., Lopez, C., Miller, S., & Engelhardt, B. (2019a). A scoping review of acupuncture as a potential intervention for neonatal abstinence syndrome. *Medical Acupuncture*, *31*(2), 69–84. https://doi.org/10.1089/acu.2018.1323

Jackson, H. J., Lopez, C., Miller, S., & Englehardt, B. (2019b). Neonatal abstinence syndrome: An integrative review of neonatal acupuncture to inform a protocol for adjunctive treatment. *Advances in Neonatal Care*, *19*(3), 165–178. https://doi.org/10.1097/ANC.0000000000000630

Jakubiak, B. K., & Feeney, B. C. (2017). Affectionate touch to promote relational, psychological, and physical well-being in adulthood: A theoretical model and review of the research. *Personality and Social Psychology Review*, *21*(3), 228–252. https://doi.org/10.1177/1088868316650307

Johnson, S. B., Riley, A. W., Granger, D. A., & Riis, J. (2013). The science of early life toxic stress for pediatric practice and advocacy. *Pediatrics*, *131*(2), 319–327. https://doi.org/10.1542/peds.2012-0469

Johnston, C., Campbell-Yeo, M., Disher, T., Benoit, B., Fernandes, A., Streiner, D., Inglis, D., & Zee, R. (2017). Skin-to-skin care for procedural pain in neonates. *Cochrane Database of Systematic Reviews*, *2*, CD006275. https://doi.org/10.1002/14651858.CD006275.pub3

Joseph, R., Wellings, A., & Votta, G. (2019). Mindfulness-based strategies: A cost-effective stress reduction method for parents in the NICU. *Neonatal Network*, *38*(3), 135–143. https://doi.org/10.1891/0730-0832.38.3.135

June, K. J. & Cho, S.-H. (2011). Low back pain and work-related factors among nurses in intensive care units. *Journal of Clinical Nursing*, *20*(3–4), 479–487. https://doi.org/10.1111/j.1365-2702.2010.03210.x

Kainu, J. P., Halmesmaki, E., Korttila, K. T., & Sarvela, P. J. (2016). Persistent pain after cesarean delivery and vaginal delivery: A prospective cohort study. *Anesthesia and Analgesia*, *123*(6), 1535–1545. https://doi.org/10.1213/ANE.0000000000001619

La Torre, G., Raffone, A., Peruzzo, M., Calabrese, L., Cocchiara, R. A., D'Egidio, V., Leggieri, P. F., Dorelli, B., Zaffina, S., Mannocci, A.; Yomin Collaborative Group. (2020). Yoga and mindfulness as a tool for influencing affectivity, anxiety, mental health, and stress among healthcare workers: Results of a single-arm clinical trial. *Journal of Clinical Medicine*, *9*(4), 1037. https://doi.org/10.3390/jcm9041037

Larson, C. P., Dryden-Palmer, K. D., Gibbons, C., & Parshuram, C. S. (2017). Moral distress in PICU and neonatal ICU practitioners: A cross-sectional evaluation. *Pediatric Critical Care Medicine*, *18*(8), e318–e326. https://doi.org/10.1097/PCC.0000000000001219

Lavand'Homme, P. (2019). Postpartum chronic pain. *Minerva Anestesiologica*, *85*(3), 320–324. https://doi.org/10.23736/S0375-9393.18.13060-4

Lavoie-Tremblay, M., Feeley, N., Lavigne, G.L., Genest, C., Robins, S., & Frechette, J. (2016). Neonatal intensive care unit nurses working in an open ward: Stress and work satisfaction. *The Health Care Manager*, *35*(3), 205–216. https://doi.org/10.1097/HCM.0000000000000122

Letvak, S. A., Ruhm, C. J., & Gupta, S. N. (2012). Nurses' presenteeism and its effects on self-reported quality of care and costs. *American Journal of Nursing*, *112*(2), 30–38. https://doi.org/10.1097/01.NAJ.0000411176.15696.f9

Lima, D. D., Pereira Alves, V. L., & Ribeiro Turato, E. (2014). The phenomenological-existential comprehension of chronic pain: Going beyond the standing healthcare model. *Philosophy, Ethics, and Humanities in Medicine*, *9*(2), 1–10. https://doi.org/10.1186/1747-5341-9-2

Lui, J. N. M. & Johnston, J. M. (2019). Working while sick: Validation of the multidimensional presenteeism exposures and productivity survey for nurses (MPEPS-N). *BMC Health Services Research*, *19*(1), 542. https://doi.org/10.1186/s12913-019-4373-x

Mangat, A. K., Oei, J.-L., Quah-Smith, I., & Schmolzer, G. M. (2018). A review of non-pharmacological treatments for pain management in newborn infants. *Children*, *5*(10), 130. https://doi.org/10.3390/children5100130

Masters, C., Robinson, D., Faulkner, S., Patterson, E., McIlraith, T., & Ansari, A. (2019). Addressing biases in patient care with the 5Rs of cultural humility, a clinician tool. *Journal of General Internal Medicine*, *34*, 627–630. https://doi.org/10.1007/s11606-018-4814-y

Maxwell, L. G., Fraga, M. V., & Malavolta, C. P. (2019). Assessment of pain in the newborn: An update. *Clinics in Perinatology*, *46*, 693–707. https://doi.org/10.1016/j.clp.2019.08.005

McClintock, A. S., McCarrick, S. M., Garland, E. L., Zeidan, F., & Zgierska, A. E. (2019). Brief mindfulness-based meditations for acute and chronic pain: A systematic review. *Journal of Alternative and Complementary Medicine*, *25*(3), 265–278. https://doi.org/10.1089/acm.2018.0351

McEwen, B. S. (1998). Stress, adaptation and disease: Allostasis and allostatic load. *Annals of the New York Academy of Sciences*, *840*(1), 33–44. https://doi.org/10.1111/j.1749-6632.1998.tb09546.x

McEwen, B. S. (2007). Physiology and neurobiology of stress and adaptation: Central role of the brain. *Physiological Reviews*, *87*, 873–904. https://doi.org/10.1152/physrev.00041.2006

McEwen, B. S. (2012). Brain on stress: How the social environment gets under the skin. *Proceedings of the National Academy of Sciences of the United States of America*, *109*(2), 17180–17185. https://doi.org/10.1073/pnas.1121254109

McGinnis, K., Murray, E., Cherven, B., McCracken, C., & Travers, C. (2016). Effect of vibration on pain response to heel lance: A pilot randomized control trial. *Advances in Neonatal Care*, *16*(6), 439–448. https://doi.org/10.1097/ANC.0000000000000315

Moen, A. (2020). If parents were drugs? *Acta Paediatrica*. https://doi.org/10.1111/apa.15306

Orovec, A., Disher, T., Caddell, K., & Campbell-Yeo, M. (2019). Assessment and management of procedural pain during the entire neonatal intensive care unit hospitalization. *Pain Management Nursing, 20*(5), 503–511. https://doi.org/10.1016/j.pmn.2018.11.061

Pados, B. F. (2019). Physiology of stress and use of skin-to-skin care as a stress-reducing intervention in the NICU. *Nursing for Women's Health, 23*(1), 59–70. https://doi.org/10.1016/j.nwh.2018.11.002

Pados, B. F., & Hess, F. (2019). Systematic review of the effects of skin-to-skin care on short-term physiologic stress outcomes in preterm infants in the neonatal intensive care unit. *Advances in Neonatal Care, 20*(1), 48–58. https://doi.org/10.1097/ANC.0000000000000596

Peng, H.-F., Yin, T., Yang, L., Wang, C., Chang, Y.-C., Jeng, M.-J., & Liaw, J.-J. (2018). Non-nutritive sucking, oral breast milk, and facilitated tucking relieve preterm infant pain during heel-stick procedure: A prospective, randomized controlled trial. *International Journal of Nursing Studies, 77*, 162–170. https://doi.org/10.1016/j.ijnurstu.2017.10.001

Pereira, T. R. C., De Souza, F. G., & Beleza, A. C. S. (2017). Implications of pain in functional activities in immediate postpartum period according to the mode of delivery and parity: An observational study. *Brazilian Journal of Physical Therapy, 21*(1), 37–43. https://doi.org/10.1016/j .bjpt.2016.12.003

Perroteau, A., Nanquette, M. C., Rousseau, A., Renolleau, A., Berard, L., Mitanchez, D., & Leblanc, J. (2018). Efficacy of facilitated tucking combined with nonnutritive sucking on very preterm infant's pain during the heel-stick procedure: A randomized controlled trial. *International Journal of Nursing Studies, 86*, 29–35. https://doi.org/10.1016/j.ijnurstu.2018.06.007

Perry, M., Tan, Z., Chen, J., Weidig, T., Xu, W., & Cong, X. S. (2019). Neonatal pain: Perceptions and current practice. *Critical Care Nursing Clinics of North America, 30*(4), 549–561. https://doi .org/10.1016/j.cnc.2018.07.013

Petteys, A. R., & Adoumie, D. (2018). Mindfulness-based neurodevelopmental care: Impact on NICU parent stress and infant length of stay; a randomized controlled pilot study. *Advances in Neonatal Care, 18*(2), e12–e22. https://doi.org/10.1097/ANC.0000000000000474

Picavet, H. S. J., Monique Verschuren, W. M., Groot, L., Schaap, L., & van Oostrom, S. H. (2019). Pain over the adult life course: 15-year pain trajectories—The Doetinchem Cohort Study. *European Journal of Pain, 23*(9), 1723–1732. https://doi.org/10.1002/ejp.1450

Pillai Riddell, R. R., Racine, N. M., Gennis, H. G., Turcotte, K., Uman, L. S., Horton, R. E., Ahola Kohut, S., Hillgrove Stuart, J., Stevens, B., & Lisi, D. M. (2015). Non-pharmacological management of infant and young child procedural pain. *Cochrane Database of Systematic Reviews, 12*, CD006275. https://doi.org/10.1002/14651858.CD006275.pub3

Polkki, T., Korhonen, A., & Laukkala, H. (2018). Nurses' perceptions of pain assessment and management practices in neonates: A cross-sectional study. *Scandinavian Journal of Caring Science, 32*(2), 725–733. https://doi.org/10.1111/scs.12503

Prouhet, P. M., Gregory, M. R., Russell, C. L., & Yaeger, L. H. (2018). Fathers' stress in the neonatal intensive care unit: A systematic review. *Advances in Neonatal Care, 18*(2), 105–120. https://doi .org/10.1097/ANC.0000000000000472

Raith, W. (2018). Auricular medicine in neonatal care. *Medical Acupuncture, 30*(3), 138–140.

Sanders, M. R., & Hall, A. L. (2018). Trauma-informed care in the newborn intensive care unit: promoting safety, security and connectedness. *Journal of Perinatology, 38*(1), 3–10. https://doi .org/10.1038/jp.2017.124

Sener Taplak, A., & Erdem, E. (2017). A comparison of breast milk and sucrose in reducing neonatal pain during eye exam for retinopathy of prematurity. *Breastfeeding Medicine, 12*, 305–310. https:// doi.org/10.1089/bfm.2016.0122

Shern, D. L., Blanch, A. K., & Steverman, S. M. (2016). Toxic stress, behavioral health, and the next major era in public health. *American Journal of Orthopsychiatry, 86*(2), 109–123. https://doi .org/10.1037/ort0000120

Shonkoff, J. P., Garner, A. S.; Committee on Psychosocial Aspects of Child and Family Health; Committee on Early Childhood, Adoption, and Dependent Care; Section on Developmental and Behavioral Pediatrics. (2012). The lifelong effects of early childhood adversity and toxic stress. *Pediatrics, 129*(1), e232–e246. https://doi.org/10.1542/peds.2011-2663

Sisson, H., Jones, C., Williams, R., & Lachanudis, L. (2015). Meta-ethnographic synthesis of fathers' experiences of the neonatal intensive care unit environ-ment during hospitalization of their premature infants. *Journal of Obstetric, Gynecologic, and Neonatal Nursing, 44*(4), 471–480. https:// doi.org/10.1111/1552-6909.12662

Skorobogatova, N., Zemaitiene, N., Smigelskas, K., & Tameliene, R. (2017). Professional burnout and concurrent health complaints in neonatal nursing. *Open Medicine, 12,* 328–334. https://doi .org/10.1515/med-2017-0047

Stanulewicz, N., Knox, E., Narayanasamy, M., Shivji, N., Khunti, K., & Blake, H. (2020). Effectiveness of lifestyle health promotion interventions for nurses: A systematic review. *International Journal of Environmental Research and Public Health, 17*(1), 17. https://doi.org/10.3390/ijerph17010017

Sun, X., Lemyre, B., Barrowman, N., & O'Connor, M. (2010). Pain management during eye exami-nation for retinopathy of prematurity in preterm infants: A systematic review. *Acta Paediatrica, 99*(3), 329–334. https://doi.org/10.1111/j.1651-2227.2009.01612.x

Talbot, K., Madden, V. J., Jones, S. L., & Moseley, G. L. (2019). The sensory and affective compo-nents of pain: Are the differentially modifiable dimensions or inseparable aspects of a unitary experience? A systematic review. *British Journal of Anaesthesia, 123*(2), e263–e272. https://doi .org/10.1016/j.bja.2019.03.033

Tan, J. B. C., Dunbar, J., Hopper, A., Wilson, C. G., & Angeles, D. M. (2019). Differential effects of the retinopathy of prematurity exam on the physiology of premature infants. *Journal of Perina-tology, 39*(5), 708–716. https://doi.org/10.1038/s41372-019-0331-z

Tan, S. Y., & Yip, A. (2018). Hans Selye (1907–1982): Founder of the stress theory. *Singapore Medical Journal, 59*(4), 170–171. https://doi.org/10.11622/smedj.2018043

UNICEF. (2020). *Convention on the Rights of the Child.* https://www.unicef.org/child-rights-convention

Vittner, D., McGrath, J., Robinson, J., Lawhon, G., Cusson, R., Eisenfeld, L., Walsh, S., Young, E., & Cong, X. (2018). Increase in oxytocin from skin-to-skin care contact enhances develop-ment of parent–infant relationship. *Biological Research for Nursing, 20*(1), 54–62. https://doi .org/10.1177/1099800417735633

Volpe, J. J. (2019). Dysmaturation of premature brain: Importance, cellular mechanisms, and potential interventions. *Pediatric Neurology, 95,* 42–66. https://doi.org/10.1016/j.pediatrneurol.2019.02.016

Watson-Singleton, N. N., Black, A. R., & Spivey, B. N. (2019). Recommendations for a culturally-responsive mindfulness-based intervention for African-Americans. *Complementary Therapies in Clinical Practice, 34,* 132–138. https://doi.org/10.1016/j.ctcp.2018.11.013

Williams, M. D., & Lascelles, B. D. X. (2020). Early neonatal pain—A review of clinical and experi-mental implications on painful conditions later in life. *Frontiers in Pediatrics, 8,* 30. https://doi .org/10.3389/fped.2020.00030

Yang, S., & Chang, C. (2019). Chronic pain: Structural and functional changes in brain structures and associated negative affective states. *International Journal of Molecular Sciences, 20*(13), 3130. https://doi.org/10.3390/ijms20133130

Yaribeygi, H., Panahi, Y., Sahraei, H., Johnston, T. P., & Sahebkar, A. (2017). The impact of stress on body function: A review. *EXCLI Journal, 16,* 1057–1072. https://doi.org/10.17179/excli2017-480

10

Activities of Daily Living

I long to accomplish a great and noble task; but it is my chief duty to accomplish small tasks as if they were great and noble.
—Helen Keller

Activities of daily living (ADL) include posture and play, eating and nourishment, skin care and hygiene; these are self-care activities that promote health, support functional capabilities, and create opportunities to cultivate attachment and build loving respectful relationships with self and other. This chapter presents the latest research and evidence-based best practices related to ADL for the hospitalized infant, the family, and the healthcare professional.

WHAT ARE ACTIVITIES OF DAILY LIVING?

Posture and Play

Postural alignment is key to optimal body function. Much like the frame of a house, our musculoskeletal system is the frame for our bodies, supporting and protecting our organs and systems from injury and/or progressive deformity (Korakakis et al., 2019). Alterations in our postural alignment can lead to pain, distress, and changes in functional integrity. In a longitudinal study looking at physical functioning trajectories among adults between the ages of 26 and 70 years, researchers discovered that over half of the population followed a stable but slightly limited level of physical functioning over the 15-year study period (Rooth et al., 2016). Risk factors for poor physical function included female gender, age, physical inactivity, being overweight or obese, poor mental health, poor self-perceived health, and having one or more chronic conditions (Rooth et al., 2016).

Posture, to include head and neck orientation, influences breathing and swallowing, with head and neck flexion or extension significantly impeding airway and esophageal diameters (Alghadir et al., 2017). In a healthy adult male cohort, the effect of body posture on swallowing was examined through videoendoscopy. The researchers discovered the

BOX 10.1 FIVE CHARACTERISTICS OF PLAYFUL EXPERIENCES

1. Play is joyful.
2. Play is meaningful.
3. Play is actively engaging.
4. Play is iterative.
5. Play is socially interactive.

Source: Data from Zosh, J. M., Hopkins, E. J., Jensen, H., Liu, C., Neale, D., Hirsh-Pasek, K., Solis, S. L., & Whitebread, D. (2017). *Learning through play: A review of the evidence* (white paper). The LEGO Foundation.

recline position prolonged the onset latency of the pharyngeal phase, or the time to swallow, creating a safer swallowing experience (Shiino et al., 2016). In addition to a reclined posture, sole–ground contact (or having your foot on the ground) during eating was found to activate trunk muscles and head posture, improving pharyngeal stability and ensuring a safe swallow (Uesugi et al., 2019).

The integrative nature of the musculoskeletal system supports systemic function and comfort. Postural deviations have been linked to episodic tension-type headaches and cervicogenic headaches (Mingels et al., 2019). In addition, slumped posture, associated with laptop, desktop, smartphone, and tablet use for greater than 3 hours per day resulted in a higher prevalence of musculoskeletal complaints such as pain in the upper extremities, neck, and head (Bubric & Hedge, 2016; Mingels et al., 2019; Osama et al., 2018). The specific postural deviation linked to these pain complaints involves the sagittal configuration of the cervical spine, or the forward head posture (FHP). Researchers have found a significant correlation between FHP and neck pain intensity and disability (Mahmoud et al., 2019). This postural deviation also alters cervical sensorimotor control and autonomic nervous system dysfunction (Moustafa et al., 2020).

Play activities can optimize musculoskeletal integrity, along with reducing stress, enriching socioemotional relationships and supporting healthy developmental trajectories across the life continuum. Historian Johan Huizinga (1955) identified play as one of the most central activities in a flourishing society. From an evolutionary perspective, play is observed across a wide range of species and as such, serves an important purpose considering the costs it entails in terms of time, energy, and risk of injury (Huizinga, 1955). We learn through play. Zosh et al. (2017) describe five characteristics of playful learning experiences (Box 10.1). Play is not just for children. In the words of George Bernard Shaw (1856–1950), "We don't stop playing because we grow old; we grow old because we stop playing."

Play is fun, supports survival, and is closely linked with exercise and stress reduction (S. Wang & Aamodt, 2012). From a survival perspective, play boosts imagination and creativity, stimulates the mind and the body, enhances problem-solving skills, develops and

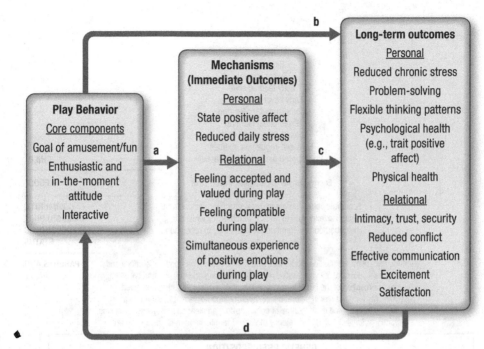

Figure 10.1 Model of the effects of play in adulthood.

Source: Van Fleet, M., & Feeney, B. C. (2015). Young at heart: A perspective for advancing research on play in adulthood. *Perspectives on Psychological Science*, *10*(5), 639–645. doi: 10.1177/1745691615596789 Reprinted with permission from Sage Publications.

improves social skills, is a source of relaxation, and relieves stress (Figure 10.1; Van Fleet & Feeney, 2015). High levels of play are associated with low levels of cortisol (S. Wang & Aamodt, 2012). Play activates the release of the neurotransmitter norepinephrine and dopamine, which rouse us to attention to facilitate learning while encoding the key component of fun: reward.

Eating and Nourishment

Eating is the process of ingesting food. *Nourishment* refers to to items, such as food, that nourish, strengthen, or build up. Eating and nourishment are supported by a myriad of physiologic and psychoemotional phenomena that influence our eating behavior and health from birth to adulthood. The consumption of food is a result of complex biopsychological and environmental factors that go beyond homeostatic energy regulation and are influenced by early-life eating experiences (Migraine et al., 2013; Moran & Ladenheim, 2016; Nicklaus, 2017; Simon et al., 2017).

Eating behaviors develop rapidly from infancy to school age and are mediated by neural mechanisms, early-life experiences, child development, parent–child interactions, and social influences (Gahagan, 2012). Many of these behaviors are the result of modifiable

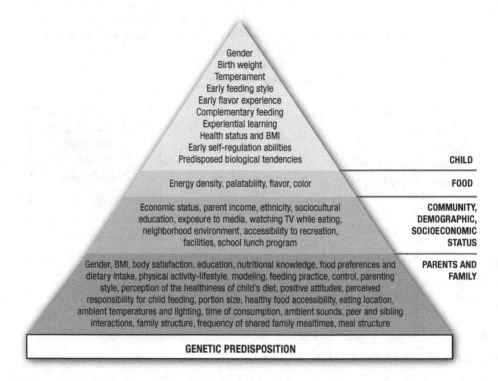

Figure 10.2 Factors that influence a child's eating behaviors.

BMI, body mass index.
Source: Scaglioni, S., De Cosmi, V., Ciappolino, V., Parazzini, F., Brambilla, P., & Agostoni, C. (2018). Factors influencing children's eating behaviours. *Nutrients, 10*(6), 706. https://doi.org/10.3390/nu10060706 Reprinted with permission under the Creative Commons Attribution License.

feeding practices (Nicklaus, 2017). Certainly, a healthy diet must be attractive and gratifying from both a homeostatic and hedonic perspective; however, the social dimensions of the eating encounter also play a role in food intake (Herman, 2015; Livovsky et al., 2020).

External factors include the social and physical environment along with specific food variables, such as temperature, color, and smell, influence food intake and food choices (Stroebele & De Castro, 2004). Ambience may be a modifiable factor to enhance the eating experience of individuals across the age spectrum (Nicklaus, 2017; Stroebele & De Castro, 2004). Understanding the mechanisms and various factors that influence eating behavior and underlie food habits is helpful to create healthy food practices (Figure 10.2; Scaglioni et al., 2018).

Healthy food practices are key to reducing obesity. Overweight and obesity are complex public health crises that continue to increase in prevalence around the globe (Figures 10.3 and 10.4; Hruby & Hu, 2015; Ritchie & Roser, 2020). Biological, behavioral, and environmental factors contribute to this disease, which is associated with high morbidity and mortality (Table 10.1; Hruby & Hu, 2015). Healthy food practices begin in infancy (Hruby & Hu, 2015).

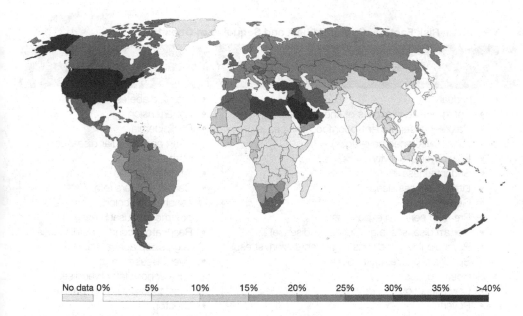

No data 0%   5%   10%   15%   20%   25%   30%   35%   >40%

Figure 10.3 Share of adults globally who are obese, 2016.

Source: Ritchie, H., & Roser, M. (2020). *Obesity.* OurWorldInData.org. https://ourworldindata.org/obesity

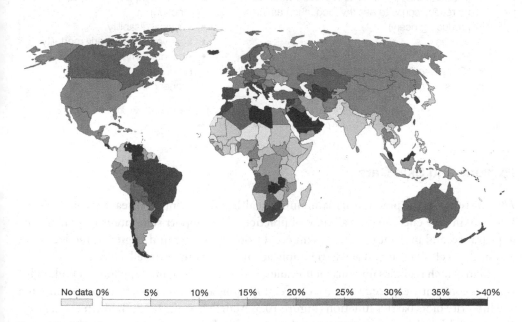

No data 0%   5%   10%   15%   20%   25%   30%   35%   >40%

Figure 10.4 Share of children ages 2 to 4 globally who are obese, 2016.

Source: Ritchie, H., & Roser, M. (2020). *Obesity.* OurWorldInData.org. https://ourworldindata.org/obesity

Table 10.1 **Risk Factors, Comorbidities, and Sequelae of Obesity**

Risk Factors (Nonexhaustive)	Comorbidities and Sequelae (Nonexhaustive)
<ul><li>Individual<ul><li>Energy intake in excess of energy needs</li><li>Calorie-dense, nutrient-poor food choices (e.g., sugar-sweetened beverages)</li><li>Low physical activity</li><li>Sedentariness</li><li>Little or excess sleep</li><li>Genetics</li><li>Pre- and perinatal exposures</li><li>Certain diseases (e.g., Cushing's disease)</li><li>Psychological conditions (e.g., depression, stress)</li><li>Specific drugs (e.g., steroids)</li></ul></li><li>Socioeconomics<ul><li>Low education</li><li>Poverty</li></ul></li><li>Environment<ul><li>Lack of access to physical activity resources/low walkability neighborhoods</li><li>Food deserts (i.e., geographic areas with little to no ready access to healthy food, such as fresh produce/grocery)</li><li>Viruses</li><li>Microbiota</li><li>"Obesogens" (e.g., endocrine-disrupting chemicals)</li><li>Obese social ties</li></ul></li></ul>	<ul><li>Type 2 diabetes</li><li>Hypertension</li><li>Dyslipidemia</li><li>Heart and vascular diseases</li><li>Osteoarthritis</li><li>Infertility</li><li>Certain cancers (e.g., esophageal, colon, postmenopausal breast)</li><li>Respiratory conditions/diseases (e.g., sleep apnea, asthma)</li><li>Liver diseases (e.g., nonalcoholic fatty liver disease, nonalcoholic steatohepatitis)</li><li>Gallstones</li><li>Trauma treatment/survival</li><li>Infection</li><li>Psychological conditions (e.g., depression, psychosocial function)</li><li>Physical disability</li><li>Lost years of life/early mortality</li><li>Absenteeism/loss of productivity</li><li>Higher medical costs</li></ul>

Source: Adapted from Hruby, A., & Hu, F. B. (2015). The epidemiology of obesity: A big picture. *Pharmacoeconomics, 33*(7), 673–689. doi: 10.1007/s40273-014-0243-x Reprinted with permission from Wolters Kluwer Health, Inc.

Hygiene and Skin Care

Hygiene refers to the practice of maintaining health and preventing disease through cleanliness. Skin care encompasses a range of practices that support skin integrity, enhance its appearance, and prevent or relieve skin conditions. Skin care and hygiene practices have physical, psychological and aesthetic implications for health and well-being.

Skin, which includes mucous membranes, is the largest organ of the human body. This organ is constantly exposed to a variety of endogenous and exogenous factors that threaten the integrity of its barrier function (Figure 10.5; Abdallah et al., 2017; Baldwin et al., 2017; Barnard & Li, 2017). Barrier function, which keeps pathogens out, limits evaporative losses and preserves skin moisture, increases with gestational age, and is generally mature by 34 weeks of gestation (Oranges et al., 2015; Visscher et al., 2015).

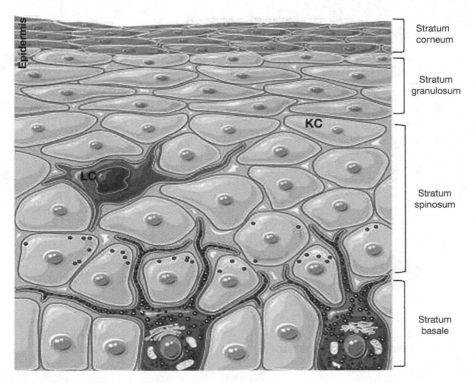

Figure 10.5 Skin anatomy and cellular constituents.

KC, keratinocyte; LC, Langerhans cell.
Source: Abdallah, F., Mijouin, L., & Pichon, C. (2017). Skin immune landscape: Inside and outside the organism. *Mediators of Inflammation.*
https://doi.org/10.1155/2017/5095293

Skin is composed of the epidermis, the dermis, and the hypodermis, or subcutaneous fat layer. The epidermis and dermis host a dynamic ecosystem, referred to as the *skin microbiota* or *microbiome*, which plays a significant role in one's physical and mental health and well-being (Abdallah et al., 2017; Butler et al., 2019; Chen et al., 2018). Although the skin microbiome is not as well studied as the gut microbiome, the shared purpose and function between these two systems highlights the relevance of evidence-based hygiene and skin care practices.

The gastrointestinal tract is an invagination of the surface of the skin and shares very similar functions with regard to the microbiome. Both systems reflect a complex network of immune and epithelial cells that continuously communicate with the external and internal environments (Abdallah et al., 2017; Salem et al., 2018). Perturbations within the microbiome as well as disruptions to tissue integrity affect health and wellness. Within this context, pathogenicity of the microbiome arises (Figure 10.6; Chen et al., 2018; Salem et al., 2018).

The skin is the first line of defense against invading pathogens and achieves its goals for defense in partnership with the microbial communities that inhabit the microbiome. Although the primary purpose for preserving and protecting skin integrity is about health maintenance, the hedonic and aesthetic aspects of skin care are equally relevant. Skin care

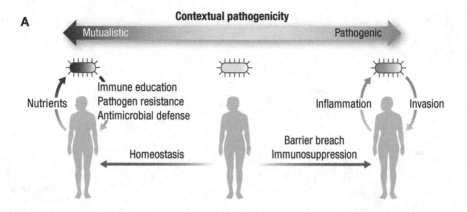

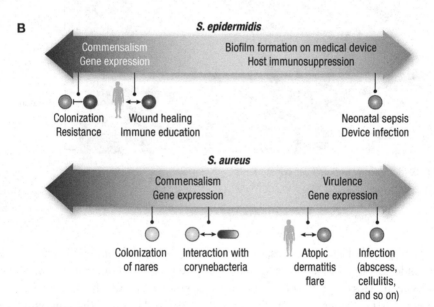

Figure 10.6 Contextual pathogenicity. (A) Represents the spectrum of the relationship between host and microbiota; (B) offers an example.

Source: Chen, Y. E., Fischbach, M. A., & Belkaid, Y. (2018). Skin microbiota-host interactions. *Nature, 553*(7689), 427–436. doi: 10.1038/nature25177 Reprinted with permission from Springer Nature.

and hygiene practices meet personal needs for comfort, soothing, and self-love that validate self-worth and realign body, mind, and spiritl.

Summary

ADL, such as posture, play, eating, and bathing, are more than indicators of functional status. ADL are opportunities to care for self and others in ways that are honorable, loving, and nurturing. A trauma-informed approach to these daily activities supports the multidimensionality of self and others, preserving health and wellness across physical, psychological, and spiritual domains. The attributes with examples of this core measure are described in Table 10.2. For additional resources on the skin and microbiome, see Reader Resources at the end of the chapter.

> *Nurturing yourself is not selfish—it's essential to your survival and your well-being.*
> —Renee Peterson Trudeau

Table 10.2 ADL Core Measure Attributes

Attributes	Examples
1. Appropriate postural alignment, mobility, and play ensure comfort, safety, and physiologic and emotional stability and support optimal neuromotor integrity.	*Infant:* Skin-to-skin care in the side-lying diagonal position promotes optimal postural alignment and facilitates play with parent. *Family:* Accessible supportive seating for parents ensures postural alignment and comfort during attachment play encounters. *Staff:* Ergonomic guidelines are established to protect musculoskeletal health; organizations provide resources/benefits that promote physical activity and well-being for staff.
2. Eating experiences are positive, pleasant, nurturing, and nourishing.	*Infant:* Direct breastfeeding is encouraged and facilitated. Oral feeding encounters are guided and directed by the infant's level of readiness and engagement, supported within an age-appropriate environmental milieu. *Family:* Parents receive education on healthy nutrition for infants and families in crisis. Families have open access to healthy, nutritious meals in a quiet, clean, and relaxed setting during the hospital stay. Food security is assessed, and appropriate resources and counseling services are activated to restore food security prior to discharge. *Staff:* Cost-conscious, nutritious food options are available to staff 24/7; vending machines provide access to healthy snack and beverage options.

(continued)

Table 10.2 **ADL Core Measure Attributes** *(continued)*

Attributes	Examples
3. Appropriate hygiene and skin care routines preserve barrier function and tissue integrity while ensuring a calming and nurturing experience.	*Infant:* Nonsterile glove use is reserved for encounters with blood and body fluids. *Family:* Swaddled bathing is provided by parents on a weekly basis. *Staff:* Staff comply with hand-hygiene protocol and the appropriate use of infection control procedures; staff have easy access to alcohol-based hand sanitizers and appropriate emollients to preserve their skin integrity.

ADL, activities of daily living.
Source: Reprinted with permission from Caring Essentials Collaborative, LLC.

Table 10.3 **Factors Associated With Musculoskeletal Disorders**

Body mass index (BMI)	Amount of time standing and walking during work
Age	Stress levels at work
Work seniority	Exercise habits
Work content	Working hours and number of hours per week

Source: Adapted from Lin, S. C., Lin, L. L., Liu, C. J., Fang, C. K., & Lin, M. H. (2020). Exploring the factors affecting musculoskeletal disorders risk among hospital nurses. *PLoS One, 15*(4), e0231319. https://doi.org/10.1371/journal.pone.0231319

ACTIVITIES OF DAILY LIVING AND THE CLINICIAN

Posture and Play

Stable posture involves complex motor skills, including the coordination of multiple body segments and sensory inputs to maintain balance. Gravitational forces, genetic predisposition, anthropometric disadvantages, and an individual's psychosocial propensity derail postural integrity and predispose the individual to work-related musculoskeletal injuries (Vasavada et al., 2015; Vieira & Kumar, 2004). Fatigue, as a consequence of physical activity, also undermines postural stability and predisposes the affected individual to injury (Thomas & Magal, 2014).

Nurses have one of the highest prevalence rates for musculoskeletal disorders (MSD; Heidari et al., 2018; Lin et al., 2020). Risk factors associated with MSD in nurses are listed in Table 10.3. Weak body posture, inappropriate movement patterns, and inadequate implementation of ergonomic work practices contribute to work-related MSD in nursing (Heidari et al., 2019; Kotcz & Jenaszek, 2020). Psychosocial elements are also linked to MSD. Nurses with low levels of job satisfaction and a perceived low quality of life are more likely to report MSD (Lin et al., 2020).

The most frequent musculoskeletal complaints reported by nurses include low-back pain, neck pain, shoulder and arm/elbow aches, as well as hand/wrist pain (Heidari et al., 2019). Nonergonomic behavior is commonplace in nursing, specifically with regard to long-term standing positions destabilizing the shoulder girdle and placing strain on cervical spine muscles (Kotcz & Jenaszek, 2020). In a recent study investigating the degree to which nurses optimize workplace ergonomics, only 36.6% of nurses indicated they adjusted the height of the patient's bed to accommodate optimal postural alignment during caregiving (Kotcz & Jenaszek, 2020).

Work-related postures have a significant impact on exertion and risk for musculoskeletal discomfort. Freitag et al. (2014) demonstrated a significant decrease in perceived exertion when care was delivered with the patient's bed height adjusted to maintain clinician's upright position. Physical ergonomics, those dimensions related to individual anthropometry, biomechanics, and physiology, affect an individual's ability to physically interact with the environment to perform lifesaving tasks (Yamada et al., 2019). These ergonomic challenges have implications for the clinician's postural integrity, procedural competence, as well as musculoskeletal and psychological well-being (Lin et al., 2020; Yamada et al., 2019).

Posture related to computer use is also linked to musculoskeletal complaints in nurses (Lin et al., 2020). Conventional computer input devices, such as keyboard and mouse, are associated with musculoskeletal symptoms (Bruno Garza & Young, 2015). Static body posture during computer use is the primary musculoskeletal risk factor (Kargar et al., 2018).

Unhealthy aspects of nurses' lifestyles, including shift work, improper dietary patterns and eating habits, sedentary lifestyles, and lower levels of physical activity or mobility, contribute to postural perturbations resulting in painful musculoskeletal complaints (Kotcz & Jenaszek, 2020). Engaging in play and physical activity optimizes physical and mental health and reduces musculoskeletal complaints by increasing flexibility and core strength and reducing stress. The physically demanding work of nursing, with long hours and rotating shifts, may contribute to low levels of leisure time, physical activity, and play (Nam et al., 2018).

There is little consensus as to what "play at work" looks like; however, the general consensus is that it increases productivity, engagement, and morale (Petelczyc et al., 2018). One form of "play at work" is Lego Serious Play (LSP; Figure 10.7). Grounded in social constructionism, LSP is a valuable tool for inquiry-based learning that facilitates creative expression, problem-solving, and meaning-making. Hayes (2016) successfully utilized LSP to facilitate affective learning in healthcare assistants around the concepts of care and compassion. Engaging in this type of play builds engagement and teamwork. Play at work opens the door for workplace fun, which is directly linked to greater employee engagement, productivity, and job satisfaction (Fluegge-Woolf, 2014; Owler & Morrison, 2020).

Figure 10.7 is an example of LSP with a team of multidisciplinary NICU clinicians. The team participated in a didactic workshop on trauma-informed care. At the end of the workshop, the team broke into small groups and built a sculpture that represented their greatest insight from the workshop. Participants experienced initial anxiety and confusion about the

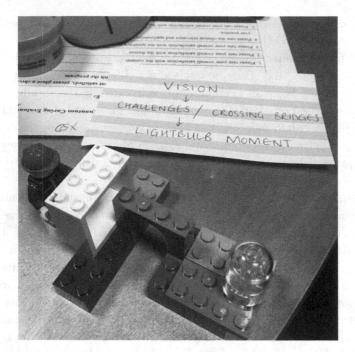

Figure 10.7 Example of Lego Serious Play at a Caring Essentials workshop.

Source: Reprinted with permission from Caring Essentials Collaborative, LLC.

play. This hesitation and confusion has been described in other LSP settings. Learners must feel safe and comfortable within the play setting before they engage in the activity, especially among colleagues and peers (Roos & Victor, 2018). The play enables participants to get out of their head and into their hands. Engaging the hand–mind connection unleashes creative and expressive ways of thinking. This method of play supports unbiased free-thinking, playful interaction, and team-building that results in shared understanding, creative problem-solving, and self-discovery (Tawalbeh et al., 2018). Additional postural resources and play resources are available in the Reader Resources section at the end of this chapter.

Eating and Nourishment

The Nurse's Health Study II reveals that more than 25% of nurses are currently obese and an additional 30% are overweight (Raney & van Zanten, 2019). Occupational factors, such as a sedentary role and working 40 hours or more per week, were significantly associated with overweight/obesity (Chin et al., 2016). Poor dietary habits put the health of 53% to 61% of U.S. nurses at risk (Priano et al., 2018). Poor diet choices coupled with inactivity increase nurses' risk for cardiovascular disease and a diminished health-related quality of life (Priano et al., 2018).

Terada et al. (2019) examined the relationship between dietary behavior and cardio-metabolic and psychological health in female nurses and compared these findings with shift work. Nurses who rotated shifts snacked more frequently, took in 400 more calories

Table 10.4 **Pender's Model for Health Promotion**

Individual Characteristics	Behavior-Specific Cognition and Affect	Behavioral Outcomes
• Prior related behavior • Personal factors	• Perceived benefits of action • Perceived barriers to action • Perceived self-efficacy • Activity-related affect • Interpersonal influences • Situational influences	• Health promoting behaviors

Source: Adapted from Ross, A., Touchton-Leonard, K., Perez, A., Wehrlen, L., Kazmi, N., & Gibbons, S. (2019). Factors that influence health-promoting self-care in registered nurses: Barriers and facilitators. *Advances in Nursing Science, 42*(4), 358–373. doi: 10.1097/ANS.0000000000000274

Table 10.5 **Barriers and Facilitators to Health-Promoting Behaviors in Nurses**

Barriers to Health-Promoting Behavior	Individuals Who Influence Health-Promoting Behaviors
• No time/overwork • Lack of adequate resources/facilities • Fatigue/lack of sleep • Outside commitments • Unhealthy food culture	• Supportive versus unsupportive individuals • Positive versus negative role models

Source: Ross, A., Touchton-Leonard, K., Perez, A., Wehrlen, L., Kazmi, N., & Gibbons, S. (2019). Factors that influence health-promoting self-care in registered nurses: Barriers and facilitators. *Advances in Nursing Science, 42*(4), 358–373. doi: 10.1097/ANS.0000000000000274

per day, and demonstrated worse mood-tension and anger-hostility scores than nurses who worked a straight day shift (Terada et al., 2019). Shift-working nurses had limited access to healthy food options and often opted for sweet food during the night shift to maintain wakefulness and energy levels (Terada et al., 2019).

Chico-Barba et al. (2019) investigated the association between metabolic syndrome and burnout, defined by the Maslach Burnout Inventory (MBI). Associations of emotional exhaustion, personal accomplishment (two subscales of the MBI), and night shift were linked to an increased waist circumference (Chico-Barba et al., 2019). Disruptions to circadian rhythms, lack of a meal routine, eating alone, having limited food options, staffing, and time constraints negatively impact dietary behavior during shift work (Saulle et al., 2018).

A. Ross et al. (2019) used qualitative content analysis to explore nurses' perceptions of barriers and facilitators to exercise, healthy eating, and stress reduction activities framed by Pender's model of health promotion (Table 10.4). Seven themes emerged (Table 10.5). Nicholls et al. (2017) corroborate Ross's findings, reporting the majority of barriers to healthy eating in the workplace are related to adverse work schedules, individual barriers, aspects of the physical environment, and social eating practices at work.

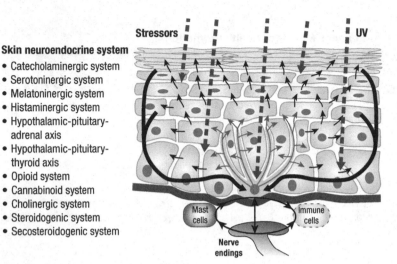

Skin neuroendocrine system
- Catecholaminergic system
- Serotoninergic system
- Melatoninergic system
- Histaminergic system
- Hypothalamic-pituitary-adrenal axis
- Hypothalamic-pituitary-thyroid axis
- Opioid system
- Cannabinoid system
- Cholinergic system
- Steroidogenic system
- Secosteroidogenic system

Figure 10.8 Skin neuroendocrine system.

Source: Slominski, A. T., Zmijewski, M. A., Skobowiat, C., Zbytek, B., Slominski, R. M., & Steketee J. D. (2012). Introduction in sensing the environment: Regulation of local and global homeostasis by the skin's neuroendocrine system. In P. Sutovsky, F. Clascá, Z. Kmiec, H.-W. Korf, M. J. Schmeisser, B. Singh, & J.-P. Timmermans (Eds.), *Advances in anatomy, embryology and cell biology* (Vol. 212, pp. 1–6). Springer Nature. Reprinted with permission from Springer Nature.

Hygiene and Skin Care

Compliance with hand-hygiene protocol is only one aspect of hygiene and skin care for the clinician. Maintaining skin integrity is critical for overall health and wellness. Skin arises from the same embryonic germ layer as the central nervous system and contains its own neuroendocrine immune system (Figure 10.8; Slominski et al., 2012). Skin, like posture and play, allows us to experience and feel the world around us.

The brain–skin connection has been linked to inflammatory skin diseases either triggered or exacerbated by stress (Figure 10.9; Arck et al., 2006). The relationship between psychosocial stress and dermatological disorders has been studied extensively within the fields of psychoneuroimmunology, molecular psychosomatics, and psychodermatology (Peters, 2016). Epidemiological evidence suggests a relationship exists between mental distress and several chronic skin conditions (Box 10.2; Martins et al., 2020; Peters, 2016; Uysal et al., 2019).

Psychological stress is also responsible for delayed wound healing and contributes to skin aging (Chen & Lyga, 2014; Martins et al., 2020). The intensity of chronic skin symptoms correlates with depression, anxiety, dysfunctional coping behaviors, dissociation, withdrawal, and feelings of helplessness in affected individuals (Peters, 2016). The complex nature of skin's immune, endocrine, and neurological functions is similar to that of the brain and explains why a holistic approach to health and wellness is so important, beginning with skin care and hygiene practices (Coleman, 2020). Within the context of nursing, understanding the psychoemotional connection between skin integrity and stress emphasizes the importance of self-care routines that optimize both physical and emotional well-being.

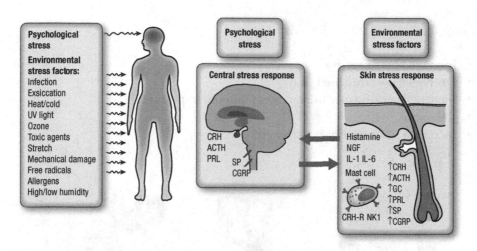

Figure 10.9 Brain–skin cross-talk with exposure to psychological and/or environmental stressors.

CGRP, calcitonin gene-related peptide; CRH, corticotropin-releasing hormone; CRH-R, corticotropin-releasing hormone receptor; GC, gluco-corticoid; IL, interleukin; NGF, nerve growth factor; NK1, neurokinin-1 antagonist; PRL, prolactin; SP, substance P.

Source: Arck, P. C., Slominski, A., Theoharides, T. C., Peters, E. M. J., & Paus, R. (2006). Neuroimmunology of stress: Skin takes center stage. *Journal of Investigative Dermatology, 126*(8), 1697–16704. doi: 10.1038/sj.jid.5700104 Reprinted with permission from Elsevier.

BOX 10.2 CHRONIC CUTANEOUS DISEASES AGGRAVATED BY STRESS

- Psoriasis
- Atopic dermatitis
- Seborrheic eczema
- Prurigo nodularis
- Chronic urticaria
- Alopecia areata

Source: Adapted from Martins, A. M., Ascenso, A., Ribeiro, H. M., & Marto, J. (2020). The brain–skin connection and the pathogenesis of psoriasis: A review with a focus on the serotonergic system. *Cells, 9*(4), 796. https://doi.org/10.3390/cells9040796

EVIDENCE-BASED STRATEGIES FOR ACTIVITIES OF DAILY LIVING FOR THE CLINICIAN

ADL are interconnected facets of self-care. Beyond the physiological benefits of good posture (Box 10.3), posture reflects an individual's internal state of mind. Research has shown that posture and mood are interrelated, and one can influence the other (Aggio

BOX 10.3 PHYSIOLOGICAL BENEFITS OF GOOD POSTURE

- Improved lung capacity
- Decreased posture-based pain
- Increased performance using correct movement posture
- Relaxation
- Increased core stability and strength

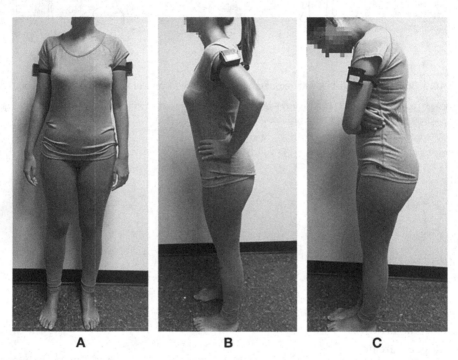

Figure 10.10 Postures adopted during Miragall et al.'s (2018) experiment. (A) Neutral posture, (B) expanded posture, (C) contracted posture.

et al., 2017; Miragall et al., 2018). The construct of embodied cognition argues that the motor system influences our cognition or how our body, movement, and posture impact our perceptions of the world and ourselves (Mahon, 2015; Miragall et al., 2018).

Aggio et al. (2017) demonstrated a 1-hour increase in daily physical activity was associated with a decreased negative effect. In a supervised group exercise program employing occupational physical therapists, participants achieved enhanced aerobic fitness, improved muscle strength, and had an increase in psychological well-being (Matsugaki et al., 2017). Miragall et al. (2018) examined the effect of posture and mood. An expansive posture (Figure 10.10)

Table 10.6 **Verbatim Instructions to Participants in the Cohen et al. (2020) Study**

Postural Instructions	Full Version	Short Version
Relax	Stand as you would if you were feeling tired and lazy; like it's the end of a day, and nobody is watching, and you do not really care about your posture. Let your head and chest feel heavy and let everything settle a bit downward.	Stand relaxed and heavy and let everything settle down.
Effortful	Use muscular effort to pull yourself up to your greatest height. Pull your head up, lift your chest, and tighten all the core muscles in your torso. You can think of holding a military posture, which *looks* really strong. Really work at it!	Pull yourself up to your greatest height, using muscular effort.
Light	Have the idea that you WANT to go up, but you are not going to do it with muscular effort. Instead, let the ground send you up through your bones, and let your head float up on top of your spine. (Remember where we touched you behind the ears when we were setting up the camera system? The top of your spine is right between those points.) Notice that at the same time as you are going up, you can also expand your width.	Allow your bones to send you up; let your head float on top of your neck.

resulted in positive emotions of happiness and self-confidence. Practitioners of Tai Chi and Qigong report not only improved postural awareness and alignment but also improved psychological health (Osypiuk et al., 2018).

Shifting one's mindset from effortful to effortless in attaining postural alignment results in less muscle activation and better balance (Table 10.6; Cohen et al., 2020). Posture is an important vehicle for communication—body language. According to Amy Cuddy, body language shapes who we are. See Reader Resources at the end of the chapter for more information. As health care professionals, recognizing how we present ourselves impacts

Table 10.7 **Subthemes and Examples of the "Supernurse" Culture**

Subthemes	Examples
Extraordinary powers used for good	Feelings of complete responsibility to care for patients and support colleagues
Cloak of invulnerability	An image of strength, invulnerability, and alignment with "supernurse" values
No sidekick	Resistant to ask for help; acs alone to handle fatigue
Kryptonite	Perception that fatigue is a sign of weakness
Alter ego	Generational differences in the perceptions of fatigue

Source: Adapted from Steege, L. M., & Rainbow, J. G. (2017). Fatigue in hospital nurses—"Supernurse" culture is a barrier to addressing problems: A qualitative interview study. *International Journal of Nursing Studies, 67,* 20–28. doi: 10.1016/j.ijnurstu.2016.11.014

how we are "seen" and the degree to which our interactions are deemed beneficial. It's about mindfulness (refer to Chapter 5).

Establishing ergonomic guidelines and ensuring the availability of ergonomically designed resources mitigates the risk of musculoskeletal injury (Richardson et al., 2019). Computer workstations must include multiple modes of input to reduce ergonomic strain at the user-interface (Bruno Garza & Young, 2015; Kargar et al., 2018). Ergonomic educational interventions improve posture and postural biomechanics and should be an integral part of new hire onboarding and annual competency review (Moazzami et al., 2016).

Workplace lifestyle interventions significantly improve dietary behaviors, body composition, physical activity, and stress reduction in nurses (Stanulewicz et al., 2020). However, these interventions are impacted by the prevailing culture regarding breaks and the adoption of self-care practices (Pearce, 2018; Power et al., 2017; Simpfel & Aiken, 2013). Steege and Rainbow (2017) introduce the concept of the "supernurse" culture when examining the concept of fatigue in nursing. Fatigue undermines healthy lifestyle choices and behaviors. Table 10.7 presents the subthemes of the "supernurse" culture and offers examples for each theme. Addressing these cultural barriers to self-care will enhance the quality of work/life balance for nurses.

Understanding the barriers and facilitators to healthy dietary behavior and self-health promotion is critical to improving the health status and job performance of nurses. Ensuring nurses have access to healthy food options while on duty and are guaranteed protected meal and rest breaks is a critical first step for a healthy workforce (refer to Chapter 6; Power et al., 2017). Employer health promotion programs are effective strategies that improve the health and wellness of staff (Gutermuth et al., 2018). Organizations committed to promoting health for their employees can assess the quality of their health promotion program using The Centers for Disease Control and Prevention (CDC) Worksite Health Score Card (www.cdc.gov/dhdsp/pubs/docs/hsc_manual.pdf; Gutermuth et al., 2018).

ACTIVITIES OF DAILY LIVING AND THE NICU FAMILY

Postural stability is altered in pregnant and postpartum women, which increases their risk of falls (Opala-Berdzik et al., 2015). Skeletal overload and biomechanical stress associated with posture and gait alterations, weight gain, and delivery compromise the integrity of the postpartum musculoskeletal system (Vassalou et al., 2019). Distortions to the recti abdominis muscles from the growing fetus and uterine capsule undermine abdominal wall strength and functionality (Werner & Dayan, 2018).

Women whose pregnancies are complicated by low-back pain and pelvic girdle pain are more likely to experience a persistence of these types of pain in the postpartum period (Sakamoto & Gamada, 2019). Postpartum postural pain can undermine maternal–infant attachment, increase psychoemotional distress and postpartum depression, and may limit maternal presence at the hospitalized infant's bedside (Angelo et al., 2014; Catena et al., 2019; refer to Chapter 9). Although posture and balance improve soon after birth, women with complications to their pregnancy outcome may continue to struggle with balance and require postural assistance.

Additional postural concerns include skin-to-skin postures and, for mothers, breast-feeding postures. The traditional parent posture for skin-to-skin holding has the parent in an upright to semi-upright position holding their infant in a chest-to-chest orientation with a receiving blanket around the infant's back. This static holding position is influenced by the force of gravity and induces fatigue to the parent's upper arms over a short period of time (Frey Law et al., 2010; Li & Chiu, 2015). The breastfeeding position is influenced by similar gravitational forces and the adoption of ergonomic principles greatly reduces musculoskeletal complaints while optimizing breastfeeding success (Afshariani et al., 2019; Colson, 2010, 2014).

Parent–infant play in the NICU facilitates bonding and attachment while validating parent role identity. Suboptimal bonding impairs hormonal, epigenetic, and neuronal development (Kommers et al., 2016). Skin-to-skin care is the perfect play activity for parents and infants in the NICU and beyond, supporting bonding and attachment. Parent–infant closeness and separation is hampered by the NICU environment (refer to Chapter 6), psychosocio-emotional factors of the family, as well as parental confidence and competence in parenting activities (Feeley et al., 2016).

Nutrition and nourishment are critical for health and well-being for the postpartum family. Increased nutritional demands can be underappreciated in times of crisis and exposure to traumatic stress. These stressors are superimposed onto the families' existing social determinants of health. Food insecurity has increased dramatically in the wake of the 2020 COVID pandemic in the United States (Figures 10.11 and 10.12; Bauer, 2020). Families with children under the age of 12 are most impacted (Bauer, 2020). Food-insecure individuals are at high risk for compromised child development and chronic illness (Health Research & Educational Trust, 2017).

Parents experience heightened states of stress and distress as a result of NICU hospitalization. This stress may manifest as skin disturbances, changes in hygiene

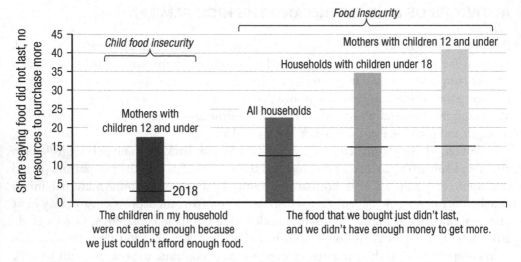

Figure 10.11 Food insecurity in the United States, April 2020.

Source: Bauer, L. (2020, May 6). *The COVID-19 crisis has already left too many children hungry in America.* https://www.brookings.edu/blog/up-front/2020/05/06/the-covid-19-crisis-has-already-left-too-many-children-hungry-in-america

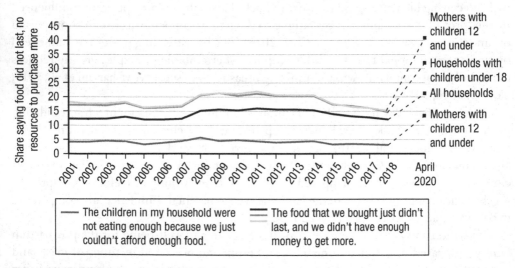

Figure 10.12 Food insecurity in the United States, 2001 to April 2020.

Source: Bauer, L. (2020, May 6). *The COVID-19 crisis has already left too many children hungry in America.* https://www.brookings.edu/blog/up-front/2020/05/06/the-covid-19-crisis-has-already-left-too-many-children-hungry-in-america

routines, and delayed wound healing (Martins et al., 2020; Peters, 2016; Uysal et al., 2019). In addition, skin integrity is compromised by sleep deficit, inadequate hydration, and poor diet.

EVIDENCE-BASED STRATEGIES FOR ACTIVITIES OF DAILY LIVING FOR THE NICU FAMILY

Understanding the musculoskeletal vulnerabilities of postpartum woman will guide NICU clinicians to support her postural alignment and comfort while caring for her hospitalized infant. Ensuring that comfortable, ergonomic seating is available for parents must be a priority. Ergonomic education for infant holding, both skin-to-skin, during breastfeeding and in arms, promotes safety in the hospital and paves the way for safe practices at home.

Mothers and their partners must be supported in playful encounters with their hospitalized infant. Infant play not only supports bonding and attachment but builds infant and parent self-efficacy while facilitating infant language skill acquisition (Gonya et al., 2017). Buil et al. (2019) investigated the use of a supported diagonal flexion (SDF) position in skin-to-skin on maternal depression risk scores and duration of skin-to-skin sessions. Mothers in the SDF group had significantly lower depression risk scores when compared to controls and spent more time in kangaroo care (Buil et al., 2019). Skin-to-skin care in the SDF position (Figure 10.13) results in a 3-time increase in infant vocalizations, when compared to the standard vertical position (Buil et al., 2020). Mothers using the SDF position spent more time vocalizing, smiling, and gazing at their infant than mothers using the standard vertical position (Buil et al., 2020).

The postpartum period is an opportunity to introduce healthy eating behaviors and well-being strategies to support family health throughout the hospital experience and at home (Faria-Schutzer et al., 2018; Lebrun et al., 2019). Improving the health of communities within a hospital's catchment area has become the mission of many hospitals (Health Research & Educational Trust, 2017). Clinical interventions include screening families for food insecurity and making healthy food choices available on site via food pharmacies, food pantries, mobile food pantries, and produce markets (Health Research & Educational Trust, 2017).

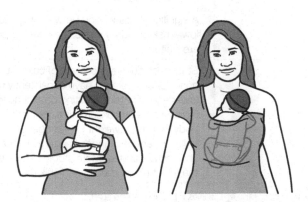

Figure 10.13 Skin-to-skin care positions. (*Left*) Standard vertical orientation, (*right*) supported diagonal flexion position.

Optimal hydration is a crucial intervention used to enhance health and wellness (Table 10.8; Liska et al., 2019). Providing families with their own water bottles and easy access to water refill stations within the unit can increase water consumption. Educational materials and staff role-modeling healthy hydration practices can also improve hydration, wellness, mood, and cognition (Liska et al., 2019).

Table 10.8 **Summary of Research on Hydration and Health Outcomes**

Health Outcomes	Summary of Literature Findings
Skin health	The effectiveness of additional water consumption on skin barrier function is unclear. A few studies suggest that increasing water consumption may improve the hydration of the stratum corneum layer of the epidermis, which plays a key role in skin barrier function. However, no changes to transepidermal water loss (measure of barrier integrity) were reported.
Cognition	Despite variability among study methodologies, dehydration impairs cognitive performance for tasks involving attention, executive function, and motor coordination when water deficits exceed 2% body mass loss. Cognitive domains involving lower order mental processing (e.g., simple reaction time) are less sensitive to changes in hydration status. In children, results from studies on hydration and cognition are mixed.
Mood and fatigue	Hypohydration is associated with increased negative emotions such as anger, hostility, confusion, depression and tension as well as fatigue and tiredness. These findings are consistent in adults, but unclear and very limited in children.
Kidney stones	A significant association between high fluid intake and a lower risk of kidney stones has been reported, but data are limited.
Body weight and body composition	Studies on fluid replacement of caloric beverages with noncaloric beverages have consistently resulted in lower energy intake. Existing data suggest that increased water consumption contributes to reductions in body fat and/or weight loss in obese adults, independent of changes in energy intake. Data in children are limited. More studies are needed to clarify the effect in both adults and children.

Source: Adapted from Liska, D., Mah, E., Brisbois, T., Barrios, P. L., Baker, L. B., & Spriet, L. L. (2019). Narrative review of hydration and selected health outcomes in the general population. *Nutrients, 11,* 70. https://doi.org/10.3390/nu11010070 Reprinted with permission Creative Commons CC BV License.

ACTIVITIES OF DAILY LIVING AND THE HOSPITALIZED INFANT

Posture and Play

Postural alignment and spontaneous mobility in the newborn period sets the stage for lifelong health and wellness. Preterm infants are at high risk for developmental delay; however, the absence of neurodevelopmental delay is not a guarantee for optimal neuromotor outcomes. Poor motor outcomes include subtle deficits in hand-eye coordination, sensory motor integration, manual dexterity, and gross motor skills and are common morbidities in this vulnerable population (Hughes et al., 2016).

The quality of general movement patterns and antigravity limb movements are markers for neurodevelopmental disorders, cognitive and behavioral outcomes in newborns (Einspieler et al., 2015, 2016; Ferrari et al., 2019; Hitzert et al., 2014; Miyagishima et al., 2016). Infants who present with abnormal general movements and concomitant motor and postural patterns had an increased risk of cerebral palsy (Ferrari et al., 2019). Preterm birth disrupts the developmental trajectory of antigravitational mechanisms of the infant's musculoskeletal system and are implicated in postural asymmetry at school age (Drzat-Grabiec et al., 2020; Walicka-Cuprys et al., 2017).

Infant orientation in skin-to-skin care has implications for postural alignment. Barriadas et al. (2006) demonstrated differences in postural findings and correlations with the Dubowitz exam comparing prone position skin-to-skin (Figure 10.14) and lateral decubitus (LD) orientation for skin-to-skin (Figure 10.15). Biomechanical analysis results are presented in Table 10.9. The LD posture supported a more flexed posture and trunk rotation that favors motor coordination (Barradas et al., 2006). The prone posture induces more postural abnormalities such as scapular retraction, external rotation of the hips, and orthopedic foot malalignment (Barradas et al., 2006). The Dubowitz examination demonstrated better development and superior performance in the LD group (Barradas et al., 2006).

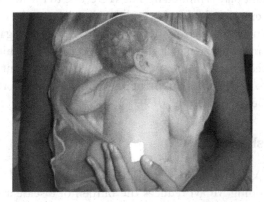

Figure 10.14 Prone position for skin-to-skin care. This image was taken to demonstrate the infant's posture yet preserve maternal modesty.

Source: Reprinted with permission from Fundação Sociedade Brasileira de Pediatria.

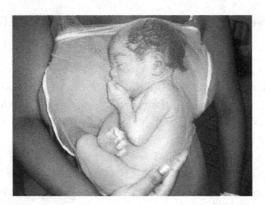

Figure 10.15 Lateral decubitus position for skin-to-skin care. This image was taken to demonstrate the infant's posture yet preserve maternal modesty.

Source: Reprinted with permission from Fundação Sociedade Brasileira de Pediatria.

Table 10.9 **Biomechanical Analysis of Skin-to-Skin Positions**

Prone Position	Lateral Decubitus Position
• Cervical extension and rotation • Shoulder extension and abduction • Scapular adduction • Hip flexion and abduction	• Cervical flexion • Shoulder flexion and adduction • Scapular abduction • Hip flexion and adduction

Source: Adapted from Barradas, J., Fonseca, A., Guimaraes, C. L. N., & Lima, G. M. D. S. (2006). Relationship between positioning of premature infants in kangaroo mother care and early neuromotor development. *Journal de Pediatria, 82*(6). https://doi.org/10.2223/JPED.1565

Newborn and infant play is limited in the NICU due to the infant's severity of illness, parental physical and emotional presence, and the clinicians' understanding of the importance of play for optimal neurosensory development. Maternal engagement is associated with infant outcomes, maternal mental health outcomes, maternal–child bonding outcomes, and breastfeeding outcomes (Klawetter et al., 2019). Time constraints and staffing impede the nurses' capacity to provide developmentally supportive and contingent responses to the infant's cues (Weber & Harrison, 2019).

Eating and Nourishment

Mother's own milk (MOM) feedings in the NICU are the gold standard for optimal infant nutrition. Providing MOM reduces the burden of disease associated with NICU hospitalization across physiologic, psychologic, and economic domains (de Halleux et al., 2019; Miller et al., 2018; Verduci et al., 2020). Studies confirm that educating NICU mothers about the benefits and superiority of MOM does not make mothers feel guilty or coerced (Meier et al., 2017). However, barriers to maternal expression of MOM, infant variables, and NICU culture and resources thwart the consistent provision of this ideal food choice (Hallowell et al., 2016; Hoban et al., 2015; Holdren et al., 2019; Ikonen et al., 2018; Maastrup et al., 2014; Mitha et al., 2019; Picaud et al., 2018).

Liu et al. (2020) report racial and ethnic disparities in human milk (HM) intake among very-low-birth weight non-Hispanic Black infants. Maternal education and country of birth were the biggest drivers for the disparity (Liu et al., 2020). Social factors to include economics, transportation challenges, and perceived support from the maternal grand-mother negatively impacted MOM feeding at discharge for Black mothers (Fleurant et al., 2017; Patel et al., 2019; Sigurdson et al., 2019).

MOM is not only the best nutrition option for preterm infants, but it also supports and promotes optimal gut microbiota, which is intimately linked to immune function, inflammatory responses to pathogenic organisms, and the regulation of gut defense systems (Xu et al., 2018). A comparison of MOM with human donor milk and formula, infants who received an exclusive MOM diet had a more balanced microbial community pattern and an increase in microbial diversity (Figure 10.16; Cong et al., 2017). Current research suggests that prematurity of the gut microbiota interferes with infant feeding success (Henderickx et al., 2019). Moreover, the levels of specific microbial groups during the first days of life compromise weight gain at 1 month of age (Figure 10.17; Arboleya et al., 2017; Henderickx et al., 2019).

Eating experiences are social encounters and require the infant to have the capacity physiologically and psychosocially to engage in the experience. Readiness for feeding is a critical element to successful oral eating encounters and is driven by the behavioral state (Table 10.10; Griffith et al., 2017). An alert state is optimal for the eating encounter. Infants may be coaxed to an alert state from drowsy or crying; however, this requires continuous assessment to ensure a safe eating experience for the infant (Griffith et al., 2017). Stress signals during eating encounters are associated with a longer transition to full oral feeding volume (Yi et al., 2018).

Hygiene and Skin Care

Hospitalized infants, both term and preterm, are at an increased risk for device-related pressure ulcers (Visscher & Taylor, 2014). Premature infants, unlike their full-term coun-terparts, have an incompetent skin barrier which increases their susceptibility to cutaneous injury, excessive transepidermal water losses, irritant exposure, skin compromise, and life-threatening infections (Visscher & Narendran, 2013). Research suggests among infants at gestational age of 24 to 27 weeks, iatrogenic skin injury rates are reported as high as 57% (Broom et al., 2019).

Skin maturation influences the development of the skin microbiome and is confounded by clinical and environmental factors (Box 10.4; Hartz et al., 2015; Pammi et al., 2017;

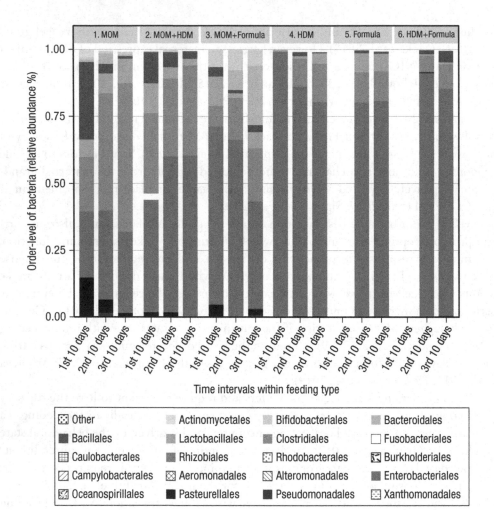

Figure 10.16 Distribution of mean relative abundance of taxa among six feeding types and development over three 10-day intervals.

Source: Cong, X., Judge, M., Xu, W., Diallo, A., Janton, S., Brownell, E. A., Maas, K., & Graf, J. (2017). Influence of infant feeding type on gut microbiome development in hospitalized preterm infants. *Nursing Research, 66*(2), 123–133. doi: 10.1097/NNR.0000000000000208 Reprinted with permission from Wolters Kluwer Health, Inc.

Underwood & Sohn, 2017; Younge et al., 2018). Skin microbiota vary by gestational age, postnatal age, and body regions and include typical skin-associated bacteria such as *Streptococcus* and *Staphylococcus* but also species associated with the gut microbiome that have pathogenic potential (Pammi et al., 2017; Underwood & Sohn, 2017; Younge et al., 2018). Alterations in skin microbiome adversely affects local skin and systemic immune development (Pammi et al., 2017; Younge et al., 2018).

Preterm and critically ill term infants are immunocompromised and highly susceptible to healthcare-associated infections (Hartz et al., 2015). The skin microbiome of infants in

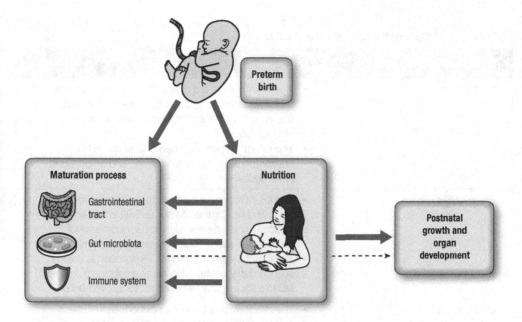

Figure 10.17 Preterm birth influences breast milk composition and affects maturation processes.

Source: Henderickx, J. G. E., Zwittink, R. D., van Lingen, R. A., Knol, J., & Belzer, C. (2019). The preterm gut microbiota: An inconspicuous challenge in nutritional neonatal care. *Frontiers in Cellular and Infection Microbiology, 9*, 85. https://doi.org/10.3389/fcimb.2019.00085

the NICU shows reduced diversity, which poses a hazard for bacterial invasion of pathogenic organisms (Pammi et al., 2017; Underwood & Sohn, 2017; Younge et al., 2018). Combined with the fragility of the infant's skin barrier and risk for iatrogenic skin injury, it is imperative that best practices to protect and preserve skin integrity is of paramount importance (Hartz et al., 2015).

Touch is the first sensory system to develop in utero around 8 weeks of gestation and plays a critical role in healthy physical and psycho-socio-emotional development. Interpersonal touch is reciprocal, you cannot touch another without being touched (Gentsch et al., 2015). Touch experiences have a valence, positive or negative, and are linked to neurobiological correlates that inform our understanding of self and the world (Bales et al., 2018; Cascio et al., 2019; Gentsch et al., 2015). Through experience-expectant and experience-dependent neuroplasticity (refer to Chapter 2), social touch shapes our brain (Bales et al., 2018; Humphreys & Zeanah, 2015). Human touch, whether from a parent or a caregiver, can be procedural or transpersonal. The misuse and overuse of nonsterile gloves in the clinical setting not only increases the risk for cross-contamination in this highly vulnerable population (Loveday et al., 2014; Wilson et al., 2015) but deprives the infant and caregiver from the shared human experience of authentic healing presence through touch (refer to Chapter 4).

Table 10.10 Description of Behavioral States

Behavioral State	Description
Alert states	• The infant's eyes are open, minimal motor activity, bright and shining appearance, visually focuses in on one person or thing in the environment, respirations are regular. • The infant's eyes are open and scanning the environment, more motor activity, and respirations are irregular.
Sleep states	• The infant's eyes are closed; respiration is regular, slow, and abdominal. Motor activity is limited to occasional startles, sigh sobs, or other brief discharges. Motor tone is maintained at a tonic level. • The infant's eyes are closed. Respiration is uneven and primarily costal. Motor movements are sporadic. Muscle tone is low between motor movements.
Drowsy states	• The infant shows behaviors of both wakefulness and sleep. There is generalized motor activity, and although the eyes are typically closed, there may be a rapid opening and closing of the eyes. Brief fussy vocalizations may occur. • The infant's eyelids are "heavy lidded." They may be opening and closing slowly, or open, but the eyes are dazed in appearance. The level of motor activity is typically low and respiration fairly even. • The infant's eyes are usually open, dull, and unfocused. Motor activity varies, but is typically high. The eyes may close during periods of high-level activity.
Crying	• The infant is either fussing or crying. The intensity of the vocalizations ranges from at least two brief fuss sounds to breathless crying.

Source: Adapted from Griffith, T., Rankin, K., & White-Traut, R. (2017). The relationship between behavioral states and oral feeding efficiency. *Advances in Neonatal Care, 17*(1), e12–e19. doi: 10.1097/ANC.0000000000000318

EVIDENCE-BASED STRATEGIES FOR ACTIVITIES OF DAILY LIVING FOR THE HOSPITALIZED INFANT

Posture and Play

Recommendations for best practice in postural alignment and mobility for hospitalized infants begin with a competent and confident staff. The Neonatal Postural Assessment Worksheet is a teaching assessment tool that alerts the clinician to optimal postural

BOX 10.4 CLINICAL AND ENVIRONMENTAL FACTORS THAT INFLUENCE THE SKIN MICROBIOTA

- Parental skin
- Feeding type
- Environmental surfaces
- Caregiving equipment
- Healthcare providers' skin
- Antibiotic use

Source: Adapted from Hartz, L. E., Bradshaw, W., & Brandon, D. H. (2015). Potential NICU environmental influences on the neonate's microbiome: A systematic review. *Advances in Neonatal Care, 15*(5), 324–335. doi: 10.1097/ANC.0000000000000220; Underwood, M. A., & Sohn, K. (2017). The microbiota of the extremely preterm infant. *Clinics in Perinatology, 44*(2), 407–427. doi: 10.1016/j.clp.2017.01.005

orientations across head, neck, scapulae, spine, hands, hips, and knees (Exhibit 10.1). The tool aims to guide the clinician in identifying optimal postural adjustments that will improve the comfort and age-appropriate alignment of the infant (Diertens & Wielenga, 2018).

Appropriate use of therapeutic positioning devices should be guided by collaboration with certified neonatal therapists with expertise in caring and supporting neuro- and musculoskeletal development (Craig & Smith, 2020; K. Ross et al., 2017). Two-person care, in which one person guides the postural activity and the other person supports the infant's self-regulation, is a clinical best practice (Weber & Harrison, 2019). The two-person technique achieves the desired care goals while mitigating the infant's stress, distress and unnecessary energy expenditure during caring encounters. For additional recommendations for postural alignment best practices refer to Coughlin (2016, p. 167).

Play with hospitalized newborns and infants focuses on sensory experiences with loving caregivers, ideally parents, but certainly includes clinicians. Engaging with soft, loving vocalizations, singing, reading, skin-to-skin contact and holding in arms are just a few examples of age-appropriate play for this fragile patient population. These social encounters teach infants about the world and help them discover their value as fellow human beings and a source of delight and awe to others.

Eating and Nourishment

NICU nurses must be educated on the importance of an exclusive HM diet for critically ill infants and achieve competence and confidence in supporting maternal milk expression and production of ample milk volumes to sustain successful breastfeeding through the hospital stay and beyond (Verduci et al., 2020). Dispelling the myth that bottle-fed

EXHIBIT 10.1 NEONATAL POSTURAL ASSESSMENT WORKSHEET (neoPAW)

Neonatal Postural Assessment Worksheet – neoPAW

Date: _____ Time: _____ AM. PM. GA @ Birth: _____; Adjusted Age @ Time of Assessment: _____   Prone   Supine   Side-lying

Indicator	0	1	2	Score	Comments / Limitations
Head	Lateral rotation > 45 degrees from midline L☐ R☐	Lateral Rotation < 45 degrees from midline L☐ R☐	Head in a midline orientation		
Neck	Neck in Extension OR Flexion Figure 1 Extension Figure 2 Flexion Ext☐ Flex☐		Neck in a neutral alignment		
Scapulae (Shoulder Blades)	Retracted L☐ R☐ Both☐	Flat L☐ R☐ Both☐	Softly Rounded L☐ R☐ Both☐		
Spine / Torso	Mal-aligned (lateral or rotational)		Aligned		
			Subtotal (page 1)		

1. Is the baby positioned in a way to support or allow for spontaneous movement?   Yes ☐   No ☐
2. Did you observe spontaneous movement during your assessment? (If yes, please describe briefly). Yes ☐   No ☐

(Describe): _____

Indicator	0	1	2	Score	Comments / Limitations
Hands	Not touching the body L☐ R☐ Both☐	Touching the torso L☐ R☐ Both☐	Touching the head / face L☐ R☐ Both☐		
Hips	Abducted with extreme external rotation (> 45 degrees) L☐ R☐ Both☐	Hips adducted & extended L☐ R☐ Both☐	Hips aligned with flexion & pelvic tilt L☐ R☐ Both☐		
Knees / ankles	Parallel legs (knees & ankles in extension) L☐ R☐ Both☐	Knees & ankles flexed but abducted L☐ R☐ Both☐	Knees & ankles aligned and softly flexed L☐ R☐ Both☐		
			TOTAL Score (Subtotal + Page 2 Score)		

SCORING LEGEND:

< 8: poor positioning – modify to provide functional and behavioral support within the medical and/or surgical limitations of the infant

8 – 10: adequate positioning – identify opportunities to modify the infant's posture within their medical and/or surgical limitations

> 10: optimal positioning for infant's behavioral and functional development

2

Source: Reprinted with permission from Caring Essentials Collaborative, LLC.

BOX 10.5 BREASTFEEDING SUPPORT FOR PREMATURE INFANTS

- Premature infants have the ability to breastfeed earlier than to bottle feed.
- Caregivers and parents must be able to support these skills.
- The time to suck varies with each child.
- Breastfeeding effectiveness should be assessed based on the child's ability to take in sufficient quantities to achieve growth that is at least equivalent to fetal growth.

Source: Adapted from Picaud, J. C., Buffin, R., Gremmo-Feger, G., Rigo, J., Putet, G., Casper, C.; Working Group of the French Neonatal Society on fresh human milk use in preterm infants. (2018). Review concludes that specific recommendations are needed to harmonize the provision of fresh mother's milk to their preterm infants. *Acta Paediatrica*, *107*(7), 1145–1155. doi: 10.1111/apa.14259

infants are discharged sooner enables clinicians to acknowledge and adopt practices that facilitate and support breastfeeding in the NICU (Briere, 2015). Key factors that support breastfeeding in preterm infants are listed in Box 10.5 (Picaud et al., 2018). Research reports a correlation between the first oral feeding at breast and the infant continuing to receive breast milk through to discharge (Casavant et al., 2015).

Standardizing the process of supporting and facilitating breastfeeding in the NICU ensures consistency for families and staff. Maternal goal setting has been identified as a core strategy to support breastfeeding in the NICU through to discharge (Briere et al., 2015; Fleurant et al., 2017; Hoban et al., 2015). Education regarding the benefits of breastfeeding and breast milk should begin prior to admission; however, if that is not possible, mothers and partners must have access to evidence-based education and resources that support discussion, exploration, and decision-making regarding the implications of breastfeeding for the mother, the infant, and the family (Casey et al., 2018). Ensuring that the first oral feeding is at the breast has the highest success of sustained breastfeeding throughout the hospital stay (Briere et al., 2015; Casey et al., 2018). When MOM is provided via feeding tube or bottle, Meier et al. (2017) identify best practices in the safe handling of MOM in the NICU (Table 10.11).

Prefeeding activities begin with early, frequent, and continuous skin-to-skin care experiences and are linked to increased milk production (Klawetter et al., 2019; Mitha et al., 2019). Policies and practices must be in place to standardize the expectation for early and frequent skin-to-skin care (Coughlin, 2016, p.179; Mitha et al., 2019). A quality experience must be the priority in order to establish successful breastfeeding. Ten steps for promoting and protecting breastfeeding for vulnerable infants have been identified and proven to significantly improve breastfeeding rates at discharge (Table 10.12; Fugate et al., 2015).

Co-regulated responsive infant feeding/eating is a best practice that has been proven to support infants' attainment of full oral dietary volume in fewer days than scheduled volume-dictated feeding approaches (Morag et al., 2019; Thoyre et al., 2013). Partnering,

Table 10.11 Safe Handling of Pumped Human Milk for Preterm Infant Feeding in the NICU

Objective	Best Practice
A. Maximize nutritive and bioactive components.	• Feed freshly pumped, never frozen, HM to greatest possible extent. • Freshly pumped, unfortified HM can be refrigerated for up to 96 hours. • Do not pasteurize mother's own HM. • Implement mechanism for identifying pumped colostrum and transitional HM so it can be fed in the order it is pumped during advancement of enteral feedings. • Alternate colostrum and transitional HM with freshly pumped HM after 72 hours postfeed initiation if colostrum and transitional HM collections have been previously frozen. • Minimize number of temperature changes (e.g., serial refrigeration + warming).
B. Optimize nutrient delivery and utilization.	• Feed freshly pumped, never frozen, HM to greatest possible extent. • Use strategies to minimize the impact of exogenous additives on the delivery and utilization of HM components. • Feed HM by intermittent rather than continuous gavage infusion to prevent lipid entrapment in infusion tubing and resultant loss of nutritional lipid and energy. • Invert syringe (bevel upward) if intermittent feedings are placed on an infusion pump to ensure HM lipid is delivered to infant. • Flush HM remaining in infusion tubing after feeding with 1–2 mL of air so that infant receives as much of trapped lipid as possible.
C. Minimize bacterial contaminants and bacterial growth	• Feed freshly pumped, never frozen, HM to greatest possible extent. • Standardize protocols for collection, storage, and transport of HM that are user friendly and easily understood by NICU families. • Ensure all HM specimens are collected and stored in sterile receptacles. • Store all pumped HM in industrial NICU refrigerators and freezers that are tamper-proof and routinely monitored for appropriate temperature maintenance. • Do not implement a routine culturing surveillance program for pumped HM as this approach has been shown ineffective in minimizing bacteria. • Use waterless warming and thawing techniques to prevent HM contamination. • Feed previously frozen HM within 24 hours of thawing.

(continued)

Table 10.11 **Safe Handling of Pumped Human Milk for Preterm Infant Feeding in the NICU** (continued)

Objective	Best Practice
D. Eliminate errors in HM fed to the wrong infant	• Implement an HM management system that minimizes the risk of HM being fed to the wrong infant, • Engage parents in the importance of accurate labeling of HM receptacles and other activities (such as checking that all pumped HM is moved from one NICU room to another with the infant) per individual NICU protocol.

HM, human milk.

Source: From Meier, P., Johnson, T. J., Patel, A. L., & Rossman, B. (2017). Evidence-based methods that promote human milk feeding of preterm infants: An expert review. Clinics in Perinatology, 44(1), 1–22. doi: 10.1016/j.clp.2016.11.005 Reprinted with permission from Elsevier.

Table 10.12 **Spatz 10 Steps**

Step	Description
1	Informed decision
2	Establishment and maintenance of milk supply
3.	Human milk management
4	Oral care and feeding of human milk
5	Skin-to-skin contact
6	Nonnutritive sucking
7	Transition to breast
8	Measurement of milk transfer
9	Preparation for discharge
10	Appropriate follow-up

Source: Adapted from Fugate, K., Hernandez, I., Ashmeade, T., Miladinovic, B., & Spatz, D. L. (2015). Improving human milk and breast-feeding practices in the NICU. Journal of Obstetric, Gynecologic & Neonatal Nursing, 44(3), 426–438. doi: 10.1111/1552-6909.12563

educating, and empowering parents in the transition from nasogastric tube feedings to oral eating experiences is associated with a shorter hospital stay and higher parent engagement (Morag et al., 2019). Utilizing a feeding readiness assessment tool supports a co-regulated and responsive feeding/eating experience while also identifying infants in need of additional interventions to support their eating and nutritional success (Pados & Fuller, 2020; Pados et al., 2016). Pados and Fuller (2020) outline foundational strategies that prepare the hospitalized infant for feeding success through the adoption and promotion of neurodevelopmentally supportive practices (Box 10.6). For additional recommendations for best practices in nurturing feeding refer to Coughlin (2016, p. 179).

BOX 10.6 FOUNDATIONAL STRATEGIES TO SUPPORT
SUCCESSFUL FEEDING IN THE NICU

- Protect sleep.
- Support postural alignment.
- Minimize and manage noxious experiences in the perioral area.
  - Avoid tight taping and CPAP positioners.
  - Avoid tension of endotracheal tubes and CPAP devices.
  - Suction only when necessary and provide nonpharmacologic support during the procedure.
  - Provide gentle oral care.
- Promote positive experiences.
  - Support skin-to-skin care.
  - Provide positive touch.
  - Provide positive gustatory and olfactory experiences with mother's own milk.
  - Provide nonnutritive sucking.

CPAP, continuous positive airway pressure.
Source: Adapted from Pados, B., & Fuller, K. (2020). Establishing a foundation for optimal feeding outcomes in the NICU. *Nursing for Women's Health.* https://doi.org/10.1016/j.nwh.2020.03.007

Hygiene and Skin Care

Routine assessment of skin integrity and skin injury risk is an evidence-based best practice. There is limited empirical evidence recommending one skin risk assessment tool over another (Kottner et al., 2011). Identifying an age-appropriate skin risk assessment tool with appropriate validity and psychometric properties is as important as consistency in performing and responding to the assessment (Broom et al., 2019; Vance et al., 2015).

The prevalence of medical adhesive-related skin injury (MARSI) ranges from 24% to 54% (D. Wang et al., 2019). Special attention to types of medical adhesive materials, surface area, and application and removal techniques minimize the pain, dermatitis, tearing, dermal stripping, and denuding associated with MARSIs. Familiarity with the properties and usage of adhesive products (Table 10.13) combined with practice guidelines aimed at preserving and protecting skin can reduce the prevalence of MARSIs in the NICU (Lund, 2014; D. Wang et al., 2019). Exploring wireless patient monitoring reduces the risk of skin injury and optimizes skin surface area for positive touch encounters creating a visually less frightening image of the infant to the parents (Abassi, 2019; Bonner et al., 2017; Chung et al., 2019).

The use of chlorhexidine gluconate (CHG) as a skin antiseptic in the NICU is not endorsed by the CDC, the U.S. Food and Drug Administration, European societies, surgical

Table 10.13 **Adhesive Used in Pediatric Settings**

Product	Backing	Adhesive	Medical Purpose
Elastic cloth tape	Elastic cloth	Acrylate	Tracheal intubation fixation
Transparent film	Polyurethane	Acrylate	Vascular access fixation/ skin protection
Paper tape	Paper	Acrylate	Vascular access fixation
Electrode pad	Foam	Acrylate/ hydrocolloid	EKG monitor
Artificial skin	Hydrophilic pads	Hydrocolloid	Skin protection

Source: Adapted from Wang, D., Xu, H., Chen, S., Lou, X., Tan, J., & Xu, Y. (2019). Medical adhesive-related skin injuries and associated risk factors in a pediatric intensive care unit. *Advances in Skin & Wound Care, 32*(4), 176–182. doi: 10.1097/01.ASW.0000553601.05196.fb

societies, the American Academy of Pediatrics, and Cochrane reviews (Boyar, 2019). The relative ubiquitous practice of CHG baths in preterm infants to reduce healthcare-associated infections must be critically and judiciously reviewed (Boyar, 2019; Kamity & Hanna, 2019). Weighing the benefits and risks of the use of CHG in this vulnerable population takes into account implications for the infant's microbiome, permeability of the infant's skin, and the susceptibility of the blood–brain barrier to CHG exposure (Boyar, 2019; Kamity & Hanna, 2019; Sathiyamurthy et al., 2016).

The adoption of immersion or tub bathing in the NICU improves temperature stability and reduces biobehavioral expressions of stress (Finn et al., 2017; Lund, 2016; Tambunan & Mediani, 2019). Swaddled bathing, a modification of tub bathing, has been shown to be the safest bathing practice for preterm infants in the NICU (Lund, 2016; Tambunan & Mediani, 2019). For additional recommendations for best practices in skin care refer to Coughlin (2016, p. 192).

Touch plays a pivotal role in developing a sense of self as separate from others, self-perception (Crucianelli & Filippetti, 2018; Longa et al., 2019; Montirosso & McGlone, 2020). Promoting parental tactile interactions, such as skin-to-skin care, in the NICU improves infant and family mental and physical health (Crucianelli & Filippetti, 2018; Weber & Harrison, 2019). Infant massage by parents is a pleasant touch experience that promotes attachment, increases weight gain, and reduces hospital length of stay (Niemi, 2017; Shoghi et al., 2018). Interpersonal affective touch plays a fundamental role in the development of the infant's bodily self-awareness and perceived sense of worth (Crucianelli & Filippetti, 2018; Longa et al., 2019).

> *Babies learn what it is to be a kind and loving presence in the world based on their experiences with kind and loving adults.*
> —Mary Coughlin

READER RESOURCES

Immunology in the skin: www.youtube.com/watch?v=_VhcZTGv0CU

Meet your microbiome: www.youtube.com/watch?v=Ybk7E7SLbWw

Posture Resources

A guide to good posture from Medline Plus: https://medlineplus.gov/guidetogoodposture.html

LifeHacker—Fix your posture with this animated guide to sitting right: https://lifehacker.com/ fix-your-posture-with-this-animated-guide-to-sitting-ri-115376

Maintaining good posture from the American Chiropractic Association: https://acatoday.org/content/ posture-power-how-to-correct-your-body-alignment

NIH news in health—Getting it straight, improve your posture for better health: https://newsinhealth .nih.gov/2017/08/getting-it-straight

U.S. Department of Labor, Occupational Safety and Health Administration—Ergonomics: www.osha.gov/ SLTC/ergonomics/

U.S. Department of Labor, Occupational Safety and Health Administration guide to good working positions at computer workstations: www.osha.gov/SLTC/etools/computerworkstations/positions .html

Play Resources

Association for Psychological Science—Playing up the benefits of play at work: www.psychologicalscience .org/news/minds-business/playing-up-the-benefits-of-play-at-work.html

HelpGuide—The benefits of play for adults: www.helpguide.org/articles/mental-health/benefits-of- play-for-adults.htm

Idealist—Why it's important to have fun at work: www.idealist.org/en/careers/important-fun-work

Lifehack—How to harness the power of play to transform your work culture: www.lifehack.org/articles/ work/how-harness-the-power-play-transform-your-work-culture.html

Swaddled bathing: www.youtube.com/watch?v=DJ3xFgNAeN0

What is LEGO Serious Play Pro: https://seriousplaypro.com/what-is-lego-serious-play

Your body language may shape who you are: Amy Cuddy: www.youtube.com/watch?v=Ks-_Mh1QhMc

REFERENCES

Abbasi, J. (2019). Wireless vital signs monitoring for the NICU. *The Journal of the American Medical Association, 321*(14), 1343. https://doi.org/10.1001/jama.2019.3243

Abdallah, F., Mijouin, L., & Pichon, C. (2017). Skin immune landscape: Inside and outside the organism. *Mediators of Inflammation.* https://doi.org/10.1155/2017/5095293

Afshariani, R., Kiani, M., & Zamanian, Z. (2019). The influence of ergonomic breastfeeding training on some health parameters in infants and mothers: A randomized controlled trial. *Archives of Public Health, 77,* 47. https://doi.org/10.1186/s13690-019-0373-x

Aggio, D., Wallace, K., Boreham, N., Shanker, A., Steptoe, A., & Hamer, M. (2017). Objectively measured daily physical activity and postural changes as related to positive and negative affect using ambulatory monitoring assessments. *Psychosomatic Medicine, 79*(7), 792–797. https://doi .org/10.1097/PSY.0000000000000485

Algghadir, A. H., Zafar, H., Al-Esa, E. S., & Iqbal, Z. A. (2017). Effect of posture on swallowing. *African Health Sciences, 17*(1), 133–137. https://doi.org/10.4314/ahs.v17i1.17

Angelo, R., Silva, D. C, Zambaldi, C. F., Cantilino, A., & Sougey, E. B. (2014). Influence of body posture on the association between postpartum depression and pain. *Trends in Psychiatry and Psychotherapy, 36*(1), 32–39. https://doi.org/10.1590/2237-6089-2013-0029

Arboleya, S., Martiniez-Camblor, P., Solis, G., Suarez, M., Fernandez, N., de Los Reyes-Gavilan, C. G., & Gueimonde, M. (2017). Intestinal microbiota and weight-gain in preterm neonates. *Frontiers in Microbiology, 8*, 183. https://doi.org/10.3389/fmicb.2017.00183

Arck, P. C., Slominski, A., Theoharides, T. C., Peters, E. M. J., & Paus, R. (2006). Neuroimmunology of stress: Skin takes center stage. *Journal of Investigative Dermatology, 126*(8), 1697–16704. https://doi.org/10.1038/sj.jid.5700104

Baldwin, H. E., Bhatia, N. D., Friedman, A., Eng, R. M., & Seite, S. (2017). The role of cutaneous microbiota harmony in maintaining a functional skin barrier. *Journal of Drugs in Dermatology, 16*(1), 12–18.

Bales, K. L., Witczak, L. R., Simmons, T. C., Savidge, L. E., Rothwell, E. S., Rogers, F. D., Manning, R. A., Heise, M. J., Englund, M., & Del Razo, R. A. (2018). Social touch during development: Long-term effects on brain and behavior. *Neuroscience and Biobehavioral Reviews, 95*, 202–219. https://doi.org/10.1016/j.neubiorev.2018.09.019

Barnard, E., & Li, H. (2017). Shaping of cutaneous function by encounters with commensals. *Journal of Physiology, 595*(2), 437–450. https://doi.org/10.1113/JP271638

Barradas, J., Fonseca, A., Guimaraes, C. L. N., & Lima, G. M. D. S. (2006). Relationship between positioning of premature infants in kangaroo mother care and early neuromotor development. *Journal de Pediatria, 82*(6). https://doi.org/10.2223/JPED.1565

Bauer, L. (2020, May 6). *The COVID-19 crisis has already left too many children hungry in America.* https://www .brookings.edu/blog/up-front/2020/05/06/the-covid-19-crisis-has-already-left-too-many-children-hungry-in-america

Bonner, O., Beardsall, K., Crilly, N., & Lasenby, J. (2017). "There were more wires than him": The potential for wireless patient monitoring in neonatal intensive care. *BMJ Innovations, 3*(1), 12–18. https://doi.org/10.1136/bmjinnov-2016-000145

Boyar, V. (2019). The use of topical antiseptics in neonates—The bad, the good, and the unknown. *Wound Management and Prevention, 65*(6), 8–13.

Briere, C.-E. (2015). Breastfed or bottle-fed: Who goes home sooner? *Advances in Neonatal Care, 15*(1), 65–69. https://doi.org/10.1097/ANC.0000000000000159

Briere, C.-E., McGrath, J. M., Cong, X., Brownell, E., & Cusson, R. (2015). Direct-breastfeeding premature infants in the neonatal intensive care unit. *Journal of Human Lactation, 31*(3), 386–392. https://doi.org/10.1177/0890334415581798

Broom, M., Dunk, A. M., & Mohamed, A.-L. E. (2019). Predicting neonatal skin injury: The first step to reducing skin injuries in neonates. *Health Services Insights, 12*, 1178632919845630. https:// doi.org/10.1177/1178632919845630

Bruno Garza, J. L., & Young, J. G. (2015). A literature review of the effects of computer input device design on biomechanical loading and musculoskeletal outcomes during computer work. *Work, 52*(2), 217–230. https://doi.org/10.3233/WOR-152161

Bubric, K., & Hedge, A. (2016). Differential patterns of laptop use and associated musculoskeletal discomfort in male and female college students. *Work*, *55*(3), 663–671. https://doi.org/10.3233/WOR-162419

Buil, A., Caeymaex, L., Mero, S., Sankey, C., Apter, G., & Devouche, E. (2019). Kangaroo supported diagonal flexion positioning: Positive impact on maternal stress and postpartum depression risk and on skin-to-skin practice with very preterm infants. *Journal of Neonatal Nursing*, *25*(2), 86–92. https://doi.org/10.1016/j.jnn.2018.10.006

Buil, A., Sankey, C., Caeymaex, L., Apter, G., Gratier, M., & Devouche, E. (2020). Fostering mother-very preterm infant communication during skin-to-skin contact through a modified positioning. *Early Human Development*, *141*, 104939. https://doi.org/10.1016/j.earlhumdev.2019.104939

Butler, M. I., Morkl, S., Sandhu, K. V., Cryan, J. F., & Dinan, T. G. (2019). The gut microbiome and mental health: What should we tell our patients? *Canadian Journal of Psychiatry*, *64*(11), 747–760. https://doi.org/10.1177/0706743719874168

Casavant, S. G., McGrath, J. M., Burke, G., & Briere, C.-E. (2015). Caregiving factors affecting breastfeeding duration within a neonatal intensive care unit. *Advances in Neonatal Care*, *15*(6), 421–428. https://doi.org/10.1097/ANC.0000000000000234

Cascio, C. J., Moore, D., & McGlone, F. (2019). Social touch and human development. *Developmental Cognitive Neuroscience*, *35*, 5–11. https://doi.org/10.1016/j.dcn.2018.04.009

Catena, R. D., Campbell, N., Wolcott, W. C., & Rothwell, S. A. (2019). Anthropometry, standing posture, and body center of mass changes up to 28 weeks postpartum in Caucasians in the United States. *Gait Posture*, *70*, 196–202. https://doi.org/10.1016/j.gaitpost.2019.03.009

Chen, Y., & Lyga, J. (2014). Brain-skin connection: Stress, inflammation and skin aging. *Inflammations & Allergy Drug Targets*, *13*(3), 177–190. https://doi.org/10.2174/1871528113666140522104422

Chen, Y. E., Fischbach, M. A., & Belkaid, Y. (2018). Skin microbiota-host interactions. *Nature*, *553*(7689), 427–436. https://doi.org/10.1038/nature25177

Chico-Barba, G., Jimenez-Limas, K., Sanchez-Jimenez, B., Samano, R., Rodriguez-Ventura, A. L., Castillo-Perez, R., & Tolentino, M. (2019). Burnout and metabolic syndrome in female nurses: An observational study. *International Journal of Environmental Research and Public Health*, *16*(11), 1993. https://doi.org/10.3390/ijerph16111993

Chin, D. L., Nam, S., & Lee, S.-J. (2016). Occupational factors associated with obesity and leisure-time physical activity among nurses: A cross sectional study. *International Journal of Nursing Studies*, *57*, 60–69. https://doi.org/10.1016/j.ijnurstu.2016.01.009

Chung, H. U., Kim, B. H., Lee, J. Y., Lee, J., Xie, Z., Ibler, E. M., Lee, K., Banks, A., Jeong, J. Y., Kim, J., Ogle, C., Grande, D., Yu, Y., Jang, H., Assem, P., Ryu, D., Kwak, J. W., Namkoong, M., Park, J. B., … Rogers, J. A. (2019). Binodal, wireless epidermal electronic systems with in-sensor analytics for neonatal intensive care. *Science*, *363*(6430), eaau0780. https://doi.org/10.1126/science.aau0780

Cohen, R. G., Baer, J. L., Ravichandra, R., Kral, D., McGowan, C., & Cacciatore, T. W. (2020). Lighten up! Postural instructions affect static and dynamic balance in healthy older adults. *Innovation in Aging*, *4*(2), igz056. https://doi.org/10.1093/geroni/igz056

Coleman, E. (2020). Treating skin conditions: A holistic approach in dermatology. *Journal of Aesthetic Nursing*, *9*(2). https://doi.org/10.12968/joan.2020.9.2.58

Colson, S. (2010). What happens to breastfeeding when mothers lie back? *Clinical Lactation*, *1*(1), 9–12. https://doi.org/10.1891/215805310807011864

Colson, S. (2014). Does the mother's posture have a protective role to play during skin-to-skin contact? *Clinical Lactation*, 5(2), 41–50. https://doi.org/10.1891/2158-0782.5.2.41

Cong, X., Judge, M., Xu, W., Diallo, A., Janton, S., Brownell, E. A., Maas, K., & Graf, J. (2017). Influence of infant feeding type on gut microbiome development in hospitalized preterm infants. *Nursing Research*, 66(2), 123–133. https://doi.org/10.1097/NNR.0000000000000208

Coughlin, M. (2016). *Trauma-informed care in the NICU: Evidence-based practice guidelines for neonatal clinicians.* Springer Publishing Company.

Craig, J. W., & Smith, C. R. (2020). Risk-adjusted/neuroprotective care services in the NICU: The elemental role of the neonatal therapist (OT, PT, SLP). *Journal of Perinatology*, 40(4), 549–559. https://doi.org/10.1038/s41372-020-0597-1

Crucianelli, L., & Filippetti, M. L. (2018). Developmental perspectives on interpersonal affective touch. *Topoi*, 39, 575–586. https://doi.org/10.1007/s11245-018-9565-1

de Halleux, V., Pieltain, C., Senterre, T., Studzinski, F., Kessen, C., Rigo, V., & Rigo, J. (2019). Growth benefits of own mother's milk in preterm infants fed daily individualized fortified human milk. *Nutrients*, 11(4), 772. https://doi.org/10.3390/nu11040772

Diertens, D. M., & Wielenga, J. M. (2018). Developmentally accurate body posture of newborn infants: A quality assessment using the neoPAW score. *Infant*, 14(1), 32–35.

Drzat-Grabiec, J., Walicka-Cuprys, K., Zajkiewicz, K., Rachwat, M., Piwonski, P., & Perenc, L. (2020). Parameters characterizing the posture of preterm children in sanding and sitting position. *Journal of Back and Musculoskeletal Rehabilitation*, 33(3), 455–462. https://doi.org/10.3233/BMR-170882

Einspieler, C., Bos, A. F., Libertus, M. E., & Marschik, P. B. (2016). The general movement assessment helps us to identify preterm infants at risk for cognitive dysfunction. *Frontiers in Psychology*, 7, 406. https://doi.org/10.3389/fpsyg.2016.00406

Einspieler, C., Marsachik, P. B., Pansy, J., Scheuchenegger, A., Krieber, M., Yang, H., Kornacka, M. K., Rowinska, E., Soloveichick, M., & Bos, A. F. (2015). The general movements optimality score: A detailed assessment of general movements during preterm and term age. *Developmental Medicine & Child Neurology*, 58, 361–368. https://doi.org/10.1111/dmcn.12923

Faria-Schutzer, D., Surita, F. G., Rodrigues, L., & Turato, E. R. (2018). Eating behaviors in postpartum: A qualitative study of women with obesity. *Nutrients*, 10(7), 885. https://doi.org/10.3390/nu10070885

Feeley, N., Genest, C., Niela-Vilen, H., Charbonneau, L., & Axelin, A. (2016). Parents and nurses balancing parent-infant closeness and separation: A qualitative study of NICU nurses' perceptions. *BMC Pediatrics*, 16, 134. https://doi.org/10.1186/s12887-016-0663-1

Ferrari, F., Plessi, C., Lucaccioni, L., Bertoncelli, N., Bedetti, L., Ori, L., Berardi, A., Della Casa, E., Iughette, L., & D'Amico, R. (2019). Motor and postural patterns concomitant with general movements are associated with cerebral palsy at term and fidgety age in preterm infants. *Journal of Clinical Medicine*, 8(8), 1189. https://doi.org/10.3390/jcm8081189

Finn, M., Meyer, A., Kirsten, D., & Wright, K. (2017). Swaddled bathing in the neonatal intensive care unit. *NeoReviews*, 18(8), e504–e506. https://doi.org/10.1542/neo.18-8-e504

Fleurant, E., Schoeny, M., Hoban, R., Asiodu, I. V., Riley, B., Meier, P. P., Bigger, H., & Patel, A. L. (2017). *Barriers to human milk feeding at discharge of very-low-birth-weight infants: Maternal goal setting as a key social factor.* Breastfeeding Medicine, 12(1), 20–27. https://doi.org/10.1089/bfm.2016.0105

Fluegge-Woolf, E. R. (2014). Play hard, work hard; fun at work and job performance. *Management Research Review*, 37(8), 682–705.

Freitag, S., Seddouki, R., Dulon, M., Kersten, J. F., Larsson, T. J., & Nienhaus, A. (2014). The effect of working position on trunk posture and exertion for routine nursing tasks: An experimental study. *Annals of Occupational Hygiene, 58*(3), 317–325. https://doi.org/10.1093/annhyg/met071

Frey Law, L. A., Lee, J. E., McMullen, T. R., & Xia, T. (2010). Relationships between maximum holding time and ratings of pain and exertion differ for static and dynamic tasks. *Applied Ergonomics, 42*(1), 9–15. https://doi.org/10.1016/j.apergo.2010.03.007

Fugate, K., Hernandez, I., Ashmeade, T., Miladinovic, B., & Spatz, D. L. (2015). Improving human milk and breastfeeding practices in the NICU. *Journal of Obstetric, Gynecologic & Neonatal Nursing, 44*(3), 426–438. https://doi.org/10.1111/1552-6909.12563

Gahagan, S. (2012). The development of eating behavior—Biology and context. *Journal of Developmental & Behavioral Pediatrics, 33*(3), 261–271. https://doi.org/10.1097/DBP.0b013e31824a7baa

Gentsch, A., Panagiotopoulou, E., & Fotopoulou, A. (2015). Active interpersonal touch gives rise to the social softness illusion. *Current Biology, 25*(18), 2392–2397. https://doi.org/10.1016/j.cub.2015.07.049

Gonya, J., Ray, W. C., Rumpf, R. W., & Brock, G. (2017). Investigating skin-to-skin care patterns with extremely preterm infants in the NICU and their effect on early cognitive and communication performance: A retrospective cohort study. *BMJ Open, 7*, e012985. https://doi.org/10.1136/bmjopen-2016-012985

Griffith, T., Rankin, K., & White-Traut, R. (2017). The relationship between behavioral states and oral feeding efficiency. *Advances in Neonatal Care, 17*(1), e12–e19. https://doi.org/10.1097/ANC.0000000000000318

Gutermuth, L. K., Hager, E. R., & Pollack Porter, K. (2018). Using the CDC's worksite health scorecard as a framework to examine worksite health promotion and physical activity. *Preventing Chronic Disease, 15*, E84. https://doi.org/10.5888/pcd15.170463

Hallowell, S. G., Rogowski, J. A., Spatz, D. L., Hanlon, A. L., Kenny, M., & Lake, E. T. (2016). Factors associated with infant feeding of human milk at discharge from neonatal intensive care: Cross-sectional analysis of nurse survey and infant outcome data. *International Journal of Nursing Studies, 53*, 190–203. https://doi.org/10.1016/j.ijnurstu.2015.09.016

Hartz, L. E., Bradshaw, W., & Brandon, D. H. (2015). Potential NICU environmental influences on the neonate's microbiome: A systematic review. *Advances in Neonatal Care, 15*(5), 324–335. https://doi.org/10.1097/ANC.0000000000000220

Hayes, C. (2016). Building care and compassion—Introducing Lego Serios Play to HCA education. *British Journal of Healthcare Assistants, 10*(3), 127–133. https://doi.org/10.12968/bjha.2016.10.3.127

Health Research & Educational Trust. (2017, June). *Social determinants of health series: Food insecurity and the role of hospitals*. Health Research & Educational Trust. https://www.aha.org/foodinsecurity

Heidari, M., Borujeni, M. G., & Khosravizad, M. (2018). Health-promoting lifestyles of nurses and its association with musculoskeletal disorders: A cross-sectional study. *Journal of Lifestyle Medicine, 8*(2), 72–78. https://doi.org/10.15280/jlm.2018.8.2.72

Heidari, M., Borujeni, M. G., Rezaei, P., & Abyaneh, S. K. (2019). Work-related musculoskeletal disorders and their associated factors in nurses: A cross-sectional study in Iran. *The Malaysian Journal of Medical Sciences, 26*(2), 122–130. https://doi.org/10.21315/mjms2019.26.2.13

Henderickx, J. G. E., Zwittink, R. D., van Lingen, R. A., Knol, J., & Belzer, C. (2019). The preterm gut microbiota: An inconspicuous challenge in nutritional neonatal care. *Frontiers in Cellular and Infection Microbiology, 9*, 85. https://doi.org/10.3389/fcimb.2019.00085

Herman, C. P. (2015). The social facilitation of eating. A review. *Appetite, 81*, 61–73. https://doi
.org/10.1016/j.appet.2014.09.016

Hitzert, M. M., Roze, E., Van Braeckel, K. N. J. A., & Bos, A. F. (2014). Motor development in
3-month-old healthy term-born infants is associated with cognitive and behavioral outcomes at
early school age. *Developmental Medicine & Child Neurology, 56*, 869–876. https://doi.org/10.1111/
dmcn.12468

Hoban, R., Bigger, H., Patel, A. L., Rossman, B., Fogg, L. F., & Meier, P. (2015). Goals for human
milk feeding in mothers of very low birth weight infants: How do goals change and are they
achieved during the NICU hospitalization? *Breastfeeding Medicine, 10*(6), 305–311. https://doi
.org/10.1089/bfm.2015.0047

Holdren, S., Fair, C., & Lehtonen, L. (2019). A qualitative cross-cultural analysis of NICU culture
and infant feeding in Finland and the U.S. *BMC Pregnancy and Childbirth, 19*, 345. https://doi
.org/10.1186/s12884-019-2505-2

Hruby, A., & Hu, F. B. (2015). The epidemiology of obesity: A big picture. *Pharmacoeconomics, 33*(7),
673–689. https://doi.org/10.1007/s40273-014-0243-x

Hughes, A. J., Redsell, S. A., & Glazebrook, C. (2016). Motor development interventions for preterm infants: A systematic review and meta-analysis. *Pediatrics, 138*(4), e20160147. https://doi
.org/10.1542/peds.2016-0147

Huizinga, J. (1955). *Homo Ludens: A study of the play-element in culture.* Beacon Press.

Humphreys, K. L., & Zeanah, C. H. (2015). Deviations from the expectable environment in early
childhood and emerging psychopathology. *Neuropsychopharmacology Reviews, 40*, 154–170. https://
doi.org/10.1038/npp.2014.165

Ikonen, R., Paavilainen, E., Helminen, M., & Kaunonen, M. (2018). Preterm infants' mothers'
initiation and frequency of breast milk expression and exclusive use of mother's breast milk
in neonatal intensive care units. *Journal of Clinical Nursing, 27*(3–4), e551–e558. https://doi
.org/10.1111/jocn.14093

Kamity, R., & Hanna, N. (2019). Chlorhexidine baths in preterm infants—Are we there yet? *Journal
of Perinatology, 39*, 1014–1015. https://doi.org/10.1038/s41372-019-0378-x

Kargar, N., Choobineh, A. R., Razeghi, M., Keshavarzi, S., & Meftahi, N. (2018). Posture and discomfort assessment in computer users while using touch screen device as compared with mouse-
keyboard and touch-pad keyboard. *Work, 59*(3), 341–349. https://doi.org/10.3233/WOR-182685

Klawetter, S., Greenfield, J. C., Speer, S. R., Brown, K., & Hwang, S. S. (2019). An integrative
review: Maternal engagement in the neonatal intensive care unit and health outcomes for U.S.-
born infants and their parents. *AIMS Public Health, 6*(2), 160–183. https://doi.org/10.3934/
publichealth.2019.2.160

Kommers, D., Oei, G., Chen, W., Feijs, L., & Bambang Oetomo, S. (2016). Suboptimal bonding
impairs hormonal, epigenetic and neuronal development in preterm infants, but these impairments can be reversed. *Acta Paediatrica, 105*(7), 738–751. https://doi.org/10.1111/apa.13254

Korakakis, V., O'Sullivan, K., O'Sullivan, P. B., Evagelinou, V., Sotiralis, Y., Sideris, A., Sakellariou, K.,
Karanasios, S., & Giakas, G. (2019). Physiotherapist perceptions of optimal sitting and standing
posture. *Musculoskeletal Science and Practice, 39*, 24–31. https://doi.org/10.1016/j.msksp.2018.11.004

Kotcz, A., & Jenaszek, K. K. (2020). Assessment of pressure pain threshold at the cervical and lum-
bar spine region in the group of professionally active nurses: A cross-sectional study. *Journal of
Occupational Health, 62*(1), e12108. https://doi.org/10.1002/1348-9585.12108

Kottner, J., Hauss, A., Schuler, A.-B., & Dassen, T. (2011). Validation and clinical impact of paediatric pressure ulcer risk assessment scales: A systematic review. *International Journal of Nursing Studies*, *50*(6), 807–818. https://doi.org/10.1016/j.ijnurstu.2011.04.014

Lebrun, A., Plante, A.-S., Savard, C., Dugas, C., Fontaine-Bisson, B., Lemieux, S., Robitaille, J., & Morisset, A.-S. (2019). Tracking of dietary intake and diet quality from late pregnancy to the postpartum period. *Nutrients*, *11*(9), 2080. https://doi.org/10.3390/nu11092080

Li, K. W., & Chiu, W.-S. (2015). Isometric arm strength and subjective rating of upper limb fatigue in two-handed carrying tasks. *PLoS One*, *10*(3), e0119550. https://doi.org/10.1371/journal.pone.0119550

Lin, S. C., Lin, L. L., Liu, C. J., Fang, C. K., & Lin, M. H. (2020). Exploring the factors affecting musculoskeletal disorders risk among hospital nurses. *PLoS One*, *15*(4), e0231319. https://doi.org/10.1371/journal.pone.0231319

Liska, D., Mah, E., Brisbois, T., Barrios, P. L., Baker, L. B., & Spriet, L. L. (2019). Narrative review of hydration and selected health outcomes in the general population. *Nutrients*, *11*, 70. https://doi.org/10.3390/nu11010070

Liu, J., Parker, M. G., Lu, T., Conroy, S. M., Oehlert, J., Lee, H. C., Gomez, S. L., Shariff-Marco, S., & Profit, J. (2020). Racial and ethnic disparities in human milk intake at NICU discharge among VLBW infants in California. *Journal of Pediatrics*, *218*, 49–56. https://doi.org/10.1016/j.jpeds.2019.11.020

Livovsky, D. M., Pribic, T., & Azpiroz, F. (2020). Food, eating, and the gastrointestinal tract. *Nutrients*, *12*(4), 986. https://doi.org/10.3390/nu12040986

Longa, L. D., Filippetti, M. L., Dragovic, D., & Farroni, T. (2019). Synchrony of caresses: Does affective touch help infants to detect body-related visual-tactile synchrony? *Frontiers in Psychology*, *10*, 2944. https://doi.org/10.3389/fpsyg.2019.02944

Loveday, H. P., Lynam, S., Singleton, J., & Wilson, J. (2014). Clinical glove use: Healthcare workers' actions and perceptions. *Observational Study*, *86*(2), 110–116. https://doi.org/10.1016/j.jhin.2013.11.003

Lund, C. (2014). Medical adhesives in the NICU. *Newborn and Infant Nursing Reviews*, *14*(4), 160–165. https://doi.org/10.1053/j.nainr.2014.10.001

Lund, C. (2016). Bathing and beyond: Current bathing controversies for newborn infants. *Advances in Neonatal Care*, *16*, s13–s20. https://doi.org/10.1097/ANC.0000000000000336

Maastrup, R., Hansen, B. M., Kronborg, H., Bojesen, S. N., Hallum, K., Frandsen, A., Kyhnaeb, A., Svarer, I., & Hallstrom, I. (2014). Breastfeeding progression in preterm infants is influenced by factors in infants, mothers and clinical practice: The results of a national cohort study with high breastfeeding initiation rates. *PLoS One*, *9*(9), e108208. https://doi.org/10.1371/journal.pone.0108208

Mahmoud, N. F., Hassan, K. A., Abdelmajeed, S. F., Moustafa, I. M., & Silva, A. G. (2019). The relationship between forward head posture and neck pain: A systematic review and meta-analysis. *Current Reviews in Musculoskeletal Medicine*, *12*(4), 562–577. https://doi.org/10.1007/s12178-019-09594-y

Mahon, B. Z. (2015). What is embodied cognition? *Language, Cognition and Neuroscience*, *30*(4), 420–429. https://doi.org/10.1080/23273798.2014.987791

Martins, A. M., Ascenso, A., Ribeiro, H. M., & Marto, J. (2020). The brain-skin connection and the pathogenesis of psoriasis: A review with a focus on the serotonergic system. *Cells*, *9*(4), 796. https://doi.org/10.3390/cells9040796

Matsugaki, R., Kuhara, S., Saeki, S., Jiang, Y., Michishita, R., Ohta, M., & Yamayo, H. (2017). Effectiveness of workplace exercise supervised by a physical therapist among nurses conducting shift work: A randomized controlled trial. *Journal of Occupational Health*, *59*(4), 327–335. https://doi.org/10.1539/joh.16-0125-OA

Meier, P., Johnson, T. J., Patel, A. L., & Rossman, B. (2017). Evidence-based methods that promote human milk feeding of preterm infants: An expert review. *Clinics in Perinatology*, *44*(1), 1–22. https://doi.org/10.1016/j.clp.2016.11.005

Migraine, A., Nicklaus, S., Parnet, P., Lange, C., Monnery-Patris, S., Des Robert, C., Darmaun, D., Flamant, C., Amarger, V., & Roze, J. C. (2013). Effect of preterm birth and birth weight on eating behavior at 2 y of age. *American Journal of Clinical Nutrition*, *97*(6), 1270–1277. https://doi.org/10.3945/ajcn.112.051151

Miller, J., Tonkin, E., Damarella, R. A., McPhee, A. J., Suganuma, M., Suganuma, H., Middleton, P. F., Makrides, M., & Collins, C. T. (2018). A systematic review and meta-analysis of human milk feeding and morbidity in very low birth weight infants. *Nutrients*, *10*(6), 707. https://doi.org/10.3390/nu10060707

Mingels, S., Dankaerts, W., & Granitzer, M. (2019). Is there support for the paradigm "spinal posture" as a trigger for episodic headache? A comprehensive review. *Current Pain and headache Reports*, *23*(3), 1–8. https://doi.org/10.1007/s11916-019-0756-2

Miragall, M., Etchemendy, E., Cebolla, A., Rodriguez, V., Medrano, C., & Banos, R. M. (2018). Expand your body when you look at yourself: The role of the posture in a mirror exposure task. *PLoS One*, *13*(3), e0194686. https://doi.org/10.1371/journal.pone.0194686

Mitha, A., Piedvache, A., Khoshnood, B., Fresson, J., Glorieux, I., Roue, J.-M., Blondel, B., Durox, M., Burguet, A., Ancel, P.-Y., Kaminski, M., & Pierrat, V. (2019). The impact of neonatal unit policies on breast milk feeding at discharge of moderate preterm infants: The EPIPAGE-2 cohort study. *Maternal Child Nutrition*, *15*(4), e12875. https://doi.org/10.1111/mcn.12875

Miyagishima, S., Asaka, T., Kamatsuka, K., Kozuka, N., Kobayashi, M., Igarashi, R., Hori, T., Yoto, Y., & Tsutsumi, H. (2016). Characteristics of antigravity spontaneous movements in preterm infants up to 3 months corrected age. *Infant Behavior & Development*, *44*, 227–239. https://doi.org/10.1016/j.infbeh.2016.07.006

Moazzami, Z., Dehdari, T., Taghdisi, M. H., & Soltanian, A. (2016). Effect of an ergonomics-based educational intervention based on transtheoretical model in adopting correct body posture among operating room nurses. *Global Journal of Health Science*, *8*(7), 26–34. https://doi.org/10.5539/gjhs.v8n7p26

Montirosso, R., & McGlone, F. (2020). The body comes first. Embodied reparation and the co-creation of infant bodily self. *Neuroscience and Biobehavioral Reviews*, *113*, 77–87. https://doi.org/10.1016/j.neubiorev.2020.03.003

Morag, I., Hendel, Y., Karol, D., Geva, R., & Tzipi, S. (2019). Transition from nasogastric tube to oral feeding: The role of parental guided responsive feeding. *Frontiers in Pediatrics*, *7*, 190. https://doi.org/10.3389/fped.2019.00190

Moran, T. H., & Ladenheim, E. E. (2016). Physiologic and neural controls of eating. *Gastroenterology Clinics of North America*, *45*(4), 581–599. https://doi.org/10.1016/j.gtc.2016.07.009

Moustafa, I. M., Youssef, A., Ahbouch, A., Tamim, M., & Harrison, D. E. (2020). Is forward head posture relevant to autonomic nervous system function and cervical sensorimotor control? Cross sectional study. *Gait & Posture*, *77*, 29–35. https://doi.org/10.1016/j.gaitpost.2020.01.004

Nam, S., Song, M., & Lee, S.-J. (2018). Relationship of musculoskeletal symptoms, sociodemographic and body mass index with leisure-time physical activity among nurses. *Workplace Health Safety*, *66*(12), 577–587. https://doi.org/10.1177/2165079918771987

Nicholls, R., Perry, L., Duffield, C., Gallagher, R., & Pierce, H. (2017). Barriers and facilitators to healthy eating for nurses in the workplace: An integrative review. *Journal of Advanced Nursing*, *73*(5), 1051–1065. https://doi.org/10.1111/jan.13185

Nicklaus, S. (2017). The role of dietary experience in the development of eating behavior during the first years of life. *Annals of Nutrition & Metabolism*, *70*(3), 241–245. https://doi.org/10.1159/000465532

Niemi, A.-K. (2017). Review of randomized controlled trials of massage in preterm infants. *Children*, *4*(4), 21. https://doi.org/10.3390/children4040021

Opala-Berdzik, A., Blaszczyk, J. W., Bacik, B., Cieslinska-Swider, J., Swider, D., Sobota, G., & Markiewicz, A. (2015). Static postural stability in women during and after pregnancy: A prospective longitudinal study. *PLoS One*, *10*(6), e0124207. https://doi.org/10.1371/journal.pone.0124207

Oranges, T., Dini, V., & Romanelli, M. (2015). Skin physiology of the neonate and infant: Clinical implications. *Advances in Wound Care*, *4*(10), 587–595. https://doi.org/10.1089/wound.2015.0642

Osama, M., Ali, S., & Malik, R. J. (2018). Posture related musculoskeletal discomfort and its association with computer use among university students. *Journal of the Pakistan Medical Association*, *68*(4), 639–641.

Osypiuk, K., Thompson, E., & Wayne, P. M. (2018). Can Tai Chi and Qigong postures shape our mood? Toward an embodied cognition framework for mind-body research. *Frontiers in Human Neuroscience*, *12*, 174. https://doi.org/10.3389/fnhum.2018.00174

Owler, K., & Morrison, R. L. (2020). "I always have fun at work": How "remarkable workers" employ agency and control in order to enjoy themselves. *Journal of Management & Organization*, *26*, 135–151. https://doi.org/10.1017/jmo.2019.90

Pados, B., & Fuller, K. (2020). Establishing a foundation for optimal feeding outcomes in the NICU. *Nursing for Women's Health*. https://doi.org/10.1016/j.nwh.2020.03.007

Pados, B., Park, J., Estrem, H., & Awotwi, A. (2016). Assessment tools for evaluation. Of oral feeding in infants less than six months old. *Advances in Neonatal Care*, *16*(2), 143–150. https://doi.org/10.1097/ANC.0000000000000255

Pammi, M., O'Brien, J. L., Ajami, N. J., Wong, M. C., Versalovic, J., & Petrosino, J. F. (2017). Development of the cutaneous microbiome in the preterm infant: A prospective longitudinal study. *PLoS One*, *12*(4), e0176669. https://doi.org/10.1371/journal.pone.0176669

Patel, A. L., Schoeny, M., Hoban, R., Johnson, T., Bigger, H., Engstrom, J. L., Fleurant, E., Riley, B., & Meier, P. P. (2019). Mediators of racial and ethnic disparity in mother's own milk feeding in very low birth weight infants. *Pediatric Research*, *85*(5), 662–670. https://doi.org/10.1038/s41390-019-0290-2

Pearce, L. (2018). Creating a "take a break" culture. *Nursing Standard*, *33*(3), 64–66. https://doi.org/10.7748/ns.33.3.64.s29

Petelczyc, C. A., Capezio, A., Wang, L., Restubog, S. L. D., & Aquino, K. (2018). Play at work: An integrative review and agenda for future research. *Journal of Management*, *44*(1), 161–190. https://doi.org/10.1177/0149206317731519

Peters, E. M. J. (2016). Stressed skin?—A molecular psychosomatic update on stress-causes and effects in dermatologic diseases. *Journal of the German Society of Dermatology*, *14*(3), 233–252. https://doi.org/10.1111/ddg.12957

Picaud, J. C., Buffin, R., Gremmo-Feger, G., Rigo, J., Putet, G., Casper, C.; Working Group of the French Neonatal Society on fresh human milk use in preterm infants. (2018). Review concludes that specific recommendations are needed to harmonize the provision of fresh mother's milk to their preterm infants. *Acta Paediatrica, 107*(7), 1145–1155. https://doi.org/10.1111/apa.14259

Power, B. T., Kiezebrink, K., Allan, J. L., & Campbell, M. K. (2017). Understanding perceived determinants of nurses' eating and physical activity behavior: A theory-informed qualitative interview study. *BMC Obesity, 4*, 18. https://doi.org/10.1186/s40608-017-0154-4

Priano, S. M., Hong, O. S., & Chen, J.-L. (2018). Lifestyles and health-related outcomes of U.S. hospital nurses: A systematic review. *Nursing Outlook, 66*, 66–76. https://doi.org/10.1016/j.outlook.2017.08.013

Raney, M., & van Zanten, E. (2019). Self-care posters serve as a low-cost option for physical activity promotion of hospital nurses. *Health Promotion Practice, 20*(3), 354–362. https://doi.org/10.1177/1524839918763585

Richardson, A., Gurung, G., Derrett, S., & Harcombe, H. (2019). Perspectives on preventing musculoskeletal injuries in nurses: A qualitative study. *Nursing Open, 6*(3), 915–929. https://doi.org/10.1002/nop2.272

Ritchie, H., & Roser, M. (2020). *Obesity*. OurWorldInData.org. https://ourworldindata.org/obesity

Roos, J., & Victor, B. (2018). How it all began: The origins of LEGO Serious Play. *International Journal of Management and Applied Research, 5*(4), 326–343. https://doi.org/10.18646/2056.54.18-025

Rooth, V., van Oostrom, S. H., Deeg, D. J. H., Verschuren, W. M. M., & Picavet, H. S. (2016). Common trajectories of physical functioning in the Doetinchem Cohort Study. *Age and Aging, 45*, 382–388. https://doi.org/10.1093/ageing/afw018

Ross, A., Touchton-Leonard, K., Perez, A., Wehrlen, L., Kazmi, N., & Gibbons, S. (2019). Factors that influence health-promoting self-care in registered nurses: Barriers and facilitators. *Advances in Nursing Science, 42*(4), 358–373. https://doi.org/10.1097/ANS.0000000000000274

Ross, K., Heiny, E., Conner, S., Spencer, P., & Pineda, R. (2017). Occupational therapy, physical therapy and speech-language pathology in the neonatal intensive care unit: Patterns of therapy usage in a level IV NICU. *Research in Developmental Disabilities, 64*, 108–117. https://doi.org/10.1016/j.ridd.2017.03.009

Sakamoto, A., & Gamada, K. (2019). Altered musculoskeletal mechanics as risk factors for postpartum pelvic girdle pain: A literature review. *Journal of Physical Therapy Science, 31*(10), 831–838. https://doi.org/10.1589/jpts.31.831

Salem, I., Ramser, A., Isham, N., & Ghannoum, M. A. (2018). The gut microbiome as a regulator of the gut-skin axis. *Frontiers in Microbiology, 9*, 1459. https://doi.org/10.3389/fmicb.2018.01459

Sathiyamurthy, S., Banerjee, J., & Godambe, S. V. (2016). Antiseptic use in the neonatal intensive care unit—A dilemma in clinical practice: An evidence-based review. *World Journal of Clinical Pediatrics, 5*(2), 159–171. https://doi.org/10.5409/wjcp.v5.i2.159

Saulle, R., Bernardi, M., Chiarini, M., Backhaus, I., & La Torre, G. (2018). Shift work, overweight and obesity in health professionals: A systematic review and meta-analysis. *La Clinica Terapeutica, 169*(4), e189–e197. https://doi.org/10.7417/T.2018.2077

Scaglioni, S., De Cosmi, V., Ciappolino, V., Parazzini, F., Brambilla, P., & Agostoni, C. (2018). Factors influencing children's eating behaviours. *Nutrients, 10*(6), 706. https://doi.org/10.3390/nu10060706

Schoghi, M., Sohrabi, S., & Rasouli, M. (2018). The effects of massage by mothers on mother–infant attachment. *Alternative Therapies in Health and Medicine, 24*(3), 34–39.

Shiino, Y., Sakai, S., Takeishi, R., Hayashi, H., Watanabe, M., Tsujimura, T., Magara, J., Ito, K., Tsukada, T., & Inoue, M. (2016). Effect of body posture on involuntary swallow in healthy volunteers. *Physiology & Behavior, 155*, 250–259. https://doi.org/10.1016/j.physbeh.2015.12.024

Sigurdson, K., Mitchell, B., Liu, J., Morton, C., Gould, J. B., Lee, H. C., Capdarest-Arest, N., & Profit, J. (2019). Racial/ethnic disparities in neonatal intensive care: A systematic review. *Pediatrics, 144*(2), e20183114. https://doi.org/10.1542/peds.2018-3114

Simon, J. J., Wetzel, A., Sinno, M. H., Skunde, M., Bendszus, M., Preissi, H., Enck, P., Herzog, W., & Friederich, H. C. (2017). Integration of homeostatic signaling and food reward processing in the human brain. *JCI Insight, 2*(15), e92970. https://doi.org/10.1172/jci.insight.92970

Simpfel, A. W., & Aiken, L. H. (2013). Hospital staff nurses' shift length associated with safety and quality of care. *Journal of Nursing Care Quality, 28*(2), 122–129. https://doi.org/10.1097/NCQ.0b013e3182725f09

Slominski, A. T., Zmijewski, M. A., Skobowiat, C., Zbytek, B., Slominski, R. M., & Steketee J. D. (2012). Introduction in sensing the environment: Regulation of local and global homeostasis by the skin's neuroendocrine system. In P. Sutovsky, F. Clascá, Z. Kmiec, H.-W. Korf, M. J. Schmeisser, B. Singh, & J.-P. Timmermans (Eds.), *Advances in anatomy, embryology and cell biology* (Vol. 212, pp. 1–6). Springer.

Stanulewicz, N., Knox, E., Narayanasamy, M., Shivji, N., Khunti, K., & Blake, H. (2020). Effectiveness of lifestyle health promotion interventions for nurses: A systematic review. *International Journal of Environmental Research and Public Health, 17*(1), 17. https://doi.org/10.3390/ijerph17010017

Steege, L. M., & Rainbow, J. G. (2017). Fatigue in hospital nurses— "supernurse" culture is a barrier to addressing problems: A qualitative interview study. *International Journal of Nursing Studies. 67*, 20–28. https://doi.org/10.1016/j.ijnurstu.2016.11.014

Stroebele, N., & De Castro, J. M. (2004). Effect of ambience on food intake and food choice. *Nutrition, 20*(9), 821–838. https://doi.org/10.1016/j.nut.2004.05.012

Tambunan, D. M., & Mediani, H. S. (2019). Bathing method for preterm infants: A systematic review. *KnE Life Sciences*, 1–11. https://doi.org/10.18502/kls.v4i13.5220

Tawalbeh, M., Riedel, R., Dempsey, M., & Emanuel, C. (2018). LEGO Serious Play as a Business Innovation enabler, 5th European Lean Educator Conference, Braga, Portugal.

Terada, T., Mistura, M., Tulloch, H., Pipe, A., & Reed, J. (2019). Dietary behavior is associated with cardiometabolic and psychological risk indicators in female hospital nurses—A post hoc, cross sectional study. *Nutrients, 11*(9), 2054. https://doi.org/10.3390/nu11092054

Thomas, K. S., & Magal, M. (2014). How does physical activity impact postural stability? *Journal of Novel Physiotherapies, 4*(2). https://doi.org/10.4172/2165-7025.1000206

Thoyre, S., Park, J., Pados, B., & Hubbard, C. (2013). Developing a co-regulated, cue-based feeding practice: The critical role of assessment and reflection. *Journal of Neonatal Nursing, 19*(4), 139–148. https://doi.org/10.1016/j.jnn.2013.01.002

Uesugi, Y., Ihara, Y., Yuasa, K.M., & Takahashi, K. (2019). Sole-ground contact and sitting leg position influence suprahyoid and sternocleidomastoid muscle activity during swallowing of liquids. *Clinical and Experimental Dental Research, 5*(5), 505–512. https://doi.org/10.1002/cre2.216

Underwood, M. A., & Sohn, K. (2017). The microbiota of the extremely preterm infant. *Clinics in Perinatology, 44*(2), 407–427. https://doi.org/10.1016/j.clp.2017.01.005

Uysal, P. I., Akdogan, N., Hayran, Y., Oktem, A., & Yalcin, B. (2019). Rosacea associated with increased risk of generalized anxiety disorder: A case-control study of prevalence and risk of anxiety in patients with rosacea. *Anais Brasileiros de Dermatologia, 94*(6), 704–709. https://doi .org/10.1016/j.abd.2019.03.002

Van Fleet, M., & Feeney, B. C. (2015). Young at heart: A perspective for advancing research on play in adulthood. *Perspectives on Psychological Science, 10*(5), 639–645. https://doi.org/10.1177/1745691615596789

Vance, D. A., Demel, S., Kirksey, K., Moynihan, M., & Hollis, K. (2015). A delphi study for the development of an infant skin breakdown risk assessment tool. *Advances in Neonatal Care, 15*(2), 150–157. https://doi.org/10.1097/ANC.0000000000000104

Vasavada, A. N., Nevins, D. D., Monda, S. M., Hughes, E., & Lin, D. C. (2015). Gravitational demand on the neck musculature during tablet use. *Ergonomics, 58*(6), 990–1004. https://doi.org/10.10 80/00140139.2015.1005166

Vassalou, E. E., Klonyzas, M. E., Tsifountoudis, I. P., Spanakis, K., & Karantanas, A. H. (2019). Spectrum of skeletal disorders during the peripartum period: MRI patterns. *Diagnostic and Interventional Radiology, 25*(3), 245–250. https://doi.org/10.5152/dir.2019.18354

Verduci, E., Gianni, M. L., & Di Benedetto, A. (2020). Human milk feeding in preterm infants: What has been done and what is to be done. *Nutrients, 12*(1), 44. https://doi.org/10.3390/nu12010044

Vieira, E. R., & Kumar, S. (2004). Working postures: A literature review. *Journal of Occupational Rehabilitation, 14*(2), 143–159. https://doi.org/10.1023/b:joor.0000018330.46029.05

Visscher, M., & Narendran, V. (2014). The ontogeny of skin. *Advances in Wound Care, 3*(4), 291–303. https://doi.org/10.1089/wound.2013.0467

Visscher, M., & Taylor, T. (2014). Pressure ulcers in the hospitalized neonate: Rates and risk factors. *Scientific Reports, 4*, 7429. https://doi.org/10.1038/srep07429

Visscher, M. O., Adam, R., Brink, S., & Odio, M. (2015). Newborn infant skin: Physiology, development, and care. *Clinics in Dermatology, 33*(3), 271–280. https://doi.org/10.1016/j.clindermatol.2014.12.003

Walicka-Cuprys, K., Drzat-Grabiec, J., Rachwat, M., Piwonski, P., Perenc, L., Przygoda, L., & Zajkiewicz, K. (2017). Body posture asymmetry in prematurely born children at six years of age. *BioMed Research International, 2017*, 9302520. https://doi.org/10.1155/2017/9302520

Wang, D., Xu, H., Chen, S., Lou, X., Tan, J., & Xu, Y. (2019). Medical adhesive-related skin injuries and associated risk factors in a pediatric intensive care unit. *Advances in Skin & Wound Care, 32*(4), 176–182. https://doi.org/10.1097/01.ASW.0000553601.05196.fb

Wang, S., & Aamodt, S. (2012). Play, stress, and the learning brain. *Cerebrum, 2012*, 12. PMCID: PMC3574776

Weber, A., & Harrison, T. M. (2019). Reducing toxic stress in the NICU to improve infant outcomes. *Nursing Outlook, 67*(2), 169–189. https://doi.org/10.1016/j.outlook.2018.11.002

Werner, L. A., & Dayan, M. (2019). Diastasis recti abdominis—Diagnosis, risk factors, effect on musculoskeletal function, framework for treatment and implications for the pelvic floor. *Current Women's Health Reviews, 15*, 86–101. https://doi.org/10.2174/1573404814666180222152952

Wilson, J., Prieto, J., Singleton, J., O'Connor, V., Lynam, S., & Loveday, H. (2015). The misuse and overuse of non-sterile gloves: Application of an audit tool to define the problem. *Journal of Infection Prevention, 16*(1), 24–31. https://doi.org/10.1177/1757177414558673

Xu, W., Judge, M., Maas, K., Hussain, N., McGrath, J. M., Henderson, W. A., and Cong, X. (2018). Systematic review of the effect of enteral feeding on gut microbiota in preterm infants. *Journal of Obstetric, Gynecologic & Neonatal Nursing, 47*(3), 451–463. https://doi.org/10.1016/j.jogn.2017.08.009

Yamada, N. K., Fuerch, J. H., & Halamek, L. P. (2019). Ergonomic challenges inherent in neonatal resuscitation. *Children* (Basel), 6(6), 74. https://doi.org/10.3390/children6060074

Yi, Y. G., Oh, B.-M., Shin, S. H., Shin, J. Y., Kim, E.-K., & Shin, H.-I. (2018). Stress signals during sucking activity are associated with longer transition time to full oral feeding in premature infants. *Frontiers in Pediatrics, 6*, 54. https://doi.org/10.3389/fped.2018.00054

Younge, N. E., Araujo-Perez, F., Brandon, D., & Seed, P. C. (2018). Early-life skin microbiota in hospitalized preterm and full-term infants. *Microbiome, 6*, 98. https://doi.org/10.1186/s40168-018-0486-4

Zosh, J. M., Hopkins, E. J., Jensen, H., Liu, C., Neale, D., Hirsh-Pasek, K., Solis, S. L., & Whitebread, D. (2017). *Learning through play: A review of the evidence (white paper)*. The LEGO Foundation.

Section IV

Application, Outcomes, and Relevance of a Trauma-Informed Paradigm

11

Quantum Caring in Action

> *Never doubt that a small group of thoughtful, committed citizens can change the world. Indeed, it is the only thing that ever has.*
> —Margaret Mead

Quantum Caring is a cultural transformation program designed and developed by Caring Essentials Collaborative, LLC. The original version of this program was presented as a pilot investigation at a Level III NICU in Rocourt, Belgium, to evaluate the impact of the adoption of the newly created core measures for developmentally supportive care (Coughlin et al., 2009). The results of this pilot program are described in the first edition of this book (Coughlin, 2014, chapter 11).

Quantum Caring in action recognizes that the tiniest, most infinitesimally smallest action makes a difference. It is the pebble in the pond, the drop of rain in the ocean. With every thought, word, action we touch lives and impact lifetimes. The work that is shared in this chapter represents the ripple effect of embracing a trauma-informed paradigm and the step-by-step engagement, education, and transformation of clinical practice in the NICU and beyond.

THE CHILDREN'S HEALTHCARE OF ATLANTA PROJECT

Studies of developmentally supportive, age-appropriate care practices traditionally exclude special patient populations. These special populations include infants with congenital or chromosomal anomalies, neurologic conditions, congenital infections, and other complex patient conditions. The patient population served in the NICU at Children's Healthcare of Atlanta (CHOA), part of the Children's Hospitals Neonatal Consortium, consists primarily of these unique and critically complex infants.

"Touch a life, impact a lifetime" was the tagline for the 3-year Quantum Caring project at CHOA. The goal of the program was to adopt and integrate the National Association of Neonatal Nurses (NANN) Guidelines for Age-Appropriate Care of the Premature and

Critically Ill Hospitalized Infant (Coughlin, 2011) as the standard for developmental care in their Level IV surgical NICU. The NANN practice guideline was adapted from the original core measures described by Coughlin et al. (2009).

A baseline assessment of staff perceptions regarding age-appropriate, developmentally supportive care was collected prior to the program start date and then reassessed annually for a total of four data points using the Quantum Caring Self-Assessment Tool (QC-SAT; this tool has since been replaced with the Trauma-informed Care Staff Perception Survey; a link to this survey can be found in the Reader Resource section of this chapter). The QC-SAT used a 5-point Likert scale ranging from 1 = never to 5 = always to examine the frequency of various age-appropriate care practices. "Not applicable" and "do not know" were included for staff who may not provide all the dimensions of care represented in the survey; these answer choices were assigned a score of zero.

The survey included questions specific to each core measure for age-appropriate care. Survey results were analyzed and compared year over year to evaluate progress and identify ongoing opportunities for quality and practice improvement. Tables 11.1 to 11.5 highlight the interval improvement in staff perceptions from baseline, January 2013, to the 3-year final assessment in January 2016. The unpaired t-test was used to determine p values and statistical significance.

Understanding staff perceptions and contrasting them to existing clinical practices related to the NANN guidelines allowed the team to identify and prioritize practice-improvement initiatives over the program period. Repeating the survey annually and sharing the results with staff and leaders kept the project top-of-mind and reinforced the work of the core measure teams. Of the four indicators that did not demonstrate a statistical change, three indicators were existing best practices in the unit prior to the program start date. These three indicators included the use of a validated pain assess-ment tool, use of a validated skin assessment tool, and weekly family meetings to share patient information updates. The fourth indicator that did not demonstrate a significant change was the assessment of family mental health and continues as an ongoing quality-improvement (QI) initiative.

A project steering committee was formed and represented the primary caregiving disciplines in the unit: medicine, nursing, rehabilitation services, respiratory therapy, and chaplaincy. The role of these managers and staff leaders was to provide project direction, facilitate operationalization, and approve budget expenditures. The initial phase of the project focused on interdisciplinary staff-wide education to establish a shared knowledge base. Self-selected interdisciplinary staff formed core measure work teams. These individuals received additional training on improvement methodologies, implementation strategies, and evidence-based practice principles. The teams were mentored by a unit-based senior staff nurse who also coordinated the project and acted as a liaison between the consultant and the clinical and administrative teams.

The "Healing Environment" was chosen as a focus for the first year. The "Quiet Time" (QT) initiative aimed to foster a quiet, healing environment while ensuring a safe work milieu for staff. QT parameters included: (a) dimmed lights to mark the onset of the QT

Table 11.1 **The Healing Environment**

Indicators for the Healing Environment	January 2013			January 2016			p value
	M	SD	N	M	SD	N	
Ambient light and sound levels in the patient care area are within recommended ranges.	3.76	1.04	127	4.11	0.78	98	.0059
RN/MD collaboration is defined, practiced, and reinforced on a daily basis.	4.28	1.06	118	4.6	0.81	87	.0195
Staff are expected and held accountable to provide developmentally supportive care (as defined by the core measures) consistently and reliably to all hospitalized infants under their care.	3.64	1.52	119	4.3	0.98	88	.0005
Annual performance appraisal includes a review of the staff member's consistent and reliable provision of age-appropriate care (aka compliance with developmental care practice standards).	4.11	1.75	116	4.68	1.03	88	.0071

Table 11.2 **Pain and Stress**

Indicators for Pain and Stress	January 2013			January 2016			p value
	M	SD	N	M	SD	N	
A valid pain assessment tool is utilized.	4.82	0.61	124	4.86	0.42	96	.5833
Nonpharmacologic and/or pharmacologic measures are utilized prior to all stressful/painful procedures.	4.47	0.72	123	4.76	0.55	96	.0012
Caregiving activities are adapted to minimize pain and stress.	4.46	0.65	124	4.67	0.55	96	.0118
Parents are involved and informed of the pain and stress management plans of care for their hospitalized infant(s).	3.97	0.97	123	4.26	0.82	96	.0198
Family is encouraged to provide comfort to their infant.	4.54	0.68	124	4.71	0.5	96	.0409

period, (b) soft voices, (c) televisions (in private rooms) turned off, and (d) the restriction of routine procedures (e.g., x-rays, echocardiograms, ultrasounds). Routine cleaning and trash removal, engineering/maintenance work, invasive lab draws, and the restocking of bedside carts were discouraged during the QT periods.

The QT initiative reduced ambient noise levels (Figure 11.1) while increasing the speech intelligibility index during the study period (SII; Figure 11.2). Increasing the SII led to greater comprehension of spoken communication despite the decrease in ambient decibel levels. Staff reported a high degree of satisfaction with the QT initiative: "*Something about when the lights dim at 1,300/0100 makes me immediately feel more relaxed. Initially I*

Table 11.3 **Protected Sleep**

Indicators for Protected Sleep	January 2013			January 2016			p value
	M	SD	N	M	SD	N	
All nonemergent caregiving is provided during wakeful states.	3.83	0.85	124	4.09	0.7	97	.0157
Scheduled caregiving is driven by and contingent on the infant's sleep/wake state.	3.48	0.95	127	3.85	0.91	98	.0035
Caregiving activities that promote sleep (i.e., facilitative tuck, swaddled bathing, and skin-to-skin care) are integrated into the patient's daily care plan.	4.26	0.88	127	4.82	0.46	98	.0001
All caregiving activities are modified according to the infant's state.	3.75	0.96	127	4.09	0.73	98	.0039

was not sold on how QT would be beneficial, but I have to say I am loving it now!" Noise levels remained lower than preintervention levels after 18 months. QT has since been adopted by other ICUs and acute care units in the facility.

The NICU team worked with the business intelligence team, using the stored vital sign data from the infants' monitors, to measure improvement in the accuracy of pain assessment scores. While staff perceptions acknowledged the use of a validated pain assessment tool, the accuracy of the pain scores were called into question when an inverse relationship was discovered between the pain scores and the stored vital sign data. A comprehensive education initiative to include one-on-one bedside training was launched to improve accuracy in the use of the Neonatal Pain, Agitation and Sedation Scale (NPASS). Chart audits (Figure 11.3) and a comparison of NPASS scores with stored vital sign data confirmed a successful education intervention (Figure 11.4).

Table 11.4 **Activities of Daily Living**

Indicators for Activities of Daily Living	January 2013			January 2016			p value
	M	SD	N	M	SD	N	
Each infant is positioned and handled in flexion, containment, and alignment during all caregiving activities.	4.06	0.89	123	4.36	0.65	96	.006
Infant position is evaluated with every infant interaction and modified to support symmetric development.	4.12	0.99	123	4.37	0.74	95	.0409
Infant position is documented with each infant interaction.	4.17	1.17	123	4.46	0.81	95	.0403
Assessment of feeding readiness cues is documented with each oral feeding encounter.	3.46	1.38	123	3.84	1.27	94	.0387
Education regarding the benefits of breast milk is provided to all families.	4.24	1.06	122	4.55	0.81	93	.0199
Skin integrity is assessed using a reliable assessment tool once per shift and documented.	4.76	0.98	122	4.91	0.58	95	.1876
The skin surface is protected during application and removal of adhesive products.	4.46	0.77	121	4.72	0.64	94	.0089

Table 11.5 **Family-Centered Care**

Indicators for Family-Centered Care	January 2013			January 2016			p value
	M	SD	N	M	SD	N	
Families are given the opportunity to be present and/or participate in medical rounds and change-of-shift report.	3.46	1.47	123	4.77	0.57	94	.0001
Families are encouraged to parent, which includes skin-to-skin care, holding, feeding activities, dressing, bathing, diapering, singing, and bonding interactions.	4.39	0.66	122	4.72	0.47	95	.0001
Families are given the opportunity to be present during invasive procedures and/or resuscitative interventions.	3.4	1.31	123	4.21	1.16	95	.0001
Family input and observations of their infant are documented in the medical record or care flowsheet.	3.64	1.53	122	4.06	1.25	95	.0311
Families are assessed weekly for their mental health status and provided appropriate resources as needed.	3.86	1.69	121	4.09	1.39	95	.285
Healthcare providers share objective infant information weekly with the family.	4.35	0.94	122	4.44	0.89	95	.4747
Families are invited to participate in a NICU family support group.	3.78	2	122	4.48	1.38	93	.0042

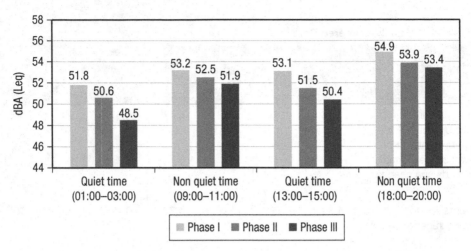

Figure 11.1 Comparison of quiet time versus nonquiet time hours.

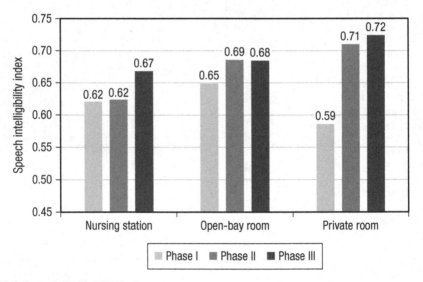

Figure 11.2 Speech intelligibility index.

Based on the QC-SAT results, the team uncovered a paucity in the documentation of developmental care interventions to support infants during caregiving encounters. The team reviewed the electronic medical record (EMR) and provided staff education to standardize documentation of stress- relieving developmental care interventions. Pre- and posteducation audits demonstrated a significant interval improvement in the documentation of developmental care interventions (Figure 11.5).

Random bedside audits of infant postural alignment were performed over the 3-year program period. Staff were encouraged to complete self-audits of their patients' postural

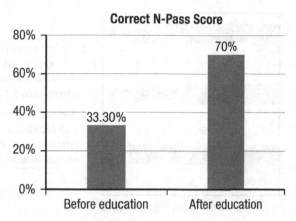

Figure 11.3 Interval improvement in Neonatal Pain, Agitation, and Sedation Scale score accuracy.

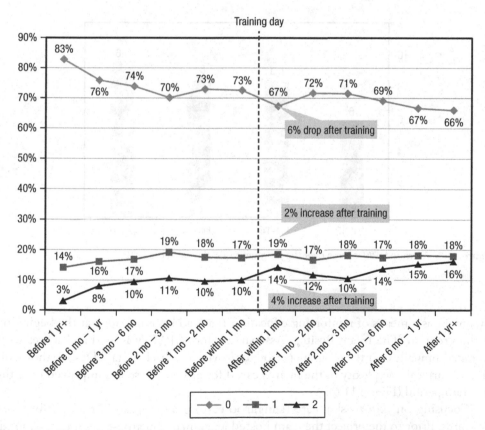

Figure 11.4 Stored vital sign data looked at the percentage of recorded Neonatal Pain, Agitation, and Sedation Scale vital sign scores of 0, 1, 2 over various time intervals before and after training. Decreases in the percentage of 0 scores, and increases in scores of 1 or 2 indicate improved correlation with actual vital sign data suggesting the training was effective.

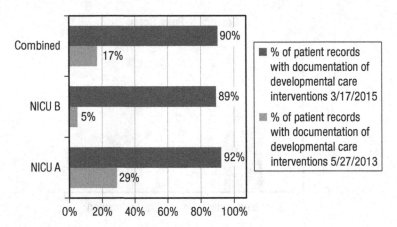

Figure 11.5 Documentation of developmental care interventions pre- and posteducation.

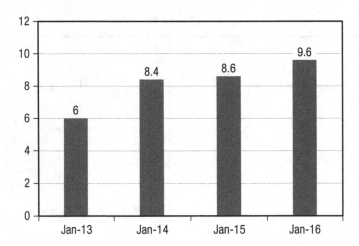

Figure 11.6. Averaged IPAT scores over the program period. Ideal score is 12.

PAT, Infant Position Assessment Tool.

alignment as a means of reinforcing education that had been provided at the beginning of the program. The Infant Position Assessment Tool (IPAT) was used and scores were averaged annually over the program period to provide feedback to staff. Despite the medical and surgical complexity of the infants cared for at CHOA, scores improved over the program period (Figure 11.6).

Focusing on skin-to-skin care (kangaroo care) practices can impact all five core measures. Prior to the project the team hosted an annual kangaroo-a-thon in the month of May. With a commitment to increase the frequency and duration of skin-to-skin care encounters, the team began a focused initiative educating parents and staff on the benefits of skin-to-skin care. Weekly reports on the frequency of skin-to-skin care encounters were

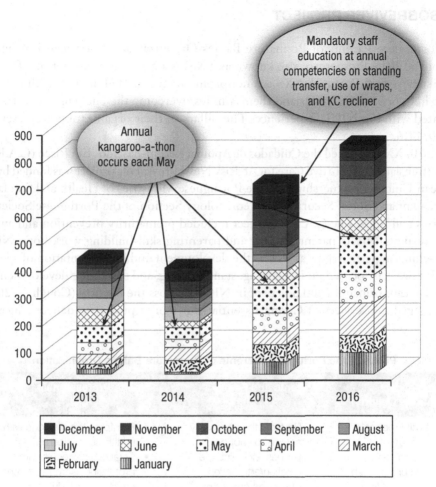

Figure 11.7 Increase in kangaroo care sessions over the program period.

KC, kangaroo care.

documented in the EMR and the team compiled monthly reports to share with staff and celebrate progress and practice improvement (Figure 11.7).

The core measure framework helped to plan and organize practice improvement initiatives. Staff perceptions shifted from viewing age-appropriate developmental care as a "nicety" to a "necessity" as staff witnessed the transformation their patients experienced with the adoption of the core measures and the NANN guidelines. As part of a sustainability plan, core measure teams now partner with the system's nursing research and evidence-based practice department to align with the organization's goals for clinician-driven practice improvement. The project inspired two funded pilot research studies and several poster and podium presentations at national and international conferences. The members of the core measure teams continue to think in evidence-based practice terms as they design ongoing practice-improvement initiatives.

THE SOBREVIVER PROJECT

The Portuguese Parents of Premature Babies Organization (Associação Portuguesa de Apoio ao Bebé Prematuro, also known as XXS) is a national organization of NICU parent survivors in Portugal. XXS is a nonprofit entity founded in 2008 with the mission to help premature babies and their families overcome the challenges and trauma associated with the NICU experience. The pillars of their organization are described in Table 11.6.

In 2014 XXS launched the Cuidados de Apoio a Recem-nascidos Em Risco (C.A.R.E.) project [translated: Supportive Care for At-Risk Newborns). This project was funded by the European Union in partnership with the Portuguese Ministries of Health and Solidarity, Employment and Social Security, the Neonatology Section of the Portuguese Society of Pediatrics and XXS. The C.A.R.E. project included prematurity prevention and awareness campaigns, NICU parent training and parenting skill-building workshops, NICU parent–clinician partnerships as well as the development and implementation of specialized pilot projects focused on integrating, standardizing, and sustaining developmentally supportive care principles and practices in NICUs across the country (Coughlin, 2015). XXS engaged the services of Caring Essentials for a pilot project to deliver education

Table 11.6 Pillars of the Portuguese Parents of Premature Babies Organization

Babies and Premature Children	Parents and Family	Health Professionals
• Submit proposals to change legislation on premature children and support for families. • Intervene with the competent entities to recognize the special needs and requirements of these children. • Collaborate in promoting child development stimulation programs.	• Promote the necessary actions to support families, including the creation/articulation of support groups at a national level, fundraising campaigns and volunteering courses. • Disseminate and share knowledge and experiences that address the issue of prematurity, including publications, explanatory leaflets, and parent forums. • Develop actions to improve the reception conditions for displaced families.	• Reinforce the dialogue with health professionals. • Establish protocols with professionals from different areas of health in child support, namely, with the Neonatology Section of the Portuguese Society of Pediatrics, promoting joint actions of prevention, awareness, and action with children and families in hospital units, health centers, and fertilization clinics. • Cooperate in prevention campaigns. • Cooperate in scientific research. • Represent Portugal as an EFCNI member.

EFCNI, European Foundation for the Care of Newborn Infants.

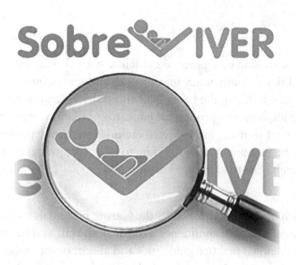

Figure 11.8 Sobreviver logo.

Source: Courtesy of XXS, Associação Portuguesa de Apoio ao Bebé Prematuro. www.xxs-prematuros.com

---

BOX 11.1 FACTORS IMPLICATED IN THE INCONSISTENT PROVISION OF SKIN-TO-SKIN CARE

1. Lack of clear practice guidelines to include eligibility criteria
2. Insufficient competency-based education and performance expectations of staff and parents
3. A paucity of consistent documentation criteria
4. A dearth of individual and systems accountability for the provision of evidence-based practice

---

and establish a standardized and sustainable approach to the provision of skin-to-skin care across three NICUs in Portugal. The program period extended from October 2014 through April 2015. The project was dubbed the Sobreviver Project; English translation: The Survive Project (Figure 11.8).

Several factors have been implicated in the inconsistency of skin-to-skin care practice (Box 11.1). Nurses' attitudes about skin-to-skin care play an intangible but key role in promoting and facilitating skin-to-skin care experiences in the NICU. Varying thresholds for the initiation of skin-to-skin care, availability of adequate or appropriate resources and workflow challenges converge to create chaos and inconsistency (Coughlin, 2015; Vittner et al., 2015).

Similar to the CHOA project, each unit developed a steering committee to guide the direction and support the work of the QI initiative. Once the leadership and direction were established, a failure modes and effects analysis with regard to the existing skin-to-skin

> **BOX 11.2** OVERARCHING PROJECT OBJECTIVES FOR EACH UNIT
>
> - Develop a skin-to-skin care practice guideline with clear eligibility criteria.
> - Establish a clinician competency for standing and seated infant transfer for skin-to-skin care (emphasizing the benefits of the standing transfer).
> - Establish and implement a process for educating and empowering NICU parents on the benefits of skin-to-skin care and include a return demonstration.
> - Standardize the documentation for skin-to-skin care to capture frequency and duration of each skin-to-skin care encounter.

care practices at each unit was performed by the Caring Essentials consultant. The analysis revealed a knowledge, skill, and confidence gap for both staff and parents regarding skin-to-skin care. Poorly defined practice guidelines and absent or inconsistent documentation criteria undermined the standardization of skin-to-skin care. Following the education intervention, the consultant met with the project leads at each of the three participating units to outline the overarching project objectives (Box 11.2).

Baseline information was collected regarding infant transfer method, obstacles to providing skin-to-skin care, perceived staff confidence in facilitating skin-to-skin care encounters as well as parent input specific to the frequency in which they provided skin-to-skin care under various conditions (Figures 11.9–11.13). Data were recollected at 3 and 6 months, compared and analyzed against the baseline data set to assess for practice improvement and statistical significance. Documentation strategies differed among the three units and were monitored and trended over time. Two of the units using EMRs adapted their documentation criteria to collect frequency, duration, and transfer mode (seated vs.

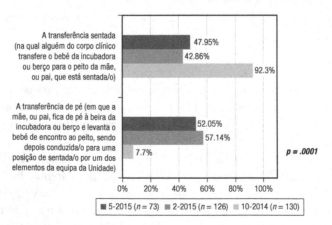

Figure 11.9 Infant transfer method (transferência sentada = seated transfer; transferência pé = standing transfer).

Source: Coughlin, M. (2015). The Sobreviver (Survive) project. *Newborn and Infant Nursing Reviews, 15*(4), 169–173. https://doi.org/10.1053/j.nainr.2015.09.010 Reprinted with permission from Elsevier.

standing). The third unit was in the process of transitioning to electronic documentation. As an intermediary strategy, this unit developed a documentation tool that was placed at each infant's bed space and parents were encouraged to document their skin-to-skin care experiences on the tool. This information was then captured into the nursing notes.

Each unit project team received sample skin-to-skin care policies, protocols and practice guidelines along with key review articles to support the development of unit-based practice guidelines with eligibility criteria for skin-to-skin care. A competency checklist for the infant transfer was developed for staff and parents. Using a simulation activity, staff and parents completed a return demonstration of a mockup infant transfer using both the seated and standing transfer methods to validate competence and confidence in the procedure.

Parent education was facilitated by a NICU staff member, a representative of the XXS organization and the Caring Essentials consultant. The XXS member, a former NICU parent, was able to relate to and support the education and the skin-to-skin care practicum with the parents. Each parent received a certificate of completion following the education sessions.

The statistical significance of the staff survey outcomes reflects the importance of integrating a systematic approach to practice improvement. The staff survey responses revealed a solid knowledge base of the benefits of skin-to-skin care. This knowledge, however, did

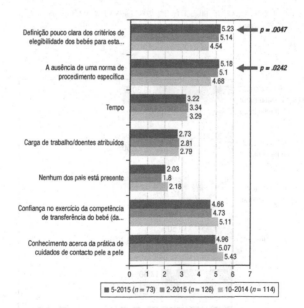

Figure 11.10 Obstacles to providing skin-to-skin care (the lower the number, the greater barrier to practice). Conhecimento acerca da prática = knowledge about the practice; Confiança no exercício da competência de transferência = confidence in the exercise of transfer competence; Nenhum dos pais está presente = neither parent is present; Carga de trabalho/doentes atribuidos = assigned workload; Tempo = time; A ausência de uma norma de procedimento especifica; absence of a specific procedure standard; Definição pouco clara dos critérios de elegebilidade = unclear eligibility criteria.

Source: Coughlin, M. (2015). The Sobreviver (Survive) project. *Newborn and Infant Nursing Reviews, 15*(4), 169–173. https://doi.org/10.1053/j.nainr.2015.09.010 Reprinted with permission from Elsevier.

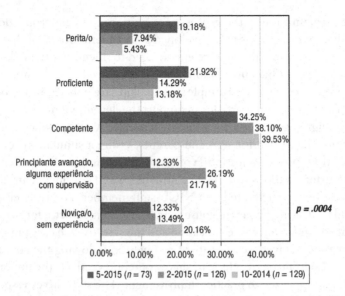

Figure 11.11 Staff confidence in facilitating skin-to-skin care using Benner's Novice (Noviça/o) to Expert (Perita/o) Scale.

Source: Coughlin, M. (2015). The Sobreviver (Survive) project. *Newborn and Infant Nursing Reviews, 15*(4), 169–173. https://doi .org/10.1053/j.nainr.2015.09.010 Reprinted with permission from Elsevier.

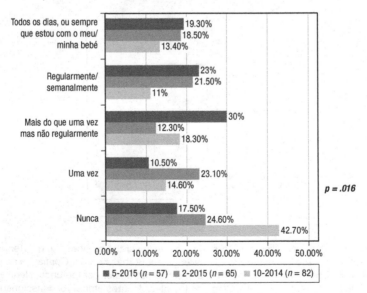

Figure 11.12 How many times parents report having skin-to-skin care experiences (Nunca—never; todos os dias = always).

Source: Coughlin, M. (2015). The Sobreviver (Survive) project. *Newborn and Infant Nursing Reviews, 15*(4), 169–173. https://doi.org/ 10.1053/j.nainr.2015.09.010 Reprinted with permission from Elsevier.

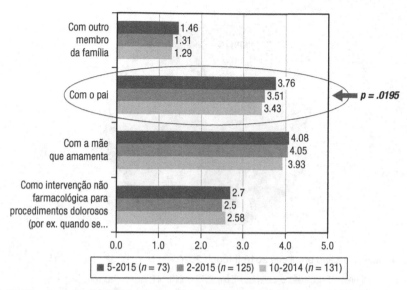

Figure 11.13 Situations in which skin-to-skin care is facilitated. Como intervenção não farmacológica para procedimentos dolorosos = as a nonpharmacologic intervention for painful procedures; Com a mãe que amamenta = with a breastfeeding mother; Com o pai = with a father; Com outro membro da familia = with another member of the family.

Source: Coughlin, M. (2015). The Sobreviver (Survive) project. *Newborn and Infant Nursing Reviews, 15*(4), 169–173. https://doi.org/10.1053/j.nainr.2015.09.010 Reprinted with permission from Elsevier.

not translate into consistent clinical practice. Addressing the staff-identified barriers (see Figure 11.10) led to a dramatic increase in skin-to-skin care encounters in all three NICUs.

Education and knowledge are not enough to ensure the adoption of evidence-based best practices. Process is critical. Engaged and empowered staff were able to share safety concerns regarding skin-to-skin care practices, explore solutions with colleagues and parents, gain consensus and build a safe, consistent, and confident approach to skin-to-skin care in the NICU.

THE QUANTUM LEAP PROJECT

The Quantum Leap program is a 12-month coaching and development program that provides the learner with a strong foundation in trauma research, evidence-based best practices in trauma-informed care, and improvement methodologies. The Quantum Leap project cultivates essential skills for program participants to become courageous, authentic, purpose-driven leaders for change. The goal of these leaders is to establish trauma-informed care as the preeminent paradigm for the care of critically ill infants, their families, and the clinicians who serve them.

The inception of the Quantum Leap program arose out of a curiosity to uncover the missing link between practice improvement and cultural transformation. Teaching clinicians about the science of early-life adversity, introducing them to evidence-based best practices in trauma-informed care, and then coaching and mentoring them to test and

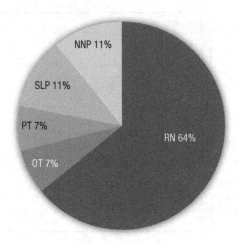

Figure 11.14 Quantum Leap enrollees 2018 through 2020.

NNP, neonatal nurse practitioner; OT, occupational therapist; PT, physical therapist; SLP, speech–language pathologist.

ultimately implement better practices did not guarantee sustainability. If knowledge and process aren't enough to sustain practice improvement, then what is?

It's not so much the "what" that gets results but the "why," specifically, the why of *you*. Why do you do the work you do? The deep, why, not the surface why. The surface why would say "it's a steady paycheck" or "I've just always wanted to be a nurse." The deep why is *THE WHY*? How does the work inspire you? How does it align with your core values? (*Do you even know what your core values are?*) By connecting your work with your sense of purpose and fulfillment you are inspired to go to work, to fully engage with improvement work and professional development, and at the end of the day you feel fulfilled and grateful to be called to this very special work.

"Leaders are the ones who have the courage to go first and open a path for others to follow" (Sinek et al., 2017, p. 32). This is what the Quantum Leap program focuses on, creating courageous authentic leaders. To date the program has enrolled 28 clinicians (Figure 11.14). These clinicians are leading change in their respective units and moving their teams toward a trauma-informed paradigm.

Expectations for Quantum Leap students include active scholarship. Several Quantum Leap students and graduates have presented poster and podium presentations of their Quantum Leap capstone projects at the 2019 and 2020 Science & Soul (S&S) Congresses (Table 11.7). These examples of leadership and scholarship highlight the individual impact that is possible when one takes a leap and believes in a vision greater than themselves. This quantum leap requires curiosity, creativity, and courage.

Curiosity, creativity, and courage are cultivated through a very thoughtful, integrated, evidence-based curriculum grounded in adult-teaching and tribe-learning principles (Table 11.8). The author of this text directs the science track. Mel MacIntyre, a certified High Performance Coach who specializes in Women's Leadership directs the soul track (https://www.melmacintyre.com).

Table 11.7 Congress Presentations by Quantum Leap Students

Format	Presenter	Topic
Podium S&S 2019	Sharon Bonifazi	H.O.P.E.
Podium S&S 2019	Sue Horner et al.	Impact of setting minimum expectations for parent participation on stress in NICU infants and parents
Poster S&S 2019	Isabelle Milette et al.	Guidelines for the institutional implementation of developmental neuroprotective care in the NICU
Poster S&S 2019	Dallyce Varty et al.	Skin-to-skin on jet ventilation: Safely bringing infants and parents together as a trauma-informed best practice
Poster S&S 2019	Beverly Walti	Our journey to improving staff engagement
Podium S&S 2020	Sharon Bonifazi	What's hope got to do with it? The science behind the virtue
Podium S&S 2020	Melinda Chacon	Standing in your courage
Podium S&S 2020	Nicole Bauwens	Quantum caring at NHS Grampian
Poster S&S 2020	Kathleen Ellis	Intimate partner violence and nurses in the neonatal ICU: Navigating safety for infants and their families
Poster S&S 2020	Sue Horner et al.	A descriptive analysis of a NICU nurse-driven IVH prevention initiative

H.O.P.E., Helping Ordinary People Be Extraordinary; IVH, intraventricular hemorrhage.

Table 11.8 The Curriculum for the Science & Soul Tracks

Science Track	Soul Track
• Introduction to the S&S of trauma stewardship • Core measures: Healing environment • Core measures: Pain and stress • Core measures: Protected sleep • Core measures: Activities of daily living • Core measures: Family collaborative care • Quality improvement • Attributes of the trauma-informed professional • Adult teaching principles • Teach back • Becoming leaders for change	• Creating clarity • Developing a vision • Setting goals and priorities • Building a strong foundation • Developing resilience and managing your energy • Getting super productive • Overcoming obstacles • Persuasion and influence • Developing your leadership • Communication and engagement

S&S, science & soul.

Learners unbundle false self-beliefs that have held them back from standing in their true power as leaders, both personally and professionally. One-on-one mentoring and coaching build confidence and competence in leading practice-improvement initiatives. Collaboration with past and present "leapers" creates a sense of solidarity, dissolves feelings of isolation, and produces a wealth of resources to facilitate growth and transformation.

Quantum Leap graduates touch the lives of infants, families, and colleagues shifting perceptions, mindsets and practice toward a trauma-informed paradigm. Built on a solid foundation of science, strategy, and soul, graduates emerge as authentic, courageous leaders continuously evolving and growing. Through role modeling, advocacy, scholarship, and personal wholeness, these knowledgeable leaders take up the call to eradicate the silent suffering of infants and families in the NICU and beyond.

If your actions inspire others to dream more, learn more,
do more and become more, you are a leader.
—John Quincy Adams

Summary

Sustainable practice change begins within; within the individual, within the team, within the unit, organization, and society at large. Becoming trauma-informed is personal. It requires introspection, acceptance, and love, of self and other. Quantum Caring in action makes manifest the true nature and essence of caring.

READER RESOURCE

Trauma-informed Care Self-Assessment: www.surveymonkey.com/r/TransformNursing2

REFERENCES

Coughlin, M. (2011). *Age-appropriate care of the premature and critically ill hospitalized infant: Guideline for practice*. National Association of Neonatal Nurses.

Coughlin, M. (2014). *Transformative nursing in the NICU: Trauma-informed, age-appropriate care*. Springer Publishing Company.

Coughlin, M. (2015). The Sobreviver (Survive) project. *Newborn and Infant Nursing Reviews, 15*(4), 169–173. https://doi.org/10.1053/j.nainr.2015.09.010

Coughlin, M., Gibbins, S., & Hoath, S. (2009). Core measures for developmentally supportive care in neonatal intensive care units: Theory, precedence and practice. *Journal of Advanced Nursing, 65*(10), 2239–2248. https://doi.org/10.1111/j.1365-2648.2009.05052.x

Sinek, S., Mead, D., & Docker, P. (2017). *Find your why: A practical guide for discovering purpose for you and your team*. Portfolio/Penguin.

Vittner, D., Casavant, S., & McGrath, J. M. (2015). A meta-ethnography: Skin-to-skin holding from the caregiver's perspective. *Advances in Neonatal Care, 15*(3), 191–200. https://doi.org/10.1097/ANC.0000000000000169

12

Trauma Stewardship

Trauma stewardship is not simply an idea. It can be defined as a daily practice through which individuals, organizations, and societies tend to the hardship, pain, or trauma experienced by humans, other living beings, or our planet itself.
—Laura van Dernoot Lipsky

EMBRACING OUR STORY

Our life experiences influence our choices, beliefs, thoughts, actions, and health. Providing trauma-informed care (TIC) and mitigating toxic stress is not only for the critically ill infant and family; this paradigm has relevance for every human being, including *you*. We are a product of our experiences. Experiences interact with our biology, impact our developmental trajectory, influence our perceptions and biases, and ultimately model our lifelong health and wellness. It's nature *and* nurture. Understanding our own story, how we became who we are, impacts how we move through life and how we engage with others.

The pervasiveness of early-life adversity leaves very few of us unscathed by adverse childhood experiences (ACEs). Sixty-one percent of Americans report at least one ACE during the first 18 years of life, with 25% reporting three or more ACEs (Table 12.1; Merrick et al., 2018, 2019). Globally, Carlson et al. (2019) report two thirds of youth experience

Table 12.1 Categories of Adverse Childhood Experiences

Abuse	Household Dysfunction	Neglect
• Physical • Emotional • Sexual	• Household member substance use • Household member incarceration • Household member mental illness • Parental divorce • Witnessing intimate partner violence	• Physical • Emotional

Table 12.2 Trauma Exposure Responses

• Feeling helpless and hopeless • A sense that one can never do enough • Hypervigilance • Diminished creativity	• Inability to embrace complexity • Minimizing • Chronic exhaustion/ physical ailments • Inability to listen/deliberate avoidance	• Dissociative moments • Sense of persecution • Guilt • Fear	• Anger and cynicism • Inability to empathize/ numbing • Addictions • Grandiosity: An inflated sense of importance related to one's work

Source: Adapted from Lipsky, L. V. D. (2009). *Trauma stewardship: An everyday guide to caring for self while caring for others.* Berrett-Koehler.

adversity in childhood regardless of where they reside around the world. ACEs are associated with significantly poorer health outcomes, risky health behaviors, and socioeconomic challenges (Crouch et al., 2019; Merrick et al., 2019).

Adversity is not restricted to the young. Many of us experience tragedy, strife, and trauma as adults, personally and professionally. Laura van Dernoot Lipsky, author of *Trauma Stewardship* and the *Age of Overwhelm*, emphasizes the importance of tending to the accumulating pain and suffering that accompanies trauma to avoid becoming saturated by it. Trauma stewardship is the careful and responsible management of the trauma exposures encountered by caring professionals in the course of caring for others. Similar to antibiotic stewardship, trauma stewardship invites us to be consciously aware of the toll bearing witness to trauma has on our day-to-day life. *An undercurrent of trauma runs through ordinary life, shot through as it is with the poignancy of impermanence* (Dr. Mark Epstein from Lipsky, 2018, p. 28). For a deeper dive on Trauma Stewardship, view Ms. Lipsky's Ted Talk; the link is available in the resource section of this chapter

Bearing witness to suffering, whether it be in the NICU or of other living beings or the planet at large, requires "metabolism" of the trauma to mitigate its consequences (Lipsky, 2009). Unmetabolized trauma leads to what Lipsky calls "trauma exposure responses" (Table 12.2). *"When we don't fully metabolize that which may accumulate within us, it tends to linger and fester and then manifest—sometimes horribly; so, we must focus on what we do have power over, even if it's only in our own mind"* (Lipsky, 2018, p. 54).

The process of metabolism has two components: anabolism and catabolism. *Catabolism* is the process of breaking down, reducing something to its most elemental forms, and *anabolism* is the building up for repair and growth. Successful metabolism of trauma supports integration of those elements of the experience that are valuable and the excretion of those elements that are not needed. Metabolizing and processing trauma can reduce our experience of overwhelm.

To overwhelm involves the action of overwhelming; the fact or state of being overwhelmed. Day-to-day life is often experienced as overwhelming. Work, school, family; caretaking for

BOX 12.1 PERSONAL AND PROFESSIONAL PRACTICES TO CULTIVATE PRESENCE

- Loving-kindness and equanimity
- Deep attentive silent listening
- Awakened heart-centered feelings
- Compassionate forgiveness
- Gratitude and deep appreciation
- Giving/receiving
- Stillness,silence
- Open to the power of one, the infinite field of universallove/source
- Manifest/radiate a caring, healing energetic loving field beyond self

Source: Adapted from Watson, D. C. (2018). Self-compassion, the "quiet ego" and materialism. *Heliyon, 4*(10), e00883. doi: 10.1016/j.heliyon.2018.e00883

self or others; engagement in social justice and advocacy; economics, world events, and the climate crisis all induce a feeling of being overwhelmed (Lipsky, 2018). Being overwhelmed erodes our capacity for empathy and compassion. As our society make an effort to metabolize the systematic oppression borne for decades by people of color amid a global pandemic, we see the caustic nature of the effects of being overwhelmed and traumatized when it is not addressed or metabolized in a timely manner. History repeats itself until the hurt has been healed, until the trauma has been resolved for the planet, society, and the individual.

Embracing one's story is to recognize our unity with humanity, nature, and all that is. Embracing one's story is an invitation to align with the authentic self. Embracing one's story takes courage, confidence, and clarity. It's not enough to survive our life, we must flourish; and to flourish we must forgive self and others. Forgiveness releases us from the shadows of our past, be they personal, generational, or societal, and enables us to step into the light of our presence.

Jean Watson refers to *presence* as an elusive and spirit-filled concept and practice; it cannot be known from the outside in but only from the inside out (J. Watson, 2018, pp. 89–90). Cultivating presence is a journey and a sacred act (Box 12.1). *From this place of presence, it is possible to aspire to do no harm, to transform whatever trauma arises, and to continue to work to dismantle systems of oppression* (Figure 12.1; Lipsky, 2009).

The pervasive nature of trauma in our lives and the world highlights the crucial importance of TIC. Understanding that maladaptive behaviors or ways of walking through the world often have their roots in traumatic experiences opens the door for compassion, empathy, and respect, for our patients, their families, each other, and ourselves (Kimberg & Wheeler, 2019). TIC holds the promise for improved health outcomes for individuals, societies, and the planet as an evidence-based vehicle to disrupt the cycle of systematic oppression and destruction in our world.

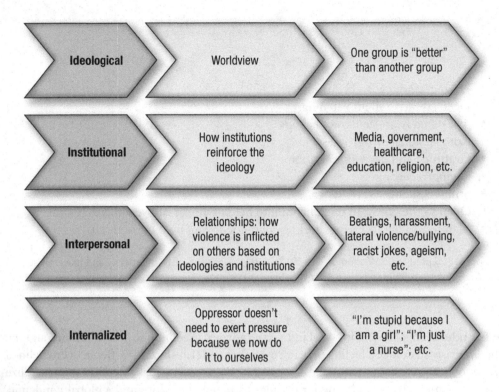

Figure 12.1 Systems of oppression.

SELF-COMPASSION AND CARE

When you begin to touch your heart or let your heart be touched, you begin to discover that it's bottomless, that it doesn't have any resolution, that this heart is huge, vast, and limitless.
—Pema Chodron

You cannot give what you do not have. You cannot give care, compassion, and love to another if you do not give it to yourself. Self-compassion is compassion for self. Where compassion is the awareness of suffering of another and a desire to alleviate it, self-compassion is a desire to alleviate the suffering of one's own self (Zessin et al., 2015). Self-compassion is comprised of three interacting components: self-kindness versus self-judgment; a sense of common humanity versus isolation; and mindfulness versus over-identification (Table 12.3; Germer & Neff, 2013; Lopez et al., 2018; Neff, 2003). Kindness is compassion in action, for others and self. Self-kindness is the degree to which one is understanding or critical toward self (Table 12.4).

Although compassion for others has not been shown to significantly influence psychological well-being, individuals who practice self-compassion report lower levels of depressive symptoms and a higher positive affect (Lopez et al., 2018). In a meta-analysis

Table 12.3 Elements of Self-Compassion and Examples

Self-kindness versus self-judgment	Being kind and understanding toward oneself rather than being self-critical, self-condemning, blaming and ruminating
Common humanity versus isolation	Seeing one's failures as part of the larger human condition rather than an isolated personal experience
Mindfulness versus over-identification	Holding one's negative thoughts and feelings in mindful awareness rather than overidentifying with them or avoiding them

Source: Adapted from Sinclair, S., Kondejewski, J., Raffin-Bouchal, S., King-Shier, K. M., & Singh, P. (2017). Can self-compassion promote healthcare provider well-being and compassionate care to others? Results of a systematic review. *Applied Psychology: Health and Well-Being*, *9*(2), 168–206. doi: 10.1111/aphw.12086

Table 12.4 Discovering Self-Compassion

How do you typically react to yourself?	• What types of things do you typically judge and criticize yourself for? (appearance, career, relationships, parenting, etc.) • What type of language do you use with yourself when you notice a flaw or make a mistake? (Do you insult yourself or encourage yourself?) • How does it make you feel when you are critical of yourself? • When you are hard on yourself, does it motivate you or do you feel discouraged? • What would it feel like if you could truly accept yourself? Is that a possibility for you?
How do you typically react to life's difficulties?	• How do you treat yourself when you encounter a challenge? Do you push through despite your pain or do you give yourself comfort and care? • Do you tend to get carried away with the drama of a difficult situation and make a bigger deal out of it or do you stay balanced? • Do you tend to feel cut off by others when things go wrong, believing that everyone else has it easier than you or do you try and remember everyone experiences hardships in their life?

Source: Adapted from Neff, K. (2011). *Self-compassion: The proven power of being kind to yourself.* HarperCollins.

examining the relationship between self-compassion and well-being, a strong correlation between the two is reported, especially with regard to psychological and cognitive well-being and reduced negative affect (Zessin et al., 2015). Benzo et al. (2017) examined the influence of self-compassion on happiness in healthcare workers. The findings indicate a significant and independent association between self-compassion and perceived happiness of healthcare workers.

Self-compassion is not the same as self-esteem. Self-esteem arises from the evaluation of self-worth based on judgments and comparisons to others. A focus on self-esteem can

BOX 12.2 QUALITIES OF THE QUIET EGO

- Forgiveness
- Gratitude
- Humility
- Generativity
- Altruism
- Interdependence
- Self-compassion
- Compassionate love

Source: Adapted from Wayment, H. A., Bauer, J. J., & Sylaska, K. (2015). The quiet ego scale: Measuring the compassionate self-identity. *Journal of Happiness Studies, 16,* 999–1033. https://doi.org/10.1007/s10902-014-9546-z

become a Pandora's box and lead to materialism or a focus on acquiring possessions or rankings as a path to happiness. *Materialism,* also referred to as the *noisy ego,* is an escape from self in search of higher aspirations that will confer worthiness on the individual (D. C. Watson, 2018).

For sure, goals and aspirations are important parts of life, but they don't bring lasting happiness. Happiness is not dictated by the ego, but by transcending the ego. Contrary to the noisy ego, the "quiet ego" reflects a self-identity neither excessively self-focused nor excessively other-focused. Instead, it is a balance between a strong sense of agency and a strong concern for the welfare of others (Box 12.2; D. C. Watson, 2018; Wayment et al., 2015). Other resources for discovering the quiet ego are available at the end of the chapter.

> I sometimes romanticized the idea of a nurse in my head, and that has occasionally led me to neglect myself in order to put others first. I was ignoring everything I was feeling; I was not giving myself permission to have human tendencies. I kept trying to convince myself that I shouldn't feel the way I do because I know that plenty of people have it worse than I do. I was feeling something parallel to "survivor's guilt," because I still had a job while others didn't. Compassion and caring [are] two-way street[s]; I (we) extend it so easily to my (our) patients and our community but easily forget to do the same for myself (ourselves). I thought that because I was a nurse, I should be able to "nurse" myself and my mental space. As a nurse, I felt like I should know what to do and how to manage stress. (Lazaro, 2020)

As Lazaro (2020) suggests, compassion and care are two-way streets. We cannot give what we do not receive from ourselves. Although we take this at face value, Sinclair et al. (2017) completed a systematic review of the literature and struggled to identify a correlation between self-compassion and compassionate care to others. Consequently Mills et al. (2018) undertook a cross-sectional survey to examine the relationship between self-care

BOX 12.3 SELF-COMPASSION BREAK

Select a place with minimum distractions where you can practice the compassion break. Approximate length of time needed for activity is 10 minutes.

1. Close your eyes. Take a few deep breaths and relax.
2. Think of a person, situation, or event that is causing you stress right now.
3. Explore your thoughts around this stress and try to gauge how bad the person or the situation makes you feel.
4. Take a deep breath and say to yourself: "This is stress." Let yourself acknowledge your pain at this stage.
5. Try to recognize your pain and understand that you are not the only one facing it. Repeat to yourself: "I am not alone in this." "Suffering is a part of human existence." "Everyone has to struggle at some point in their lives," and so forth.
6. Put your hands on your heart and feel the warmth of your skin touching your body. Allow yourself to explore all the love and kindness you have within and whisper positive self-statements: "I can make peace with myself." "I can overcome this." "May I be patient and strong," and so forth.
7. Open your eyes and release yourself with a long deep breath.

Source: Adapted from Neff, K., & Germer, C. (2018). *The mindful self-compassion workbook.* Guilford Press.

ability, self-compassion, and compassion among palliative care nurses and doctors in Australia. As self-care ability increased, self-compassion also increased and as compassion for others increased self-compassion decreased (Mills et al., 2018).

Burridge et al. (2017) call for compassion literacy to be an integral component to nursing education and practice. Although compassion is an expectation for healthcare workers, self-compassion is often stigmatized as being self-indulgent and selfish (Mills et al., 2015). Compassion literacy embraces self-compassion and compassion for others, protects against compassion fatigue, and enables the consistently reliable provision of compassionate care (Burridge et al., 2017).

Suffering, failure, and feelings of inadequacy are part of the human experience. All people—the tiny babies in the NICU, their families, our colleagues, the checkout person at the supermarket, the bus driver, the hospital chief executive officer, and you—are worthy of compassion. Self-compassion is an invitation to be present to yourself. Try a simple mindfulness-based compassion exercise developed by Dr. Kristin Neff, called the self-compassion break (Box 12.3). Additional resources on self-compassion are available in the resource section of this chapter.

A RETURN TO PASSION AND PURPOSE

The best day of your life is the one on which you decide your life is your own. No apologies or excuses. No one to lean on, rely on, or blame. The gift is yours—it is an amazing journey—and you alone are responsible for the quality of it. This is the day your life really begins.
—Bob Moawad

People with a purpose in life experience better health outcomes, are better at overcoming stress, have increased happiness and greater longevity (Schippers & Ziegler, 2019). The health benefits of having a purpose in life are thought to be secondary to focused attention and engagement in healthier behaviors (Kang et al., 2019). Self-endorsed goals enhance well-being while pursuing goals directed or dictated by external factors will leave an individual wanting (Schippers & Ziegler, 2019).

Eudaemonia, a sense of meaning or purpose in life, is intimately linked to happiness and is a core criterion of the United Nation's World Happiness Report. Purpose in life has consequences for happiness and performance at the individual and societal levels. "I alone cannot change the world, but I can cast a stone across the waters to create many ripples" (Mother Theresa).

Purpose is fueled by passion. Passion is more than something you like to do. Choosing to do something important and meaningful, that's what ignites passion. Passion that aligns with one's values fuels more passion. However, one's passion must be balanced.

Obsessive passion leads to more conflict with other areas of one's life and is often linked to perceptions of low self-worth (Schippers & Ziegler, 2019). Obsessive passion is when the "work" takes over your life—you may enjoy the work, but it has now consumed you. Obsessive passion doesn't make room for self-compassion or self-care. Harmonious passion is a balanced passion and results in enhanced performance and positive outcomes (Schippers & Ziegler, 2019).

Engagement, passion, and meaning of work reduce burnout in nurses (Gomez-Salgado et al., 2019). Using a positive psychology approach, these three constructs reflect occupational health in nursing (Figure 12.2). Engagement comes from a sense of job performance satisfaction, confidence in one's ability to do the work without fear of reprisals of negative consequences, and the availability of physical resources to fully engage in the work (Gomez-Salgado et al., 2019; Keyko et al., 2016). Keyko et al. (2016) identified 77 factors that influence nurse engagement. These factors are categorized into six themes represented in Box 12.4.

Passion is linked with motivation and can be promoted. Passion is often associated with *grit*, which is defined as a perseverance and passion for long-term impact. Grit is associated with an increased sense of personal accomplishment and a decrease in burnout (Seguin, 2019). Successful nurses are passionate about their work and this passion often translates into more stable and effective relationships with peers and a reduced staff turnover (Gomez-Salgado et al., 2019). Check out Angela Lee Duckworth's Ted Talk on Grit; the link is in the resource section of this chapter.

Meaning of work describes the value, relevance, and presence that work has in one's life. Meaning of work embraces the joy one experiences in service to others. Lee (2015)

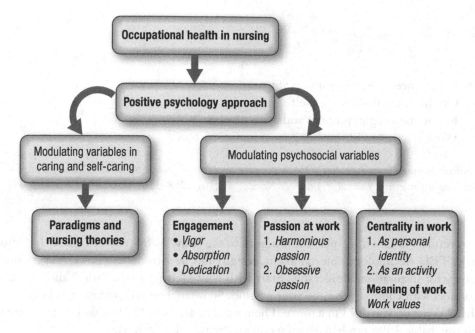

Figure 12.2 Concepts flowchart.

Source: Gomez-Salgado, J., Navarro-Abal, Y., Lopez-Lopez, M. J., Romero-Martin, M., & Climent-Rodriguez, J. A. (2019). Engagement, passion and meaning in work as modulating variables in nursing: A theoretical analysis. *International Journal of Environmental Research and Public Health, 16*(1), 108. doi: 10.3390/ijerph16010108 Reprinted with permission under the Creative Commons License.

BOX 12.4 SIX THEMES ASSOCIATED WITH NURSE ENGAGEMENT

- Organizational climate
- Job resources
- Professional resources
- Personal resources
- Job demands
- Demographic variables

Source: Adapted from Keyko, K., Cummings, G. C., Yonge, O., & Wong, C. A. (2016). Work engagement in professional nursing practice: A systematic review. *International Journal of Nursing Studies, 61*, 142–164. doi: 10.1016/j.ijnurstu.2016.06.003

---

undertook a concept analysis of *meaning in work* and identified four critical attributes of this concept (Box 12.5). We find meaning in what we give to the world, in our relationships with others, and how we engage with suffering (Malloy et al., 2015). Courage and dignity in the face of adversity, difficult situations, and even death brings meaning to the work of nurses.

BOX 12.5 CRITICAL ATTRIBUTES OF THE CONCEPT
MEANING IN WORK

- Experienced positive emotion at work
- Got meaning from work itself
- Found meaningful purpose and goals of work
- Work is a part of life enabling meaningful existence

Source: Adapted from Lee, S. (2015). A concept analysis of "meaning in work" and its implications for nursing. *Journal of Advanced Nursing, 71*(10), 2258–2267. doi: 10.1111/jan.12695

A return to passion and purpose brings us to the "why." Why are you a nurse? In Simon
Sinek's TED (technology, entertainment, design) Talk he introduces a powerful yet simple
strategy for inspirational leadership. Start with why. Getting to the "why" allows you to
reconnect with your purpose and your passion. So often, however, many of us begin with
"what." What do you do? I'm a nurse. Then, we may ask "how"? How do you take care of
such tiny babies? But rarely does someone ask "why." The deep why.

Why?

Why are you a neonatal nurse? Why do you care for infants and families in crisis? Why
does this service mean so much to you? Why do you tolerate the long shifts, the rotating
weekends, the short staffing, and all the other challenges you face day to day?

Write your "why" down, commit it to memory, wrap a blessing and gratitude around
it. It is a special soul who can bear witness to such tragedy as is experienced in the NICU.
Your "why" keeps you grounded to your purpose; it fuels your passion. Your "why" becomes
your beacon that carries you through the difficult times. Your "why" gives you courage,
confidence, and clarity to do the right thing not just sometimes but every time!

Remember YOU MAKE A DIFFERENCE. YOU touch lives and impact lifetimes.

Step into your power as a nurse, a healer, an advocate, and a leader. What will your
legacy be?

> *Plain and simple, passion is a commitment without condition. It requires*
> *intensity for caring about something without regard to difficulty.*
> —Laura van Dernoot Lipsky

READER RESOURCES

To discover your "quiet ego" visit this link: quiet-ego.bleeker.co/ to answer 14 questions and gain
a general awareness of your relationship with the four attributes of the quiet ego: (a) detached
awareness, (b) inclusive identity, (c) perspective taking, and (d) growth.

Angela Lee Duckworth—Grit: The power of passion and perseverance: www.ted.com/talks/angela_lee_duckworth_grit_the_power_of_passion_and_perseverance?language=en#t-180899

Beyond the cliff, TED Talk with Laura van Dernoot Lipsky: www.youtube.com/watch?v=uOzDGrcvmus

Boundaries with Brené Brown: www.youtube.com/watch?v=5U3VcgUzqiI

15 most interesting self-compassion research findings: positivepsychology.com/self-compassion-research/

How great leaders inspire action, TED Talk with Simon Sinek: www.ted.com/talks/simon_sinek_how_great_leaders_inspire_action?language=en

The power of self-compassion: www.youtube.com/watch?v=BTQP7XzDxjI

What trauma taught me about resilience, TED Talk with Charles Hunt: www.youtube.com/watch?v=3qELiw_1Ddg

REFERENCES

Benzo, R. P., Kirsch, J. L., & Nelson, C. (2017). Compassion, mindfulness and the happiness of health care workers. *Explore, 13*(3), 201–206. https://doi.org/10.1016/j.explore.2017.02.001

Burridge, L. H., Winch, S., Kay, M., & Henderson, A. (2017). Building compassion literacy: Enabling care in primary health nursing. *Collegian, 24*(1), 85–91. https://doi.org/10.1016/j.colegn.2015.09.004

Carlson, J. S., Yohannan, J., Darr, C. L., Turley, M. R., Larez, N. A., & Perfect, M. M. (2019). Prevalence of adverse childhood experiences in school-aged youth: A systematic review (1990–2015). *International Journal of School & Educational Psychology.* https://doi.org/10.1080/21683603.2018.1548397

Crouch, E., Probst, J. C., Radcliff, E., Bennett, K. J., & Hunt McKinney, S. (2019). Prevalence of adverse childhood experiences (ACEs) among US children. *Child Abuse and Neglect, 92,* 209–218. https://doi.org/10.1016/j.chiabu.2019.04.010

Germer, C. K., & Neff, K. D. (2013). Self-compassion in clinical practice. *Journal of Clinical Psychology: In Session, 69*(8), 856–867. https://doi.org/10.1002/jclp.22021

Gomez-Salgado, J., Navarro-Abal, Y., Lopez-Lopez, M. J., Romero-Martin, M., & Climent-Rodriguez, J. A. (2019). Engagement, passion and meaning in work as modulating variables in nursing: A theoretical analysis. *International Journal of Environmental Research and Public Health, 16*(1), 108. https://doi.org/10.3390/ijerph16010108

Kang, Y., Strecher, V. J., Kim, E., & Falk, E. B. (2019). Purpose in life and conflict-related neural responses during health decision-making. *Health Psychology, 38*(6), 545–552. https://doi.org/10.1037/hea0000729

Keyko, K., Cummings, G. C., Yonge, O., & Wong, C. A. (2016). Work engagement in professional nursing practice: A systematic review. *International Journal of Nursing Studies, 61,* 142–164. https://doi.org/10.1016/j.ijnurstu.2016.06.003

Kimberg, L., & Wheeler, M. (2019). Trauma and trauma-informed care. In M. R. Gerber (Ed.), *Trauma-informed healthcare approaches* (pp. 25–56). Springer Nature Switzerland AG.

Lazaro, R. (2020, June 12). *Caring for the caregiver: My story and lessons learned.* Reflections on Nursing Leadership. https://www.reflectionsonnursingleadership.org/features/more-features/caring-for-the-caregiver-my-story-and-lessons-learned?utm_source=4.16.20&utm_medium=email&utm_term=&utm_content=Read%20more&utm_campaign=RNL-digest

Lee, S. (2015). A concept analysis of "meaning in work" and its implications for nursing. *Journal of Advanced Nursing, 71*(10), 2258–2267. https://doi.org/10.1111/jan.12695

Lipsky, L. V. D. (2009). *Trauma stewardship: An everyday guide to caring for self while caring for others.* Berrett-Koehler Publishers Company.

Lipsky, L. V. D. (2018). *The age of overwhelm: Strategies for the long haul.* Berrett-Koehler.

Lopez, A., Sanderman, R., Ranchor, A. V., & Schroevers, M. J. (2018). Compassion for others and self-compassion: Levels, correlates, and relationship with psychological well-being. *Mindfulness, 9*(1), 325–331. https://doi.org/10.1007/s12671-017-0777-z

Malloy, D. C., Fahey-McCarthy, E., Murakami, M., Lee, Y., Choi, E., Hirose, E., & Hadjistavropoulos, T. (2015). Finding meaning in the work of nursing: An international study. *The Online Journal of Issues in Nursing, 20*(3). https://doi.org/10.3912/OJIN.Vol20No03PPT02

Merrick, M. T., Ford, D. C., Ports, K. A., & Guinn, A. S. (2018). Prevalence of adverse childhood experiences from 2011–2014 behavioral risk factor surveillance system in 23 states. *JAMA Pediatrics, 172*(11), 1038–1044. https://doi.org/10.1001/jamapediatrics.2018.2537

Merrick, M. T., Ford, D. C., Ports, K. A., Guinn, A. S., Chen, J., Klevens, J., Metzler, M., Jones, C. M., Simon, T. R., Daniel, V. M., Ottley, P., & Mercy, J. A. (2019). *Vital signs:* Estimated proportion of adult health problems attributable to adverse childhood experiences and implications for prevention—25 states, 2015–2017. *Morbidity and Mortality Weekly Report, 68*(44), 999–1005. https://doi.org/10.15585/mmwr.mm6844e1

Mills, J., Wand, T., & Fraser, J. (2018). Examining self-care, self-compassion and compassion for others: A cross-sectional survey of palliative care nurses and doctors. *International Journal of Palliative Nursing, 24*(1), 4–11. https://doi.org/10.12968/ijpn.2018.24.1.4

Mills, J., Wand, T., & Fraser, J. A. (2015). On self-compassion and self-care in nursing: Selfish or essentials for compassionate care? *International Journal of Nursing Studies, 52*(4), 791–793.

Neff, K. (2003). Self-compassion: An alternative conceptualization of a healthy attitude toward oneself. *Self & Identity, 2,* 85–101. https://doi.org/10.1080/15298860309032

Schippers, M. C., & Ziegler, N. (2019). Life crafting as a way to find purpose and meaning in life. *Frontiers in Psychology, 10,* 2778. https://doi.org/10.3389/fpsyg.2019.02778

Seguin, C. (2019). A survey of nurse leaders to explore the relationship between grit and measures of success and well-being. *Journal of Nursing Administration, 49*(3), 125–131. https://doi.org/10.1097/NNA.0000000000000725

Sinclair, S., Kondejewski, J., Raffin-Bouchal, S., King-Shier, K. M., & Singh, P. (2017). Can self-compassion promote healthcare provider well-being and compassionate care to others? Results of a systematic review. *Applied Psychology: Health and Well-Being, 9*(2), 168–206. https://doi.org/10.1111/aphw.12086

Watson, D. C. (2018). Self-compassion, the "quiet ego" and materialism. *Heliyon, 4*(10), e00883. https://doi.org/10.1016/j.heliyon.2018.e00883

Watson, J. (2018). *Unitary caring science: The philosophy and praxis of nursing.* University Press of Colorado.

Wayment, H. A., Bauer, J. J., & Sylaska, K. (2015). The quiet ego scale: Measuring the compassionate self-identity. *Journal of Happiness Studies, 16,* 999–1033. https://doi.org/10.1007/s10902-014-9546-z

Zessin, U., Dickhauser, O., & Garbade, S. (2015). The relationship between self-compassion and well-being: A meta-analysis. *Applied Psychology: Health and Well-Being, 7*(3), 340–364. https://doi.org/10.1111/aphw.12051

13

Attributes of the Trauma-Informed Professional

Trauma, by definition, is unbearable and intolerable ... Nobody wants to remember trauma ... We all want to live in a world that is safe, manageable, and predictable, and victims remind us that this is not always the case.
—Van der Kolk (2015)

BECOMING TRAUMA INFORMED

Becoming trauma informed must be a self-endorsed goal (refer to Chapter 12). Self-endorsed goals arise out of a calling, a sense of deep purpose, a desire to make a difference in the world. When one chooses to do that which is worth doing, one creates congruence with one's deeply held values and true self. From this place of alignment springs purpose and feelings of fulfillment.

To become trauma informed one must:

1. Realize the pervasiveness of trauma in everyday life.
2. Recognize the signs and symptoms of trauma in patients, families, colleagues, and self.
3. Respond to trauma by integrating knowledge and evidence-based best practices that mitigate and prevent trauma into policies, procedures, and annual performance appraisals.
4. Resist retraumatization by ensuring consistency in service delivery.

The infinitive "to become" has an aspirational connotation; it indicates an understanding that to become trauma informed isn't a destination. Becoming trauma informed is a continuous journey of self-discovery and growth that moves one toward excellence. Each moment is an invitation to become more trauma informed, more openhearted, more knowledgeable, more courageous than the moment before. "Becoming" represents

EXHIBIT 13.1 MATRIX OF MASTERY

Attributes	Levels				
	Level 1—Core	Level 2—Advanced	Level 3—Organizational focus	Level 4—Community/regional Focus	Level 5—National/global focus
Knowledgeable					
Healing intention	Each level has specific competencies the applicant must submit proof of in order to advance a level at each recertification cycle.				
Personal wholeness					
Courage					
Advocacy					
Role model/mentor					
Scholar					
Leader for change					

Source: Reprinted with permission from Caring Essentials Collaborative, LLC.

an ongoing transformation and evolution both personally and professionally. Becoming trauma informed is indeed the road less traveled.

Pursuing certification as a trauma-informed professional (TIP) is the starting point for this journey. To become a certified TIP requires more than a box tick. It's not about simply passing a test and then maintaining some level of ongoing professional education. Pursuing certification as a TIP is about walking the talk. It's making your knowledge of the science and soul of trauma-informed care (TIC) live and breathe every day, with every encounter (refer to Chapters 4 and 5).

Becoming a TIP demands action, both internally and externally. Expectations for recertification include participation and completion in quality-improvement initiatives aimed at integrating a trauma-informed approach into the clinical setting and beyond. Prospective certificants submit exemplars reflecting their insights and competence across the eight attributes of the TIP; letters of recommendation corroborate these exemplars. TIPs continually grow and develop across the matrix of mastery to become global leaders for transformation, creating a kinder, more compassionate, and loving world (Exhibit 13.1).

Clarity of vision and dogged determination are necessary to realize a trauma-free world. This journey is not for the faint of heart or the alphabet soup gang (the folks that love to collect credentials to place on their signature line). When the going gets tough, the "why" behind becoming trauma informed is a core motivator (Ntoumanis et al., 2014).

WHY FOCUS ON MENTAL HEALTH?

Chapters 2 and 3 present the consequences associated with early-life adversity and the value proposition of a trauma-informed approach to care. As you read through Chapters 4 and 5 you were introduced to the science and soul underpinning the relevance of a trauma-informed paradigm. This knowledge base creates the fundamental building blocks for a TIP. Creating a tribe of TIPs is required to eradicate the many modes of trauma endured by vulnerable populations around the world.

Mitigating the trauma experience for hospitalized infants and their families goes beyond the day-to-day hospital care. The impact of a trauma-informed approach changes the developmental trajectory of the infant and the family, touching lives, impacting lifetimes. The birth of a baby and becoming a family is a defining moment in one's life. How clinicians show up to these special moments defines the clinician and the healthcare organization—a single encounter can change a life forever.

In the fast-paced world of neonatal intensive care, with everyone focused on "saving lives," the thought of weaving mental health into the existing paradigm may seem ludicrous. However noble and exhilarating it is to save lives, nurses cannot lose sight of their core mission, their core purpose. Nurses protect, promote, and optimize health, prevent illness and injury, facilitate healing, and alleviate suffering (American Nurses Association, 2015a). The suffering we alleviate goes beyond the physical; it is the emotional, psychological, and spiritual suffering humans experience in crisis that must be alleviated. Mental health encompasses emotional, psychological, social, and spiritual well-being. Mental health is the foundation for overall health and well-being (McLoughlin, 2017a, 2017b).

The American Psychiatric Nurses Association (APNA) issued a position statement in March 2017 titled: "Whole Health Begins with Mental Health." The organization posits that *mental health promotion, through prevention, recognition and adequate care and treatment must be the starting point comprehensively woven throughout the delivery of services ... [and] our definition of health must be transformed to recognize mental health as a foundation for all health*. Supporting points to endorse the APNA's position statement are listed in Box 13.1; access to the position statement is available in the resource section of this chapter.

Zarse et al. (2019) published a comprehensive literature review of two decades of research using the Adverse Childhood ExperienceQuestionnaire. The results highlight the dose-dependent, causal relationship between ACEs and mental illness, addictions, adult noncommunicable diseases, disrupted parenting, and insecure child rearing (Zarse et al., 2019). The perturbations in family integrity leave a transgenerational footprint of the burden of disease associated with early-life adversity (Figure 13.1; Zarse et al., 2019).

BOX 13.1 EVIDENCE BASE IN SUPPORT OF AMERICAN PSYCHIATRIC NURSES ASSOCIATION POSITION STATEMENT

- Health is a state of physical, mental, and social well-being and not merely the absence of disease.
- There is a broad consensus among health care experts that it is necessary to transform healthcare systems to be proactive and to promote health and wellness [*salutogenic—refer to Chapter 6*] rather than reactively treating illness.
- Mental illnesses are risk factors that affect the incidence and prognosis of NCDs; addressing mental illnesses delays progression, improves survival outcomes, and reduces healthcare costs associated with NCDs.
- Research demonstrates a strong link between ACEs and long-term negative health and well-being.

ACE, adverse childhood experience; NCD, noncommunicable diseases.
Source: Adapted from American Psychiatric Nurses Association. (2017). *Whole health begins with mental health* [position statement]. https://www.apna.org/files/public/Whole-Health-Begins-With-Mental-Health-Position-Paper.pdf

More than 1 billion individuals globally were affected by mental illness and addictive disorders in 2016 (Rehm & Shield, 2019). Depression and anxiety disorders cost the global economy $1 trillion in lost productivity each year, with depression identified as the leading cause of disability worldwide (National Alliance on Mental Illness, 2019). Recent data and statistics from the U.S. Centers for Disease Control and Prevention reveal that one in six children aged 2 to 8 years is diagnosed with a mental, behavioral, or developmental disorder (Figure 13.2; Centers for Disease Control and Prevention, 2020). A comprehensive meta-analysis of six preterm-born adult cohorts from five countries reveals a heightened risk for internalizing problems (depression, sadness, anxiety and fear) and socially avoidant personality traits in this highly susceptible population (Pyhala et al., 2017).

Controlling for fetal growth, Apgar score, maternal characteristics and sociodemographic status, infants born between 32 and 36 weeks' gestation are 60% more likely to have nonaffective psychosis, 34% more likely to have depression, and more than twice as likely to have bipolar disorder than their term counterparts (Nosarti et al., 2012). Individuals born at less than 32 weeks' gestation doubled their risk of nonaffective psychosis, tripled their risk of depression, and had a more than 7 times higher risk of bipolar affective disorder (Nosarti et al., 2012). In addition to a three- to fourfold increased risk of psychiatric disorders, NICU survivors are also at an increased risk for attention deficit hyperactivity disorder and autism spectrum disorder (Ream & Lehwald, 2018). The prevalence of autism in the general populations is 1.5%;, however, for infants born between 23 and 27 weeks, the prevalence is 7.1% (Ream & Lehwald, 2018).

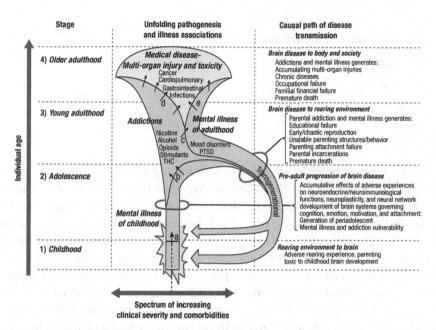

Figure 13.1 Neuroscience-informed causal pathway to adverse childhood experiences comorbidities.

Source: Zarse, E. M., Neff, M. R., Yoder, R., Hulvershorn, L., Chambers, J. E., & Chambers, R. A. (2019). The adverse childhood experiences questionnaire: Two decades of research on childhood trauma as a primary cause of adult mental illness, addiction, and medical diseases. *Cogent Medicine, 6*, 1581447. Reprinted with permission under the Creative Commons Attribution (CC-BY) 4.0 license.

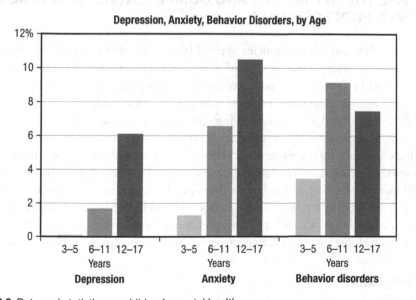

Figure 13.2 Data and statistics on children's mental health.

Source: Centers for Disease Control and Prevention. (2020). *Data and statistics on children's mental health.* https://www.cdc.gov/childrens-mentalhealth/data.html

Table 13.1 **Attributes of the Trauma-Informed Professional**

Knowledgeable	Role model/mentor
Healing intention	Advocacy
Personal wholeness	Scholarship
Courage	Leader for change

The body keeps score with early-life adversity leaving molecular scars (refer to Chapter 5; Lucero, 2018; Van der Kolk, 2015). Brains shaped by toxic stress are wired to survive, not thrive. Complex trauma describes the developmental ripple effect of early-life adversity across the infant's attachment, biology, affect, psychology, behavior control, cognition, and sense of self (Lucero, 2018). *"Social support is a biological necessity, not an option, and this reality should be the backbone of all prevention and treatment"* (Van der Kolk, 2015, p. 169).

Showing up with patience, compassion, presence, and a healing intention is the antidote to complex trauma and toxic stress for the infant, family, and the professional. Environments characterized by safe, stable,and nurturing relationships foster resiliency. We are being called to transform the NICU culture from a focus on pathology and technology to a focus on ecology and healing. The attributes of the TIP translate into core competencies and performance expectations that humanize the healthcare experience in the NICU and beyond.

WHAT ARE THE ATTRIBUTES AND COMPETENCIES OF A TRAUMA-INFORMED PROFESSIONAL?

The eight attributes and competencies of the TIP were identified in collaboration with an international and interdisciplinary board of neonatal clinicians and academicians (Table 13.1). The board co-created a unique process to certify professionals as trauma informed that not only assesses core knowledge regarding TIC, but also challenges the applicant to exemplify how knowledge is translated into practice across the eight attributes of a TIP. These attributes then become competencies that guide the growth and developmental trajectory of the certificant on their journey to becoming a global leader in the TIC movement.

An *attribute* is a quality or characteristic that can be learned over time. A *competency* is a combination of a skill and behavior that is easily identified and can be measured or validated. Each attribute represents a quality and a skill the board deemed critical to a leader for TIC and that's the point of the assessment-based certificate program, to qualify leaders for this global movement. Each attribute is described in the following paragraphs.

Knowledgeable

Core knowledge regarding the science and soul underpinning early-life adversity and the biologic and existential sequelae associated with it is primal. Relevant research crosses all

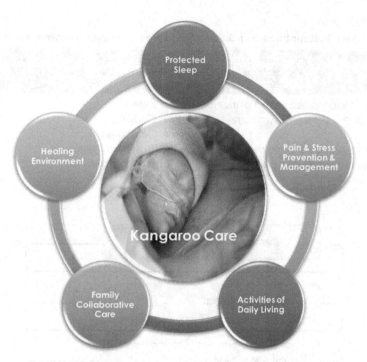

Figure 13.3 Core measures for trauma-informed care.

Source: Reprinted with permission from Caring Essentials Collaborative, LLC.

scientific realms from molecular biology to psychology; from genetics to metaphysics. Unitary caring science is a critical cornerstone of TIC. This cornerstone brings about an awakening of humans and science to an evolved worldview, a cosmology of one humanity, one heart, one world, one planet Earth (Watson, 2018, p. xix).

Knowledge of the latest evidence specific to each core measure (Figure 13.3) is fundamental for the TIP (refer to Chapters 6–10). The TIP must also be familiar with the key assumptions of TIC and its five guiding principles (Table 13.2). Knowledge and skill in articulating what TIC looks like in clinical practice through exemplars across each of the eight attributes are part of the credentialing process. For example, what does knowledge in TIC look like in practice? The answer: Examples of providing two-person care during a heel stick and observing the infant's response, guiding a colleague in facilitating a skin-to-skin care encounter with an intubated infant, supporting the first oral feeding encounter at the breast,. As the certificant advances through the matrix of mastery, knowledge requirements will progress to more complex concepts. This progression is part of the journey to becoming a global leader in TIC.

Healing Intention

Healing means to become whole, involves an integrated wholeness of body, mind, and spirit. Healing is about transcendence, a movement toward wholeness and well-being over time

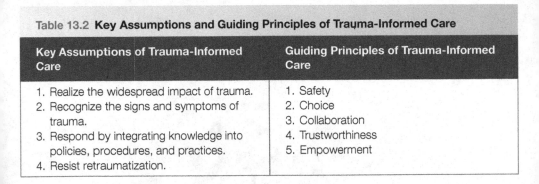

Table 13.2 Key Assumptions and Guiding Principles of Trauma-Informed Care

Key Assumptions of Trauma-Informed Care	Guiding Principles of Trauma-Informed Care
1. Realize the widespread impact of trauma. 2. Recognize the signs and symptoms of trauma. 3. Respond by integrating knowledge into policies, procedures, and practices. 4. Resist retraumatization.	1. Safety 2. Choice 3. Collaboration 4. Trustworthiness 5. Empowerment

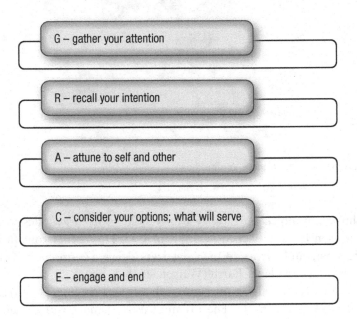

G – gather your attention

R – recall your intention

A – attune to self and other

C – consider your options; what will serve

E – engage and end

Figure 13.4 GRACE: acronym for cultivating compassion.

Source: Adapted from Halifax, J. (2014). G.R.A.C.E. for nurses: Cultivating compassion in nurse/patient interactions. *Journal of Nursing Education and Practice, 4*(1), 121–128. https://doi.org/10.5430/jnep.v4n1p121

(Zahourek, 2012). *Intention* is distinct and purposeful, defined as the action of directing one's mind or attention to something. Healing intention requires presence and conscious alignment with the divine essence of self in order to create a sense of oneness or wholeness with others during the caring moment (Sofhauser, 2016; Zahourek, 2019)

Healing intention in practice may include practicing GRACE. before a caring encounter (Figure 13.4; Halifax, 2014). One may set an intention for healing at the beginning of one's shift, either as an individual or as a team. This may be a silent prayer or moment before laying hands on the patient. Practicing healing intention includes a reflective component. What did you notice about yourself and others during the caring interaction when you took

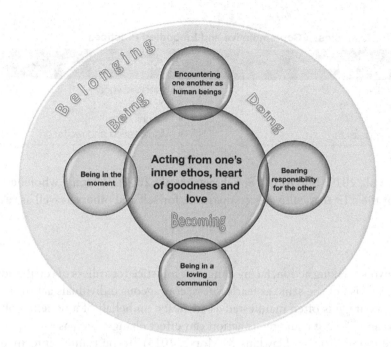

Figure 13.5 Mediating compassion from becoming to belonging.

Source: Hemberg, J., & Wiklund Gustin, L. (2020). Caring from the heart as belonging—The basis for mediating compassion. *Nursing Open, 7,* 660– 668. https://doi.org/10.1002/nop2.438 Reprinted with permission from John Wiley and Sons.

the time to be present with your healing intention? Keeping a journal of these moments will support your success in submitting exemplars during your matriculation through the certificate program and the recertification process. Journaling also supports your growth and development as an ever evolving human being "becoming and belonging" a TIP (Figure 13.5; Hemberg & Wiklund Gustin, 2020).

Personal Wholeness

Personal wholeness involves the congruence of one's sense of self with one's ideal self (Ananth, 2009). Personal wholeness is a journey toward physical, psychological, social, spiritual, and existential well-being. The self-healing dimensions of personal wholeness seek to mitigate the corrosive effects of stress-reactive habits and support health-promoting activities (Loizzo et al., 2009). The whole person is able to embrace their perceived imperfections, honor and celebrate their unique contribution to humanity.

The absence of personal wholeness leads to suffering. Cultivating behaviors that realign the multiple dimensions of "self" creates personal wholeness. Self-care is key to gaining congruence and acceptance of the beauty and grace that is uniquely and only you. Self-care strategies include contemplative and embodied practices, adequate sleep, optimal nutrition, and engaging with supportive and loving social networks(Table 13.3; Dorjee,

Table 13.3 Examples of Contemplative and Embodied Practices

Contemplative Practices	Embodied Practices
• Meditation • Simple yoga • Prayer • Self-compassion	• Kundalini yoga • Qigong • Tai-chi • Visualization and recitation

2016; Ge et al., 2019; Loizzo, 2018; Schmalzl et al., 2014). Personal wholeness is a core attribute of the TIP that cultivates compassion, for self and others as well as resilience.

Courage

Courage involves taking action, facing danger or injustice regardless of retribution (Figure 13.6). Courage is not the same as fearlessness; courageous individuals act in spite of fear. In nursing, courage is often manifested as advocacy on behalf of a patient, colleague, or moral situation. Taking courageous action can effect change, increase self-actualization, and reduce moral distress (Hawkins & Morse, 2014). To be trauma informed requires courage, respectful courage, but courage nonetheless, to challenge the status quo, to be a change-maker.

Courageous action is speaking up on rounds regarding a pain management concern, respectfully addressing and intervening during an invasive clinical practice (e.g., offering to be the second person to support the patient or provide a nonpharmacologic therapy), assisting a colleague to facilitate a skin-to-skin care encounter using the standing transfer method. Nurses must have the courage to question physician orders, report errors, and advocate for safe working environments (Hawkins & Morse, 2014). Courage fosters nurse integrity and advocacy reducing patient suffering and ensuring the delivery of safe, compassionate, quality care.

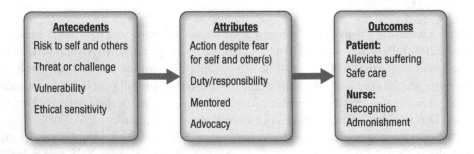

Figure 13.6 Components of the concept of courage.

Source: Hawkins, S. F., & Morse, J. (2014). The praxis of courage as a foundation for care. *Journal of Nursing Scholarship, 46*, 263–270. https://doi.org/10.1111/jnu.12077 Reprinted with permission from John Wiley and Sons.

Table 13.4 **Attributes of a Role Model and Qualities of a Mentor**

Attributes of a Role Model	Qualities of a Mentor
• Approachable • Trustworthy • Empathetic • Adaptable • Knowledgeable • Good communicator • Clinically skilled • Friendly • Professional • Inspires confidence • Motivated	• Communication skills:Listening, questioning, and the wise use of silence • Being a sounding board for ideas and a reality check for plans • Giving guidance without being directive • Providing feedback, suggestions, and options • Time and willingness to contribute • Confidentiality, respecting personal privacy

Source: Adapted from Rolfe, A. (2017). What to look for in a mentor. *Korean Journal of Medical Education, 29*(1), 41–43; Vinales, J. J. (2015). The mentor as a role model and the importance of belongingness. *British Journal of Nursing, 24*(10), 532–535.

Role Model and Mentor

A role model is someone looked to by others as an example to be emulated. A mentor is an experienced and trusted advisor. As a TIP you are a role model for best practice in TIC and a mentor to your colleagues who wish to pursue certification (Table 13.4). Mentoring is most effective when the mentor and mentee share similar values and interests (Burgess et al., 2018).

Mentor–mentee rapport plays a pivotal role in a successful mentorship exchange (Pham et al., 2019). Mentorship is a bidirectional learning experience. As the mentee builds confidence the mentor expands their breadth of knowledge and insight. As the TIP is mentored through the matrix of mastery they mentor others on their journey.

Advocacy

Advocacy is any action that speaks in favor of, recommends, argues for a cause, supports or defends, or pleads on behalf of another/others. Nightingale set the precedent for advocacy in nursing as she championed safe, clean environments and basic human rights for all (Gerber, 2018). The American Nurses Association (ANA) identifies advocacy as a key tenet of nursing in its Code of Ethics, Provision 3: "The nurse promotes, advocates for, and protects the rights, health, and safety of the patient" (ANA, 2015b). Preserving human dignity, patient equality, and freedom from suffering form the basis of nursing advocacy.

TIPs advocate for care that mitigates the experience of trauma for infants and families in hospital and at home. Advocating for continuous, unrestricted parental presence during the intensive care stay, for unencumbered skin-to-skin care experiences, and addressing policies that create additional burdens of stress and trauma on families

Table 13.5 Leadership Theories

Transformational leadership	Connects with shared values; involves the team; inspires, motivates, and empowers others to reach a shared vision; learns from failures; effective with innovation and organizational change.
Servant leadership	Serves others first; develops others to build empowerment and trust.
Emotional intelligence	Gets results through relationships and the effective use of emotional awareness; manages one's personal competence through self-awareness, self-regulation, and motivation and social competence through empathy and social skills.
Authentic leadership	Being your own person; true to one's values to guide action; serves others through leadership; empowers others to make a difference.
Thought leadership	Inspires, innovates, promotes ideas, and convinces others to consider new ideas for sustained change.
Quantum leadership	Adaptable and flexible in systems that are dynamic and nonlinear; identifies common goals; empowers staff and supports efficiency and job performance by assessing systems, processes, and relationships to achieve goals.

Source: Adapted from Smith, C. M., & Johnson, C. S. (2018). Preparing nurse leaders in nursing professional development. *Journal for Nurses in Professional Development, 34*(1), 38–40.

is the role of the TIP clinician. In these unprecedented times of COVID-19 and civil disobedience, advocacy is in great need and the TIP clinician is called to champion the underserved and vulnerable.

Scholarship

Scholarship is the pursuit of academic study or academic achievement. In nursing, scholarship includes research, quality-improvement work, educational innovations, mentoring, and more. Scholarly endeavors advance the science and praxis of nursing.

Pursuing scholarship in TIC invites the clinician to investigate, evaluate and disseminate the impact of a trauma-informed approach across clinical, psychosocio-emotional, spiritual, and economic domains. Presenting at local, national, and international conferences is one example of scholarship. Collaborating and publishing research findings and/or quality improvement work is another example.

Leader for Change

Although there are some individuals with natural leadership abilities, effective leadership skills are grounded in theory (Table 13.5). Recognizing the elements and philosophy of the various leadership styles, prospective leaders can hone their skill to align with a style

BOX 13.2 ATTRIBUTES AND CHARACTERISTICS OF A SUCCESSFUL CLINICAL LEADER

1. Clinical competence/good clinical practice
2. Effective communicator
3. Supportive
4. Values/belief focused
5. Focus on clinical excellence/quality care
6. Role model for others
7. Motivator of others
8. Mentor
9. Decision maker
10. Visible
11. Team focused
12. Approachable
13. Clinical knowledge
14. Empowered
15. Participates in staff development/education

Source: Adapted from Stanley, D., & Stanley, K. (2018). Clinical leadership and nursing explored: A literature search. *Journal of Clinical Nursing, 27*(9–10), 1730–1743. doi: 10.1111/jocn.14145

that resonates with their values and beliefs about leadership. Stanley and Stanley (2018) uncovered 15 core attributes and characteristics of a successful clinical leader (Box 13.2). Leaders may be formal, bearing a title in a hierarchical organization or they may be informal, as frontline clinicians.

As the TIP moves through the matrix of mastery they will grow and develop their leadership skills. Beginner leadership activities may include leading or co-leading on a quality-improvement initiative, enrolling in a leadership development program, or becoming a mentor, role model, or expert in the field of TIC. At the expert level the TIP may be leading systemwide initiatives to adopt TIC, and may be authoring guidelines or white papers discussing cultural transformation in TIC.

Summary

Becoming trauma informed is both a personal and professional journey of discovery and enlightenment. The attributes provide a road map for growth and development that unleash the potential to change the world, one baby, one family at a time. Adopting a trauma-informed approach to healthcare requires a tribe of like-minded, heart-centered professionals. Join the movement. Visit the Caring Essentials Collaborative website to learn more about becoming a TIP. The link can be found in the resource section of this chapter.

> *We ourselves feel that what we are doing is just a drop in the ocean.*
> *But the ocean would be less because of that missing drop.*
> —Mother Theresa

READER RESOURCES

APNA position statement: www.apna.org/files/public/Whole-Health-Begins-With-Mental-Health-Position-Paper.pdf

Caring Essentials Collaborative, LLC website: www.caringessentials.net

Centers for Health Care Strategies, Inc.: www.chcs.org/what-does-it-take-to-become-trauma-informed-lessons-from-early-adopters/

Harvard Health Publishing, Harvard Medical School: www.health.harvard.edu/blog/trauma-informed-care-what-it-is-and-why-its-important-2018101613562

Trauma tool box from American Academy of Pediatrics: www.aap.org/en-us/advocacy-and-policy/aap-health-initiatives/healthy-foster-care-america/Pages/Trauma-Guide.aspx

REFERENCES

American Nurses Association. (2015a). *Code of ethics with interpretative statements.* Author.

American Nurses Association. (2015b). *Nursing: Scope and standards of practice.* Author.

Ananth, S. (2009). Experiencing personal wholeness. *Explore, 5*(5), 304–305. https://doi.org/10.1016/j.explore.2009.06.009

Burgess, A., Diggele, C., & Mellis, C. (2018). Mentorship in the health professions: A review. *Clinical Teacher, 15*(3), 197–202. https://doi.org/10.1111/tct.12756

Centers for Disease Control and Prevention. (2020). *Data and statistics on children's mental health.* https://www.cdc.gov/childrensmentalhealth/data.html

Dorjee, D. (2016). Defining contemplative science: The metacognitive self-regulatory capacity if the mind, context of meditation practice and modes of existential awareness. *Frontiers in Psychology, 7,* 1788. https://doi.org/10.3389/fpsyg.2016.01788

Ge, J., Wu, J., Li, K., & Zheng, Y. (2019). Self-compassion and subjective well-being mediate the impact of mindfulness on balanced time perspective in Chinese college students. *Frontiers in Psychology, 10,* 367. https://doi.org/10.3389/fpsyg.2019.00367

Gerber, L. (2018). Understanding the nurse's role as a patient advocate. *Nursing 2018, 48*(4), 55–58. https://doi.org/10.1097/01.NURSE.0000531007.02224.65

Halifax, J. (2014). G.R.A.C.E. for nurses: Cultivating compassion in nurse/patient interactions. *Journal of Nursing Education and Practice, 4*(1), 121–128. https://doi.org/10.5430/jnep.v4n1p121

Hawkins, S. F., & Morse, J. (2014). The praxis of courage as a foundation for care. *Journal of Nursing Scholarship, 46,* 263–270. https://doi.org/10.1111/jnu.12077

Hemberg, J., & Wiklund Gustin, L. (2020). Caring from the heart as belonging—The basis for mediating compassion. *Nursing Open, 7,* 660– 668. https://doi.org/10.1002/nop2.438

Loizzo, J., Charleson, M., & Peterson, J. (2009). A program in contemplative self-healing: Stress, allostasis, and learning in the Indo-Tibetan tradition. *Annals of the New York Academy of Sciences, 1172,* 123–147. https://doi.org/10.1111/j.1749-6632.2009.04398.x

Loizzo, J. J. (2018). Can embodied contemplative practices accelerate resilience training and trauma recovery? *Frontiers in Human Neuroscience, 12,* 134. https://doi.org/10.3389/fnhum.2018 .00134

Lucero, I. (2018). Written in the body? Healing the epigenetic molecular wounds of complex trauma through empathy and kindness. *Journal of Child & Adolescent Trauma, 11*(4), 443–455. https:// doi.org/10.1007/s40653-018-0205-0

McLoughlin, K. A. (2017a). Five steps to engage in the concept of whole health begins with mental health. *Journal of the American Psychiatric Nurses Association, 23*(3), 230. https://doi .org/10.1177/1078390317706510

McLoughlin, K. A. (2017b). The importance of purpose in whole health and well-being. *Journal of the American Psychiatric Nurses Association, 23*(5), 375. https://doi.org/10.1177/1078390317728481

National Alliance on Mental Illness. (2019). *Mental health by the numbers.* http://www.nami.org/ Learn-More/MentalHealth-By-the-Numbers

Nosarti, C., Reichenberg, A., Murray, R. M., Cnattingius, S., Lambe, M. P., Yin, L., MacCabe, J., Rifkin, L., & Hultman, C. M. (2012). Preterm birth and psychiatric disorders in young adult life. *JAMA Psychiatry, 69*(6), 610-617. https://doi.org/10.1001/archgenpsychiatry.2011.1374

Ntoumanis, N., Healy, L. C., Sedikides, C., Duda, J., Stewart, B., Smith, A., & Bond, J. (2014). When the going gets tough: The "why" of goal striving matters. *Journal of Personality, 82*(3), 225–236. https://doi.org/10.1111/jopy.12047

Pham, T. T. L., Teng, C.-I., Friesner, D., Li, K., Wu, W.-E., Liao, Y.-N., Chang, Y.-T., & Chu, T.-L. (2019). The impact of mentor-mentee rapport on nurses' professional turnover intention: Perspectives of social capital theory and social cognitive career theory. *Journal of Clinical Nursing, 28*(13–14), 2669–2680. https://doi.org/10.1111/jocn.14858

Pyhala, R., Wolford, E., Kautiainen, H., Andersson, S., Bartmann, P., Baumann, N., Brubakk, A.-M., Evensen, K. A. I., Hovi, P., Kajantie, E., Lahti, M., Van Lieshout, R. J., Saigal, S., Schmidt, L. A., Indredavik, M. S., Wolke, D., & Raikkonen, K. (2017). Self-reported mental health problems among adults born preterm: A meta-analysis. *Pediatrics, 139*(4), e20162690. https://doi .org/10.1542/peds.2016-2690

Ream, M., & Lehwald, L. (2018). Neurologic consequences of preterm birth. *Current Neurology and Neuroscience Reports, 18*(8), 48. https://doi.org/10.1007/s11910-018-0862-2

Rehm, J., & Shield, K. D. (2019). Global burden of disease and the impact of mental and addictive disorders. *Current Psychiatry Reports, 21*(2), 10. https://doi.org/10.1007/s11920-019-0997-0

Rolfe, A. (2017). What to look for in a mentor. *Korean Journal of Medical Education, 29*(1), 41–43.

Schmalzl, L., Crane-Godreau, M. A., & Payne, P. (2014). Movement-based embodied contemplative practices: Definitions and paradigms. *Frontiers in Human Neuroscience, 8,* 205. https://doi .org/10.3389/fnhum.2014.00205

Smith, C. M., & Johnson, C. S. (2018). Preparing nurse leaders in nursing professional development. *Journal for Nurses in Professional Development, 34*(1), 38–40.

Sofhauser, C. (2016). Intention in nursing practice. *Nursing Science Quarterly, 29*(1), 31–34. https:// doi.org/10.1177/0894318415614629

Stanley, D., & Stanley, K. (2018). Clinical leadership and nursing explored: A literature search. *Journal of Clinical Nursing, 27*(9–10), 1730–1743. https://doi.org/10.1111/jocn.14145

Van der Kolk, B. (2015). *The body keeps the score: Brain, mind, and body in the healing of trauma*. Penguin Books.

Vinales, J. J. (2015). The mentor as a role model and the importance of belongingness. *British Journal of Nursing, 24*(10), 532–535.

Watson, J. (2018). Unitary caring science: The philosophy and praxis of nursing. University Press of Colorado.

Zahourek, R. P. (2012). Healing through the lens of intentionality. *Holistic Nursing Practice, 26*(1), 6–21. https://doi.org/10.1097/HNP.0b013e31823bfe4c

Zahourek, R. P. (2019). Intentionality the matrix of healing: A theory revised with nonnurse care providers. *Journal of Holistic Nursing*. https://doi.org/10.1177/0898010119892093

Zarse, E. M., Neff, M. R., Yoder, R., Hulvershorn, L., Chambers, J. E., & Chambers, R. A. (2019). The adverse childhood experiences questionnaire: Two decades of research on childhood trauma as a primary cause of adult mental illness, addiction, and medical diseases. *Cogent Medicine, 6*, 1581447. https://doi.org/10.1080/2331205X.2019.1581447

Index

Printed in the United States
by Baker & Taylor Publisher Services

Printed in the United States
by Baker & Taylor Publisher Services